RADIOFREQUENCY CATHETER ABLATION FOR THE TREATMENT OF CARDIAC ARRHYTHMIAS

A Practical Atlas with Illustrative Cases

RETAC

Réseau Européen pour le Traitement des Arythmies Cardiaques
Reunion of European countries for the Treatment of Arrhythmias in Cardiology

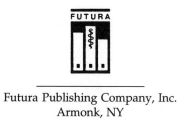

Futura Publishing Company, Inc.
Armonk, NY

Library of Congress Cataloging-in-Publication Data

Radiofrequency catheter ablation for the treatment of cardiac arrhythmias: a practical atlas with illustrative cases / RETAC, Reunion of European countries for the Treatment of Arrhythmias in Cardiology.
    p. ; cm.
Includes bibliographical references and index.
ISBN 0-87993-710-6 (hardcover: alk. paper)
    1. Catheter ablation—Atlases. 2. Arrhythmia—Surgery—Atlases. I. Réseau Européen pour le Traitement des Arythmies Cardiaques.
    [DNLM: 1. Arrhythmia—surgery—Atlases. 2. Arrhythmia—surgery—Case Report. 3. Catheter Ablation—methods—Atlases. 4. Catheter Ablation—methods—Case Report. WG 17 R129 2002]
RD598.35.C39 R325 2002
617.4'12—dc 21   2002024359

Published by
Futura Publishing Company, Inc.
135 Bedford Road
Armonk, New York 10504
www.futuraco.com

ISBN #:0-87993-710-6

Every effort has been made to ensure that the information in this book is as up to date and accurate as possible at the time of publication. However, due to the constant developments in medicine, neither the author, nor the editor, nor the publisher can accept any legal or other responsibility for any errors or omissions that may occur.

Printed in the United States of America on acid-free paper.

History of the RETAC

The concept of the RETAC (Réseau Européen pour le Traitement des Arythmies Cardiaques/Reunion of European countries for the Treatment of Arrhythmias in Cardiology) was at first an idea born in the early 1990s in the mind of colleagues from Barcelona (Spain) and Limoges (France) in order to improve the quality in the treatment of cardiac arrhythmias, especially in the field of radiofrequency catheter ablation. The main objective was to share mutual experiences and to discuss difficult or original cases in the field of arrhythmology. After a few live and video-transmitted procedures, the practical interest of such meetings appeared clearly. Soon after, colleagues from Geneva (Switzerland), Grenoble (France), and Bad Krozingen (Germany) joined this venture and the first meeting supported by a grant from the European Community took place in Limoges in 1995. It was in fact a very original meeting with live cases and a lot of discussions about original case reports. All members then decided enthusiastically to continue the experience: the RETAC was born. Since the beginning, Biotronik and ELA Medical strongly supported the project. Every 6 months, a meeting based on the same characteristics took place in the various institutions included into the RETAC. The second phase of the project, in 1997, included five new members: Gent (Belgium), Meyrin (Switzerland), Toulouse (France), Mont-Godinne (Belgium), and Venezia (Italy). At the same time, RETAC obtained a grant for permanent medical education from the "Leonardo da Vinci Program" of the European Community. Since 1995, RETAC has organized meetings in every institution of the network with the same interest for education and therapeutic improvement. It immediately became an incomparable tool to constantly improve knowledge in such a rapidly evolving field as arrhythmology mainly by exchanging different ways of working and different ways of solving problems in our daily practice. This "little baby called RETAC is growing fast" as Professor Bayés de Luna said. We sincerely thank him for his unconditional support, and we all hope that the group will continue his venture for a very long time following important future evolutions in the treatment of cardiac arrhythmias.

Patrick Blanc, MD
Serge Boveda, MD

* RETAC is supported by Grant N°F/97/2/00225/PI/II.1.1.c/FPC of the Leonardo da Vinci Program of the European Union.

Introduction

Since its introduction in 1987, radiofrequency catheter ablation (RFCA) of both supraventricular and ventricular arrhythmias has become an accepted treatment modality and a first-line treatment option for a variety of different arrhythmia mechanisms. The success rate is high and the efficacy and safety of RFCA depend on the particular type of arrhythmia and on the physician's own experience. At present, RFCA is considered an accepted treatment modality for patients with atrioventricular nodal reentrant tachycardia (AVRNT), atrioventricular reentrant tachycardia (AVRT) in the presence of an accessory pathway and for different types of atrial and ventricular tachycardias.

Atrioventricular nodal reentrant tachycardia is the most common form of recurrent, paroxysmal tachycardia and accounts for about 65% of all paroxysmal supraventricular tachycardias. The AVNRT circuit consists of two pathways, the "fast" and "slow" AV nodal pathways, each with different conduction velocities and refractory periods. In clinical practice, the most common form is the slow-fast type of AV nodal tachycardia, which is observed in about 80% of cases. The fast-slow and slow-slow forms are observed in about 10% each. Because slow pathway ablation has been associated with a lower risk of inducing AV block than fast pathway ablation it has become the prefered procedure for patients with AVNRT. Long-term success rates range from 96% to 98% and the incidence of inadvertent complete AV block is less than 2%.

Atrioventricular reentrant tachycardia in the setting of an accessory pathway accounts for about 30% of all paroxysmal supraventricular tachycardias. Accessory AV pathways were the primary targets to validate the new technique of RFCA in the late 1980s. Presently, RFCA is the treatment of choice in the management of accessory AV pathways, including left freewall, right sided, posteroseptal, anteroseptal, and midseptal accessory pathways. Accessory AV pathways may be located at any point along the tricuspid or mitral valve rings where the atria and ventricles are in direct continuity. The most common location for accessory pathways is along the lateral portion of the mitral annulus joining the left atrium to the left ventricle. Left-sided accessory AV pathways are most frequently ablated in retrograde fashion across the aortic valve into the left ventricle by delivering RF current along the mitral annulus. Right-sided accessory AV pathways can be ablated along the tricuspid annulus, at either the atrial or ventricular insertion of the accessory pathway. The probability of successful ablation is lower in the presence of anomalies of the tricuspid annulus, such as Ebstein's anomaly. Ablation of accessory pathways located in the anteroseptal or midseptal regions and close to the AV conduction system, may be technically difficult and present a risk of inducing complete AV block. Posteroseptal accessory pathways need a careful mapping for determining a right-sided, left-sided or coronary sinus approach. Long-term success rate of RFCA of accessory pathways ranges between 76% to 100%, with a recurrence rate of 3% to 9%. The overall rate of complications of accessory pathway ablation is low.

Atrial tachycardias have been recently subdivided into macroreentrant atrial tachycardias, including different forms of atrial flutter, focal atrial tachycardias originating from a single focus, the syndrome of inappropriate sinus tachycardia and atrial fibrillation. This subdivision was performed according to the geometry of the tachycardia substrate, the relationship of the substrate to the atrial anatomy, and the geometry of atrial lesions required to ablate the substrate in the specific tachycardia. The different mechanisms involved in the genesis of focal atrial tachyardias include microreentry, focus automaticity, and triggered activity. Atrial tachycardias can effectively be eliminated by RFCA in 80% to 100% of cases and the rate of complications is somewhat lower than with either ablation of accessory pathways or AVNRT.

The mechanism of typical *atrial flutter* is macro-reentry within the right atrium. An important part of the macroreentrant circuit lies between the inferior vena cava and the tricuspid annulus (i.e., the cavotricuspid isthmus). Ablation of common-type atrial flutter was initially performed by delivering focal RF pulses within the cavotricuspid isthmus for termination of the arrhythmia with inability of reinduction. Presently, the endpoint of the procedure consists of creating a cavotricuspid bidirectional electrical conduction block by means of point-to-point RF linear lesions along the cavotricuspid isthmus. The acute success rate of RFCA of the common atrial flutter is high, ranging between 90% to 95%. The bidirectional isthmic conduction block has resulted in a substantial reduction of recurrence during long-term follow-up, from 10% to 25% to less than 10%.

Atrial fibrillation is the most common arrhythmia and there is presently no ideal treatment for this arrhythmia. In patients with atrial fibrillation and disabling symptoms refractory to drug treatment, a palliative approach has been used consisting of AV nodal modification or ablation. Atrioventricular nodal ablation requires a permanent pacemaker implantation, VVIR for chronic atrial fibrillation and DDDR with automatic switch-mode to DDIR or VVIR pacing mode for patients with paroxysmal atrial fibrillation. The goal of this technique is to control ventricular rate and is reserved for patients with atrial fibrillation that are both highly symptomatic and poorly responsive to drug therapy. Successful ablation of the AV conduction system can be achieved in nearly all patients and the rate of complications is low. Sudden death has been reported in patients with poor left ventricular function and congestive heart failure. A proarrhythmic effect of ablation cannot be excluded. The long-term efficacy of AV nodal ablation is greater than 95%. Recurrence of symptoms occurs in less than 5%. Improvement of both quality of life and exercise tolerance has been demonstrated.

An alternative strategy for AV nodal ablation is to modify AV nodal conduction by slowing the ventricular response rather than to intentionally create complete heart block. Catheter modification of AV nodal conduction is achieved by the application of radiofrequency current to the base of Koch's triangle in the region typically targeted for ablation of the slow AV nodal pathway. This procedure may result in slowing of the AV nodal conduction without requiring permanent pacemaker implantation. However, patients may continue to experience palpitations due to an irregular cardiac rhythm.

Curative treatment of atrial fibrillation is still under investigation. Replication of the Maze procedure using RF catheter technique is a potentially curative treatment option. However, a large number of RF pulses is commonly required and duration of the procedure is rather long. The long-term efficacy of this procedure remains to be determined. Recently, intra-atrial mapping has allowed identification of focal mechanisms initiating and perpetuating atrial fibrillation. Such foci may originate from one or more pulmonary veins in more than 90% of cases. Radiofrequency pulses can be successfully delivered at discrete sites presenting the earliest activation during spontaneous extra beats or at time of onset of atrial fibrillation. The prevalence of a focal mechanism as a trigger of paroxysmal atrial fibrillation remains to be determined. Ostial pulmonary venous stenosis with hemodynamic impairment has been reported as a possible complication during follow-up.

Ventricular tachycardias may be divided into focal and macroreentrant forms according to the geometry of the arrhythmogenic substrate. Because of their influence on the hemodynamic balance, RF ablation of ventricular tachycardias can only be performed in presence of hemodynamic stability. Focal ventricular tachycardias are more commonly encountered in patients without underlying organic heart disease, and include two forms: one originating from the right ventricular outflow tract and one from the septal wall of the left ventricle (idiopathic left ventricular tachycardia).

Right ventricular outflow tract ventricular tachycardia is characterized by a left bundle branch block QRS morphology in ECG lead V_1 with an inferior frontal plane QRS axis. Catheter ablation is accomplished by localizing the site of earliest ventricular activation during tachycardia, usually in the right ventricle immediately below the pulmonic valve.

Idiopathic left ventricular tachycardia is often characterized by a right bundle branch block QRS morphology with a superior frontal plane QRS axis. It originates most commonly from the posteroinferior left ventricular septum, close to the left posterior fascicle. Successful RFCA may be performed at the recording site of a high frequency deflection suggestive of the specialized intraventricular conduction system termed "Purkinje potential." Long-term success rates of 85% to 100% have been reported, with a recurrence rate lower than 10% in focal ventricular tachycardia.

Macroreentrant ventricular tachycardias are usually found in patients with underlying disease, particularly in association with prior myocardial infarction. Other conditions may include patients with dilated or hypertrophic cardiomyopathy, valvular heart disease, and arrhythmogenic right ventricular dysplasia. In patients with coronary artery disease, monomorphic ventricular tachycardia is most often generated by macroreentry around areas of prior myocardial necrosis. The efficacy of radiofrequency energy to ablate ventricular tachycardia following myocardial infarction may be limited by endocardial scarring overlying the region of infarction, by multiple morphologies of the tachycardia and by the possible occurrence of hemodynamic compromise during ventricular tachycardia. The long-term success rate of RF ablation ranges between 60% and 90%, with a recurrence rate up to 40% and an acute complication rate of about 2%. Recent studies report a high acute success rate and a reasonable long-term result after RFCA using a cooled tip ablation catheter system.

Bundle branch reentrant tachycardia is a rare form of ventricular tachycardia presenting generally with a left bundle branch block morphology on the 12-lead ECG. Right bundle branch or interfascicular block morphology may also be found, but are less frequent. RF ablation of the one bundle responsible for anterograde conduction provides curative treatment of this type of tachycardia in more than 95% of patients.

Radiofrequency catheter ablation is a safe and presently a routine method for the treatment of arrhythmias related to accessory AV pathways, AVNRT, atrial flutter, atrial tachycardias, and idiopathic ventricular tachycardia. The curative way to treat atrial fibrillation or ventricular tachycardia due to coronary artery disease should be considered investigational at present. In the near future, the combined use of new diagnostic and therapeutic tools will further improve the efficacy and expand the indications of RFCA. The use of *saline-irrigated tip electrodes or internally perfused saline-cooled catheters* has proven to be effective for the ablation of common-type atrial flutter not treatable with conventional techniques, for the ablation of atrial fibrillation (acquisition of a linear multicompartmentalized model), and of post-myocardial infarction ventricular tachycardia. *Two mapping systems* recently introduced in clinical practice have allowed three-dimensional reconstruction of electrical activation within a target area: *a nonfluoroscopic and a noncontact mapping system*. These two new strategies are useful to guide mapping and RF ablation of cardiac arrhythmias such as macroreentrant atrial or ventricular tachycardias, and atrial fibrillation.

Interventional electrophysiology is a fascinating experience, and for a little bit more than a decade now electrophysiologists are not only able to elucidate the mechanism of most cardiac arrhythmias but are also able cure the patient during the same procedure. Experience cannot be replaced by lectures and books, but we sincerely hope that the cases presented in this atlas will help our colleagues for the management of their patients.

Selected Reading

Huang SK, Bharati S, Graham AR, et al. Closed chest catheter desiccation of the atrioventricular junction using radiofrequency energy: A new method of catheter ablation. *J Am Coll Cardiol* 1987;9:349-358.

Jackman WM, Beckman KI, McClelland JH, et al. Treatment of supraventricular tachycardia due to atrioventricular nodal reentry by radiofrequency catheter ablation of slow-pathway conduction. *N Engl J Med* 1992;327:313-318.

Haissaguerre M, Gaita F, Fischer B, et al. Elimination of atrioventricular nodal reentrant tachycardia using discrets slow potentials to guide application of radiofrequency energy. *Circulation* 1992;85:2162-2175.

Jazayeri M, Hempe S, Sra J, et al. Selective transcatheter ablation of the slow pathway for the treatment of atrioventricular nodal reentrant tachycardia. *Circulation*. 1992;85:1318-1328.

Kay GN, Epstein AE, Dailey SM et al. Selective radiofrequency ablation of the slow pathway for the treatment of atrioventricular nodal reentrant tachycardia: Evidence for involvement of perinodal myocardium within the reentrant circuit. *Circulation* 1992; 85: 1675-1688.

Kuck KH, Schlüter M, Geiger M, et al. Radiofrequency current catheter ablation of accessory atrioventricular pathways. *Lancet* 1991;337:1567-1661.

Kuck KH, Schluter M. Single-catheter approach to radiofrequency current ablation of left-sided accessory pathways in patients with Wolff-Parkinson-White syndrome. *Circulation* 1991;84:2366-2375.

Lesh MD, Van Hare GF, Schamp DJ, et al. Curative percutaneous catheter ablation using radiofrequency energy for accessory pathways in all locations: Results in 100 consecutive patients. *J Am Coll Cardiol* 1992;19:303-1309.

Kay GN, Cheng F, Epstein AE et al. Radiofrequency ablation of primary atrial tachycardias. *J Am Coll Cardiol* 1993; 21:901-909.

Cosio FG, Lopez-Gil M, Goicolea A, et al. Radiofrequency ablation of the inferior vena cava-tricuspid valve isthmus in common atrial flutter. *Am J Cardiol* 1993;71:705-709.

Cauchemez B, Haissaguerre M, Fischer B, et al. Electrophysiological effects of catheter ablation of the cavo-tricuspid annulus isthmus in common atrial flutter. *Circulation* 1996;93:284-294.

Cosio FG, Goicolea A, Lopez-Gil M, et al. Catheter ablation of atrial flutter circuits. *Pacing Clin Electrophysiol* 1993; 16:637-642.

Williamson BID, Mari KC, Daoud E, et al. Radiofrequency catheter modification of atrioventricular conduction to control the ventricular rate during atrial fibrillation. *N Engl J Med* 1994;331:910-917.

Chen SA, Lee SH, Chiang CE, et al. Electrophysiological mechanisms in successful radiofrequency catheter modification of atrioventricular junction for patients with medically refractory paroxysmal atrial fibrillation. *Circulation* 1996;93:1690-1701.

Morady F, Hasse C, Strickberger SA, et al. Long-term follow-up after radiofrequency modification of the atrioventricular node in patients with atrial fibrillation. *J Am Coll Cardiol* 1997;29:113-121.

Haissaguerre M, Jais P, Shah D, et al. Spontaneous initiation of atrial fibrillation by ectopic beats originating from the pulmonary veins. *N Engl J Med* 1999;339:659-666.

Klein LS, Shih HT, Hackett FK, et al. Radiofrequency catheter ablation of ventricular tachycardia in patients without structural heart disease. *Circulation.* 1992;85:1666-1674.

Nakagawa H, Beckman KJ, McClelland JH, et al. Radiofrequency catheter ablation of idiopathic left ventricular tachycardia guided by a Purkinje potential. *Circulation* 1993;88:2607-2617.

Coggins DL, Lee RJ, Sweeney J, et al. Radiofrequency catheter ablation as a cure for idiopathic tachycardia of both right and left ventricular origin. *J Am Coll Cardiol* 1994; 23:1333-1341.

Morady F, Harvey M, Kalbfleisch SJ, et al. Radiofrequency catheter ablation of ventricular tachycardia in patients with coronary artery disease. *Circulation* 1993;87:363-372.

Stevenson WG, Friedman PL, Kocovic D, et al. Radiofrequency catheter ablation of ventricular tachycardia after myocardial infarction. *Circulation* 1998;98:308-314.

Cohen TJ, Chien WW, Lune KG, et al. Radiofrequency catheter ablation for treatment of bundle branch reentrant ventricular tachycardia: Results and long-term follow-up. *J Am Coll Cardiol* 1991;18:1767-1773.

Hindricks G. The Multicentre European Radiofrequency Survey (MERFS): Complications of radiofrequency catheter ablation of arrhythmias. *Eur Heart J* 1993;14:1644-1653.

Calkins H, Yang P, Miller JM, et al. Catheter ablation of accessory pathways, atrioventricular nodal reentrant tachycardia, and the atrioventricular junction: Final results of a prospective, multicenter clinical trial. *Circulation* 1999;99:262-270.

Wharton JM, Wilber DJ, Calkiris H, et al. Utility of tip thermometry during radiofrequency ablation in humans using an internally perfused saline cooled catheter. *Circulation* 1997;96:13-18.

Schilling RJ, Peters NS, Davies DW. Simultaneous endocardial mapping in the human left ventricle using a noncontact catheter: Comparison of contact and reconstructed electrograms during sinus rhythm. *Circulation* 1998; 98:887-898.

Contributors

Richard Adamec, MD, Internal Medecine Department, Hôpital Universitaire Cantonal, Geneve, Switzerland
Concepcion Alonso, MD, Cardiology Department, Hospital de Sant Pau, Barcelona, Spain
Thomas Arentz, MD, Cardiology Department, Herz-Zentrum de Bad Krozingen, Bad Krozingen, Germany
Patrick Blanc, MD, Cardiology Department, Centre Hospitalier Universitaire Dupuytren, Limoges, France
Dominique Blommaert, MD, Cardiology Department, UCL de Mont-Godinne, Yvoir, Belgium
Thomas Blum, MD, Cardiology Department, Herz-Zentrum de Bad Krozingen, Bad Krozingen, Germany
Aldo Bonso, MD, Cardiology Department, Ospedale Umberto I, Mestre Venezia, Italy
Gerd Bürkle, MD, Cardiology Department, Herz-Zentrum de Bad Krozingen, Bad Krozingen, Germany
Serge Boveda, MD, Cardiology Department, Centre Hospitalier Universitaire de Rangueil, Toulouse, France
Benoît Collet, Cardiology Department, UCL de Mont-Godinne, Yvoir, Belgium
Claudine Coudert, Cardiology Department, Centre Hospitalier Universitaire Dupuytren, Limoges, France
Pascal Defaye, MD, Cardiology Department, Centre Hospitalier Universitaire Michallon, Grenoble, France
Luc De Roy, MD, Cardiology Department, UCL de Mont-Godinne, Yvoir, Belgium
Johan de Sutter, MD, Cardiology Department, Universitair Ziekenhuis, Gent, Belgium
Francesco Di Pede, MD, Cardiology Department, Ospedale Umberto I, Mestre Venezia, Italy
Winoc Fonteyne, MD, Cardiology Department, Universitair Ziekenhuis, Gent, Belgium
Gianni Gasparini, MD, Cardiology Department, Ospedale Umberto I, Mestre Venezia, Italy
Dietrich Kalusche, MD, Cardiology Department, Herz-Zentrum de Bad Krozingen, Bad Krozingen, Germany
Philippe Lagrange, MD, Cardiology Department, Centre Hospitalier Universitaire Dupuytren, Limoges, France
Anahita Lagrange-Kowsar, MD, Cardiology Department, Centre Hospitalier Universitaire Dupuytren, Limoges, France
Georges Mairesse, MD, Cardiology Department, UCL de Mont-Godinne, Yvoir, Belgium
Ramon Oter, MD, Cardiology Department, Hospital de Sant Pau, Barcelona, Spain
Antonio Raviele, MD, Cardiology Department, Ospedale Umberto I, Mestre Venezia, Italy
Juan Sztajzel, MD, Internal Medecine Department, Hôpital Universitaire Cantonal, Geneve, Switzerland
René Tavernier, MD, Cardiology Department, Universitair Ziekenhuis, Gent, Belgium
Sakis Themistoclakis, MD, Cardiology Department, Ospedale Umberto I, Mestre Venezia, Italy
Pelayo Torner, MD, Cardiology Department, Hospital de Sant Pau, Barcelona, Spain
Xavier Viñolas, MD, Cardiology Department, Hospital de Sant Pau, Barcelona, Spain
Jörg von Rosenthal, MD, Cardiology Department, Herz-Zentrum de Bad Krozingen, Bad Krozingen, Germany
Marc Zimmermann, MD, Cardiology Department, Hôpital de la Tour, Meyrin, Switzerland

Contents

Chapter 1

Atrioventricular Junction Ablation for Refractory Atrial Fibrillation

Medical History

A 76-year-old patient had presented with extensive anterior myocardial infarction some years ago with a residual ejection fraction of 32%. He developed atrial fibrillation in 1998, which was converted to sinus rhythm three times by external direct current (DC) shock. An early recurrence was observed 2 weeks after the third cardioversion, and atrial fibrillation was then maintained. The mean ventricular rate without drugs was 150 beats/min during atrial fibrillation, and atrioventricular conduction was decreased by an association of digoxin, amiodarone, and diltiazem. Despite this treatment, the mean heart rate was 118 beats/min over the 24-hour period during Holter recording. After 3 months, the patient developed congestive heart failure and the ventricular rate was still 120 beats/min. It was then decided to perform an ablation of the AV junction after having implanted a VVI-R pacemaker.

Comments

Atrioventricular node ablation is only a palliative procedure, but it may be very useful in some cases of atrial fibrillation when ventricular rate remains rapid despite adequate pharmacological treatment, especially in patients with a low left ventricular ejection

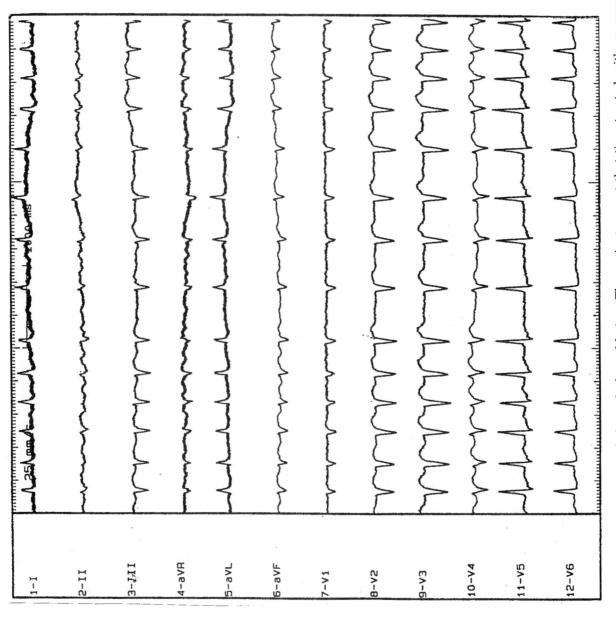

Figure 1. Twelve-lead ECG (25 mm/s) recorded just before ablation. The patient was at that time treated with an association of digoxin, amiodarone, and diltiazem. Minimal RR interval during atrial fibrillation was 360 ms.

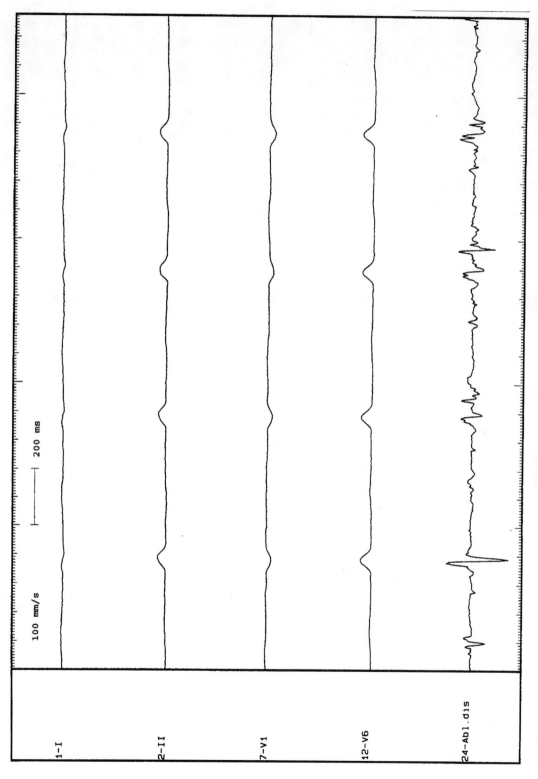

Figure 2. Here are represented four surface ECG leads (I, II, V_1, V_6) and an endocardial recording at the successful site (Abl dis): a discrete His potential is present and the A/V ration is almost equal to 1 on the ablation catheter. Recording speed 100 mm/s.

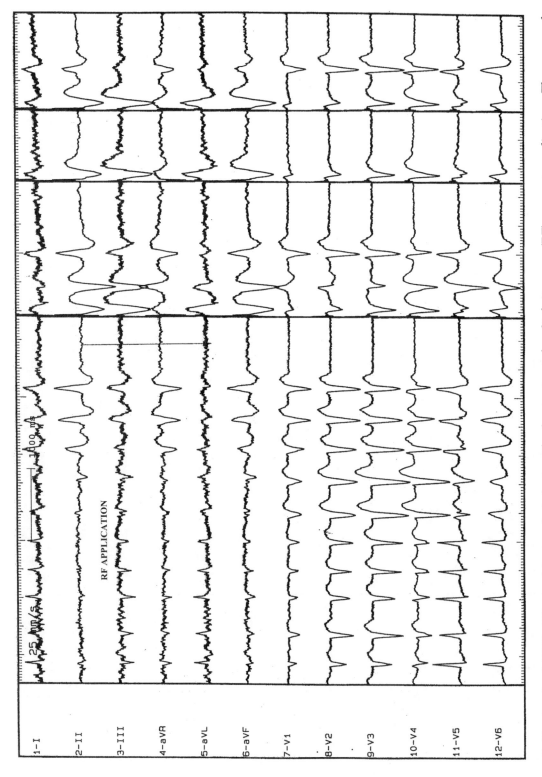

Figure 3. Twelve-lead ECG (25 mm/s) recorded during the beginning of radiofrequency (RF) current application. The pacemaker was programmed in VVI mode with a rate of 60 beats/min. The site of ablation was on the atrial side, in the proximal zone of the His bundle. Ablation was successful after a few seconds with the occurrence of atrioventricular block and intervention by the pacemaker. Of note is the presence of ventricular premature beats just after ablation, with an R on T phenomenon and a high risk of Torsade de Pointes. The ventricular premature beats disappeared shortly after ablation.

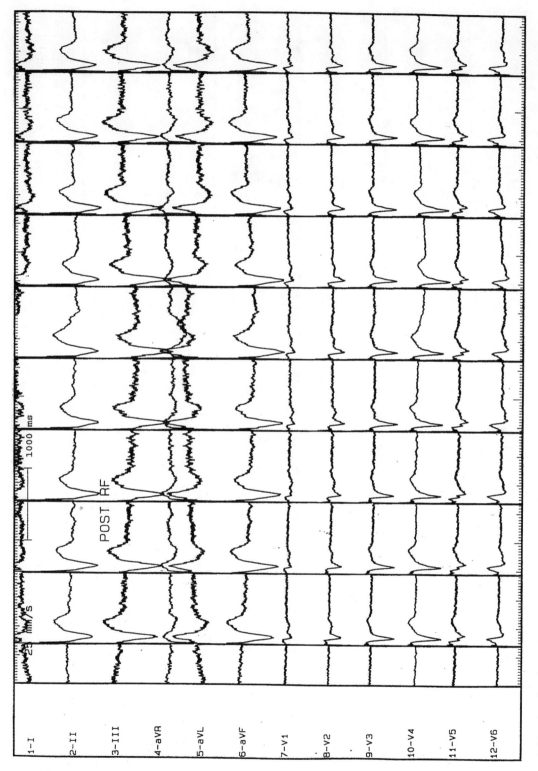

Figure 4. Twelve-lead ECG (25 mm/s) showing the regular ventricular rate at 60 beats/min due to the pacemaker function just after the radiofrequency application. The QT interval is about 460 ms, probably because of amiodarone therapy (withdrawn immediately after the ablation procedure) but also in relation with the major decrease in ventricular rate and with pacing. Because of the risk of malignant ventricular arrhythmias like Torsade de Pointes, the pacemaker minimal rate should be programmed between 80 and 90 beats/min during the first few weeks after ablation.

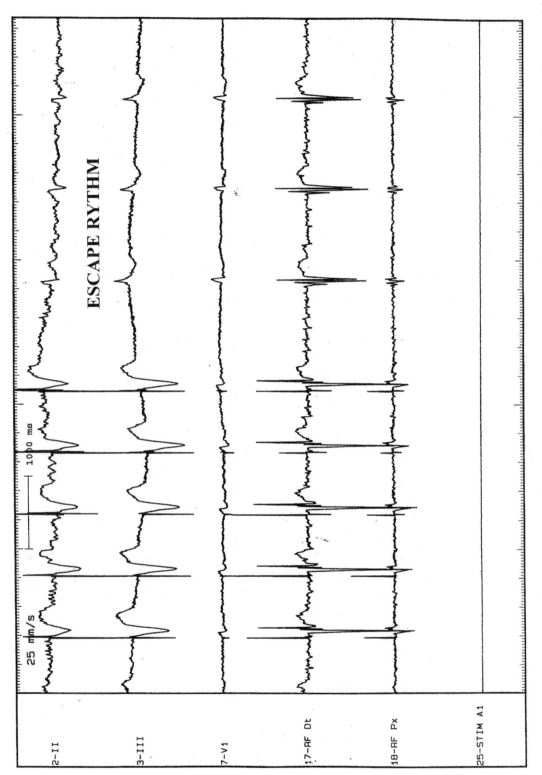

Figure 5. Intracardiac tracing (25 mm/s) showing an escape ventricular rhythm at a rate of 48 beats/min when the pacemaker is suddenly inhibited after ablation. The presence of such an escape rhythm is essential to avoid asystole in case of pacemaker dysfunction. The regular ventricular spontaneous rhythm confirms the complete atrioventricular block.

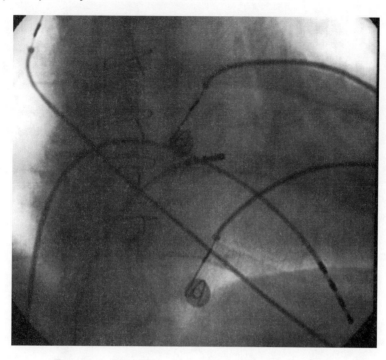

Figure 6. Chest X-ray showing catheter position.

fraction. Atrioventricular junction ablation is usually easy and fast to perform. The main drawback of this procedure is the necessity to implant a permanent pacemaker before or just after ablation. Implantation of the pacemaker before ablation is preferable in order to obtain a good stability of the ventricular lead. The target for ablation should be the proximal zone of the atrioventricular node to obtain an acceptable ventricular escape rhythm in case of pacemaker dysfunction or lead dislocation. Another important feature is the risk of malignant ventricular arrhythmias after ablation of the atrioventricular junction. To avoid this type of potentially lethal complication, it is necessary to pace the ventricle at a minimal rate of 80 beats/min during the first few weeks after ablation and it appears mandatory to closely monitor the patient for at least 24 hours after the ablation procedure.

Suggested Reading

Scheinmann MM, Morady F, Hess DS, Gonzalez R. Catheter induced ablation of the atrioventicular junction to control refractory supraventricular arrhythmias. *JAMA* 1982;248: 851-855.

Gallagher JJ, Svensen RH, Kasell JH, et al. Catheter technique for closed chest ablation of the atrioventricular conduction system. A therapeutic alternative for the treatment of refractory supraventricular tachycardia. *N Engl J Med* 1982;306: 194-200.

Williamson BD, Man KC, Daoud E, et al. Radiofrequency catheter modification of atrioventricular conduction to control the ventricular rate during atrial fibrillation. *N Engl J Med* 1994;331:910-917.

Touboul P. Atrioventricular nodal ablation and pacemaker implantation in patients with atrial fibrillation. *Am J Cardiol* 1999;83:241D-245D.

Brignole M, Menozzi C, Gianfranchi L, et al. Assessment of atrioventricular junction ablation and VVI-R pacemaker versus pharmacological treatment in patients with heart failure and chronic atrial fibrillation. *Circulation* 1998;98:953-960.

Darp B, Walfridsson H, Aunes M, et al. Incidence of sudden death after radiofrequency ablation of the atrioventricular junction for atrial fibrillation. *Am J Cardiol* 1997;80:1174-1177.

Chapter 2

Atrial Tachycardia and Tachycardiomyopathy

Medical History

A 23-year-old man was admitted after a generalized epileptic attack. He had a history of generalized seizures since childhood treated with valproic acid and was known to have an irregular pulse. Before admission he was in good general condition (NYHA class I) and exercised regularly without complaints. The physical examination was unremarkable except for an irregular heartbeat of 140 beats/min with pulse deficit. The ECG showed bursts of atrial tachycardia interrupted by isolated sinus beats. A chest X-ray showed the presence of cardiomegaly with a cardiothoracic index of 60%. The left ventricular end diastolic diameter was 77 mm, the end systolic diameter 68 mm. Hypokinaesia of all segments was present. There was a secondary mitral valve insufficiency grade 1. The left ventricular

ejection fraction as measured with Tc^{99} was 24%. A treatment with lisinopril, digoxin, and atenolol was initiated. Despite rate control with 2:1 atrioventricular (AV) block, cardiac enlargement persisted and an ablation of the arrhythmia focus was performed. A quadripolar catheter was positioned in the high right atrium, a quadripolar catheter over the His bundle and a decapolar catheter in the coronary sinus. A quadripolar ablation catheter was positioned transseptally and used as a roving catheter. The tachycardia could not be initiated or terminated with programmed atrial stimulation but showed overdrive suppression. The earliest atrial activation occurred 30 ms before the onset of the P wave, with the roving catheter positioned between the ostia of the left and right inferior pulmonary veins. At this site a QS pattern was observed in the unipolar recording, and the activation sequence during tachycardia and pacing from this site was comparable. During the second application of radiofrequency energy, the incessant automatic atrial tachycardia terminated with restoration of normal sinus rhythm. Six months after ablation the patient was still in normal sinus rhythm. Only the ACE-inhibitor was continued. The cardiothoracic index decreased to 44%, the left ventricular end diastolic diameter decreased to 57 mm, and the end systolic diameter to 37 mm. The left ventricular ejection fraction measured with Tc^{99} 3 months and 6 months after ablation increased to 43% and 64%, respectively. ACE-inhibition was stopped.

Comments

Incessant atrial tachycardia is an uncommon type of supraventricular tachycardia but is clinically important because it can lead to a tachycardia-induced cardiomyopathy that may be reversible with tachycardia rate control or rhythm control. This arrhythmia generally occurs in children or young adults and may be asymptomatic until signs of heart failure develop. Although this patient had clear evidence of cardiomyopathy as reflected in the cardiothoracic index of 60%, the increased end systolic and end diastolic diameter of the left ventricle, and the low left ventricular ejection fraction, he had no complaints of congestive heart failure.

The mechanisms leading to a tachycardia-induced contractility dysfunction are unknown, but several hypotheses have been presented. They include an energy depletion of the myocardium, an impaired energy utilization, ischemia of the myocardium, cardiac calcium handling abnormalities, and remodelling of myocytes and the extracellular matrix.

Electrocardiographically incessant atrial tachycardia is characterized by an acceleration during initiation and deceleration before termination. The P wave, with a rate between 120 and 240 beats/min, has a morphology different from the sinus P wave depending upon the site of origin. The tachycardia cannot be initiated or terminated by atrial stimulation but it may exhibit overdrive suppression. Premature atrial beats may reset the tachycardia, suggesting abnormal automaticity, although triggered activity as a mechanism has also been reported.

The treatment of this arrhythmia is focused on ventricular rate control or suppression of the arrhythmogenic focus. Rate control can be obtained with AV node blocking agents or with AV junction ablation followed by pacemaker insertion. These procedures, however, do not restore AV synchrony and can lead to pacemaker dependency. Therefore suppression of the focus is more desirable. Class I or III drugs have been used, but with moderate success. In the early 1990s, surgical resection and cryoablation was suggested as a curative treatment of this arrhythmia, but this requires a thoracotomy and recurrences are rather frequent. Therefore, as for most supraventricular tachyarrhythmias, transvenous catheter ablation techniques have been developed. Mapping of the focus of origin is based on identification of the site of earliest activation relative to the onset of the P wave, pace mapping from the tip of the ablation catheter, analysis of pacing activation sequences and the presence of a QS configuration at site of earliest activation in the unipolar recording.

Suggested Reading

Olsson SB, Glomstrom P, Sabel KG, et al. Incessant ectopic atrial tachycardia: Successful surgical treatment with regression of dilated cardiomyopathy picture. *Am J Cardiol* 1984;53:1465-1466.

Shinbane JS, Wood MA, Jensen DN, et al. Tachycardia-induced cardiomyopathy: A review of animal models and clinical studies. *J Am Coll Cardiol* 1997;29:709-715.

De Pauw M, Vincent A, Hodeige D, et al. Ca++ responsiveness after 48 hours of rapid pacing in conscious dogs (abstract). *Circulation* 1994;90:Suppl I: I-38.

Goldreyer BN, Gallagher JJ, Damato AN. The electrophysiologic demonstration of atrial ectopic tachycardia in man. *Am Heart J* 1973;85:205-215.

Wellens HJJ, Brugada P. Mechanisms of supraventricular tachycardia. *Am J Cardiol* 1988;62:10D-15D.

Langberg JJ, Chin MC, Rosengrist M, et al. Catheter ablation of the atrioventricular junction with radiofrequency energy. *Circulation* 1989;80:1527-1535.

Gillette PC, Wampler DG, Garson A, et al. Treatment of atrial automatic tachycardia by ablation procedures. *J Am Coll Cardiol* 1985;6:405-409.

Walsh EP, Saul JP, Hulse JE, et al. Transcatheter ablation of ectopic atrial tachycardia in young patients using radiofrequency current. *Circulation* 1992;86:1138-1146.

Fenelon G, Wijns W, Andries E, et al. Tachycardiomyopathy: Mechanisms and clinical implications. *Pacing Clin Electrophysiol* 1996;19:95-106.

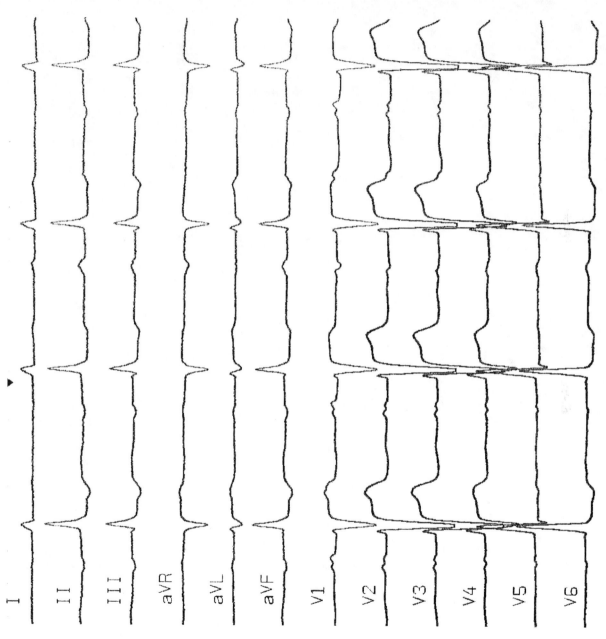

Figure 1. Twelve-lead ECG during tachycardia. Bursts of atrial tachycardia (2:1 atrioventricular conduction) with negative P″ waves in I, II, III, aVF and V₆ are interrupted by single sinus beats.

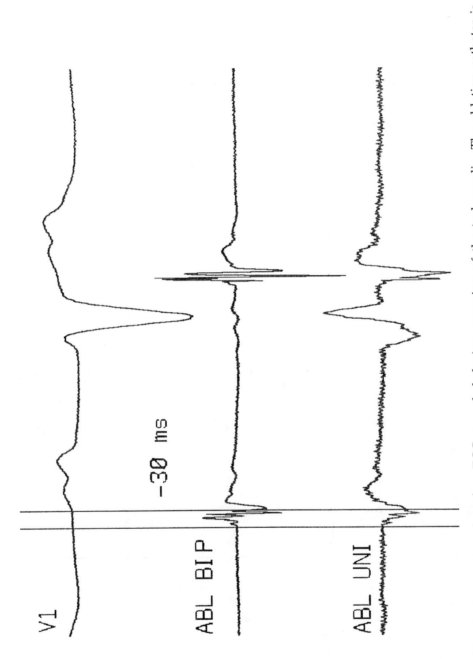

Figure 2. Intracardiac electrograms and surface ECG recorded during mapping of the tachycardia. The ablation catheter is positioned transseptally and located at the site where successful ablation was achieved. Local atrial activation precedes the onset of the P wave (vertical line) by 30 ms. The unipolar recording shows a QS configuration at this site. (ABL bip = bipolar recording on ablation catheter; ABL uni = unipolar recording on ablation catheter).

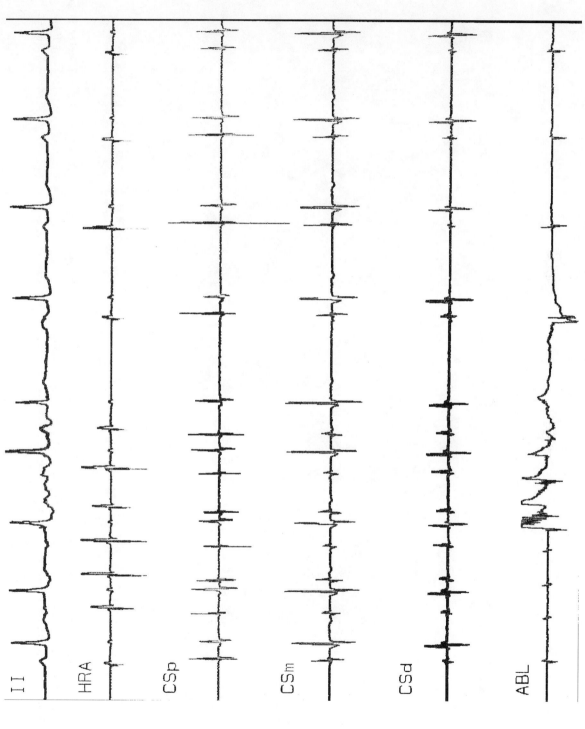

Figure 3. Radiofrequency energy delivery results in an abrupt termination of the tachycardia. (HRA = high right atrium; CSD = distal coronary sinus; CSM = middle coronary sinus; CSP = proximal coronary; ABL = signal on ablation catheter).

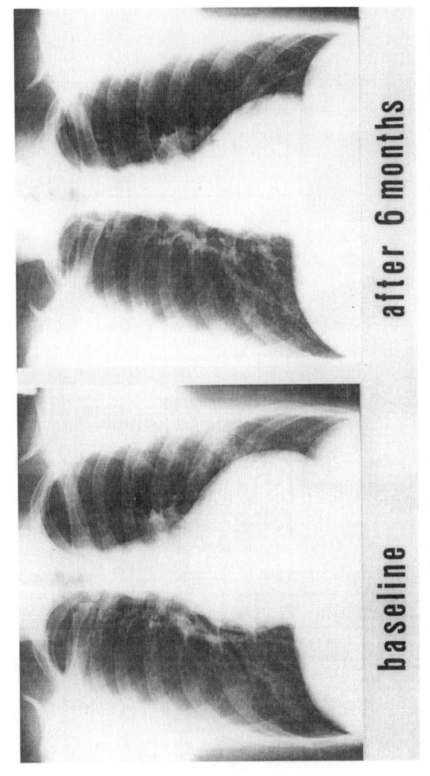

Figure 4. Chest X-ray before (**A**) and 6 months after ablation (**B**). The cardiothoracic index decreases from 60% to 44%.

Chapter 3

Permanent Right Atrial Tachycardia

Medical History

A 37-year-old female flight attendant presented with permanent palpitations. Symptoms were so disabling that the patient had to stop working for the last 18 months, complaining of asthenia and shortness of breath.

Several antiarrhythmic drugs (including sotalol, flecainide, and verapamil) had been prescribed, but no beneficial effect was observed.

Comments

Atrial tachycardia is an uncommon form of supraventricular tachycardia that can be caused by abnormal automaticity, triggered activity, or atrial reentry. Atrial tachycardia is often drug-resistant and may become incessant or permanent leading to tachycardiomyopathy. Radiofrequency catheter ablation is an effective mode of treatment, but precise mapping techniques are essential to localize the site for ablation. Analysis of P wave morphology on the 12-lead ECG has been shown to be helpful in differentiating right from left atrial foci, and inferior leads have been shown to be helpful in differentiating superior from inferior foci. However, the 12-lead ECG may only serve as an indicator and the site for successful ablation should be assessed using the earliest local atrial depolarization during tachycardia and unipolar atrial recordings.

Suggested Reading

Chen SA, Chiang CE, Yang CJ, et al. Sustained atrial tachycardia in adult patients: Electrophysiological characteristics,

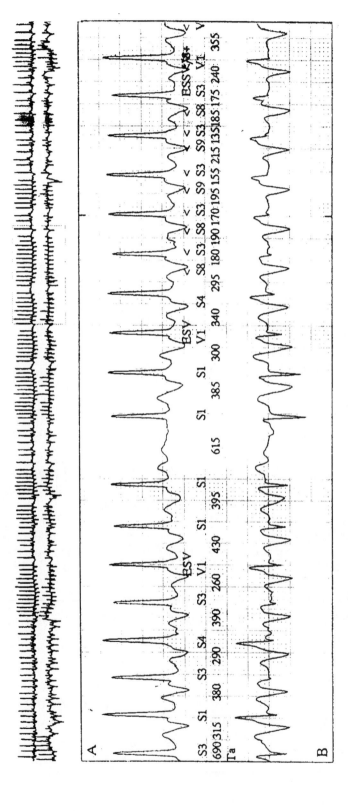

Figure 1. Twenty-four hour ambulatory ECG recording (Holter) showing incessant atrial tachycardia at a rate of 160 beats/min with 1:1 AV conduction. Paper speed 25 mm/s.

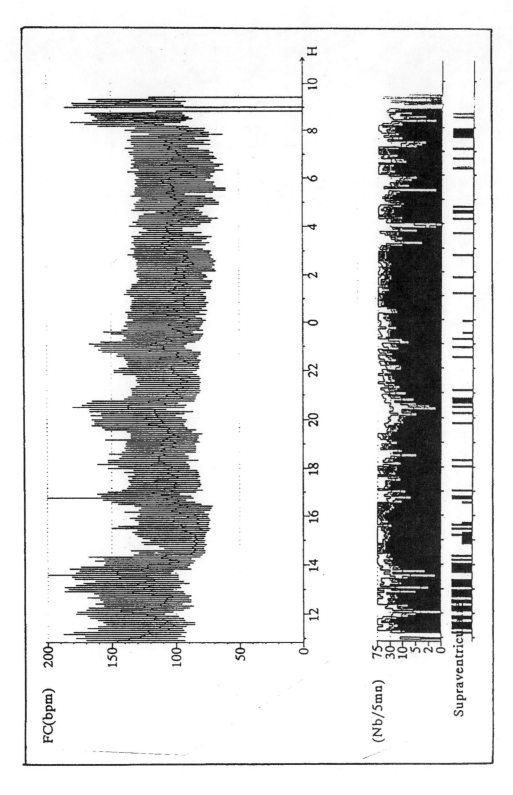

Figure 2. Heart rate histogram (upper panel) and graphic representation of supraventricular ectopic beats and salvoes (lower panel) obtained from the 24-hour Holter recording showing permanent tachycardia with a ventricular rate between 100 and 170 beats/min.

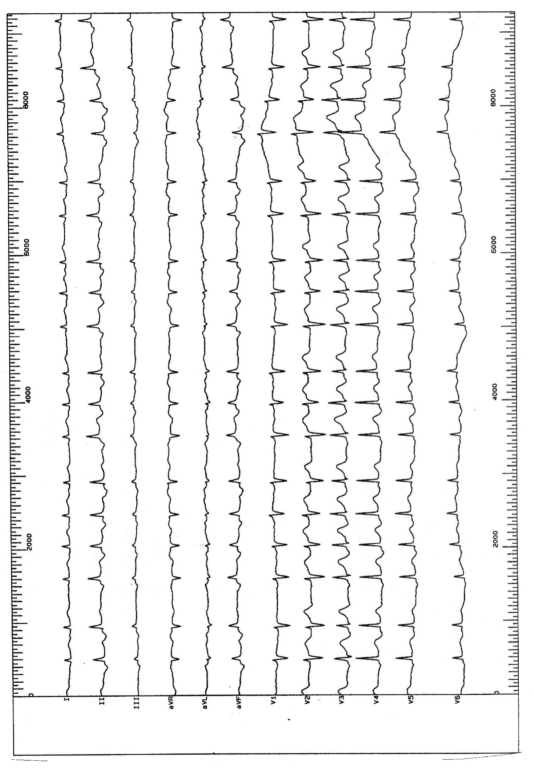

Figure 3. Twelve-lead ECG (25 mm/s) before the ablation procedure showing permanent atrial tachycardia. Note that the P wave is negative in lead DII, DIII and aVF.

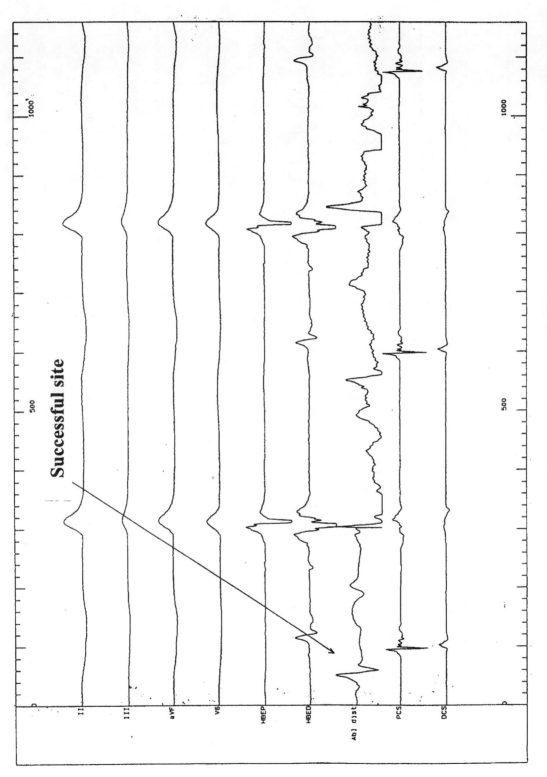

Figure 4. Intracardiac recordings before the ablation procedure. Paper speed 200 mm/s. The figure shows four surface ECG leads (II, III, aVF, V₆) together with five bipolar intracardiac recordings. A very early atrial potential is recorded from the tip of the ablation catheter which is located in the close vicinity of the coronary sinus os. (HBEP – HBED : proximal and distal His bundle recording, Abl dist : bipolar recording obtained from the distal poles of the ablation catheter, PCS and DCS : proximal and distal coronary sinus.)

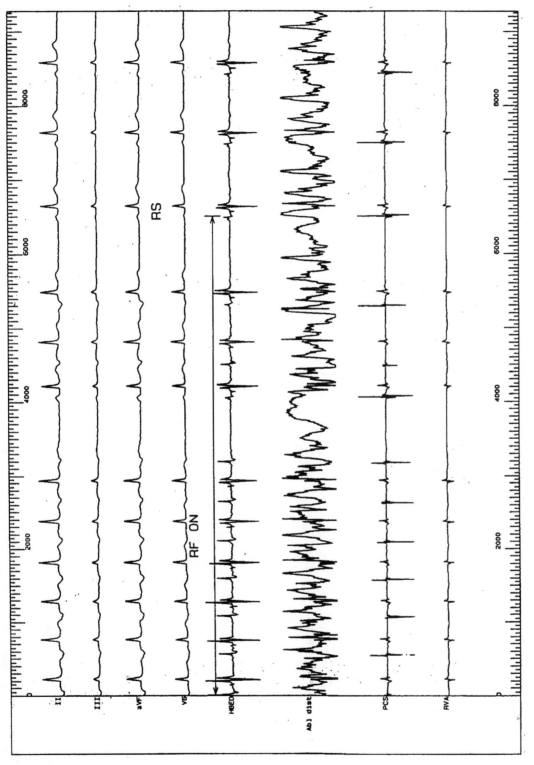

Figure 5. Intracardiac recordings during radiofrequency current application. Paper speed 25 mm/s. The figure shows four surface ECG leads (II, III, aVF, V$_6$) together with four bipolar intracardiac recordings. The permanent atrial tachycardia is interrupted by radiofrequency current application and sinus rhythm (RS) is restored with normal atrioventricular conduction. (HBED = distal His bundle recording; Abl dist = bipolar recording obtained from the distal poles of the ablation catheter; PCS = proximal coronary sinus; RVA = right ventricular apex.)

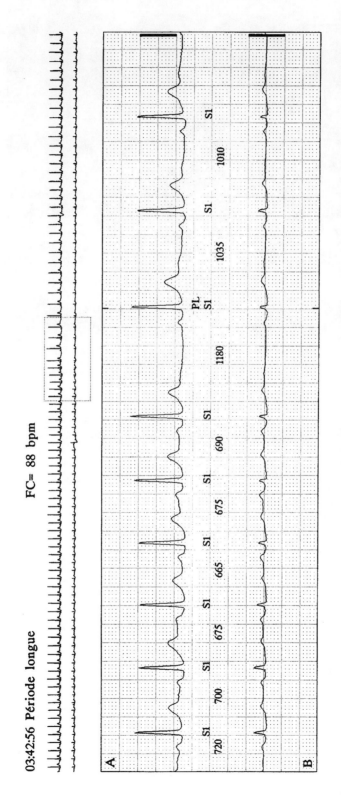

Figure 6. Twenty-four hour ambulatory ECG recording (Holter) showing stable sinus rhythm (with sinus arrhythmia) 6 months after the ablation procedure. Paper speed 25 mm/s.

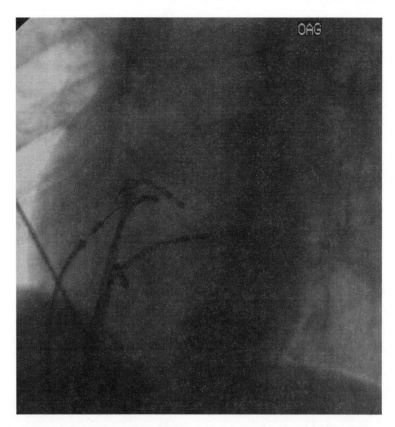

Figure 7. Chest X-ray showing catheter position in the LAO position (OAG).

pharmacological response, possible mechanisms, and effects of radiofrequency ablation. *Circulation* 1994;90:1262-1278.

Walsh EP, Saul JP, Hulse JE, et al. Transcatheter ablation of ectopic atrial tachycardia in young patients using radiofrequency current. *Circulation* 1992;86:1138-1146.

Tang CW, Scheinman MM, Hare GFV, et al. Use of P wave configuration during atrial tachycardia to predict site of origin. *J Am Coll Cardiol* 1995;26:1315-1324.

Tada H, Nogami A, Naito S, et al. Simple electrocardiographic criteria for identifying the site of origin of focal right atrial tachycardia. *Pacing Clin Electrophysiol* 1998;21(Part II):2431-2439.

Chapter 4

Catheter Ablation of a Right Atrial Incisional Tachycardia

Medical History

An 85-year-old female patient had mitral valve repair 5 years ago for severe mitral regurgitation related to mitral valve prolapse. Paroxysmal atrial fibrillation was intermittently observed during the first 2 postoperative months but evolution thereafter was uneventful. Four years after surgery, she complained of palpitations and shortness of breath, and she was found to have prolonged incessant episodes of supraventricular tachycardia at a rate of 120 beats/min. Because the arrhythmia was resistant to digitalis, verapamil and amiodarone, the patient was referred for electrophysiologic evaluation.

Comments

Although it is impossible to assess the exact mechanism of an atrial arrhythmia during an electrophysio-logic investigation, reentry within the atrium is typically initiated and terminated by programmed atrial stimulation which was the case in this patient. Reentry occurred in the region of the scar related to the previous atriotomy, and marked local conduction delay was observed in that region. The atrial activation sequence was slightly different from the atrial activation sequence observed during sinus rhythm (allowing distinction from sinus node reentry), and P-R interval was related to the tachycardia rate with atrioventricular (AV) block occurring sometimes without affecting the tachycardia (proving the atrial origin of the tachycardia). The type of arrhythmia is usually drug-resistant, especially when major intra-atrial conduction delays are present. Drugs such as digitalis, verapamil, β-blockers or adenosine typically cause AV block with atrial reentry persisting. When the arrhythmia is permanent or incessant, radiofrequency catheter ablation is the treatment of choice. When focal ablation is not

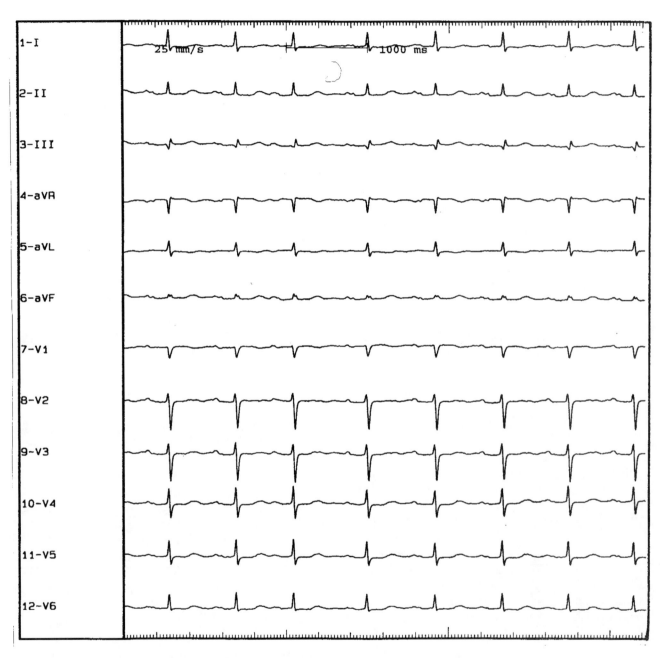

Figure 1. Twelve-lead resting ECG (25 mm/s) during sinus rhythm. P waves are notched and enlarged (P wave duration 120 ms), with a marked decrease in amplitude.

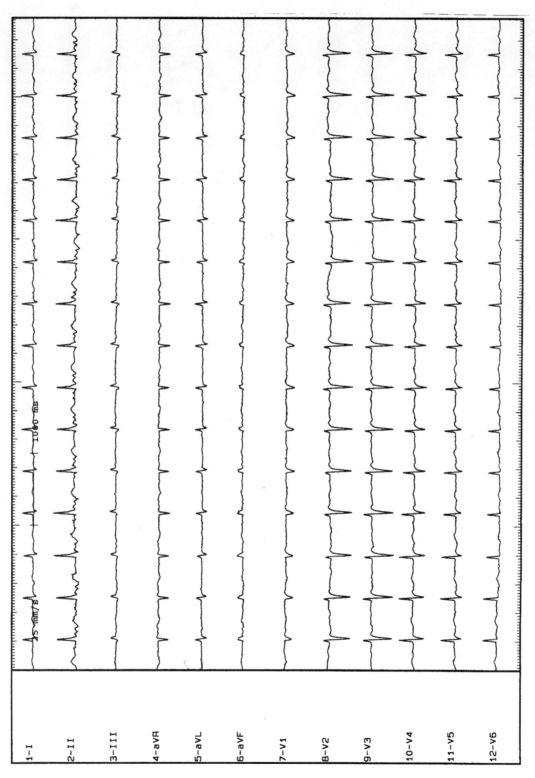

Figure 2. Twelve-lead ECG (25 mm/s) recorded during an episode of palpitations showing a regular narrow QRS complex tachycardia (rate 115 beats/min) with visible P waves just after the QRS complex. P waves are notched and positive in lead II and aVF.

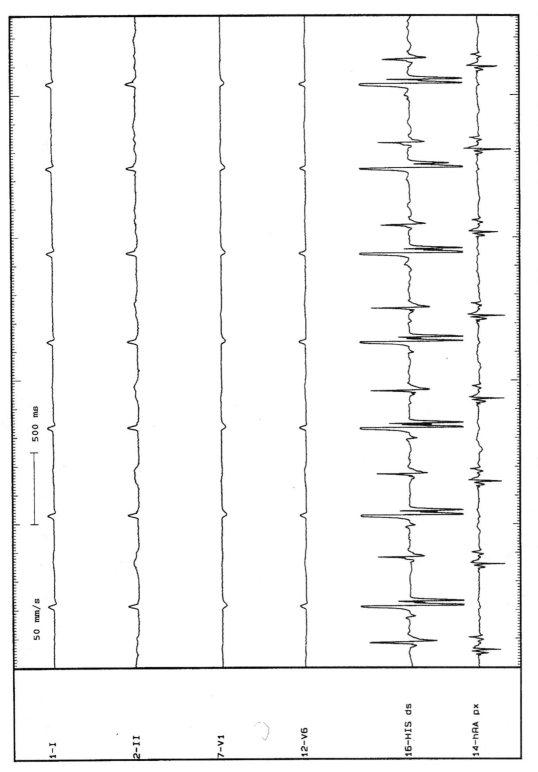

Figure 3. Intracardiac recordings (50 mm/s) during tachycardia. Here are represented four surface ECG leads (I, II, V_1, V_6), one bipolar recording from the His bundle region (His ds), and one bipolar recording from the high right atrium (hRA px). Fragmentation of the local electrogram is observed in the high right atrial region. During tachycardia, A-H interval is progressively increasing and there are major changes in the relationship between V and A (atrial tachycardia).

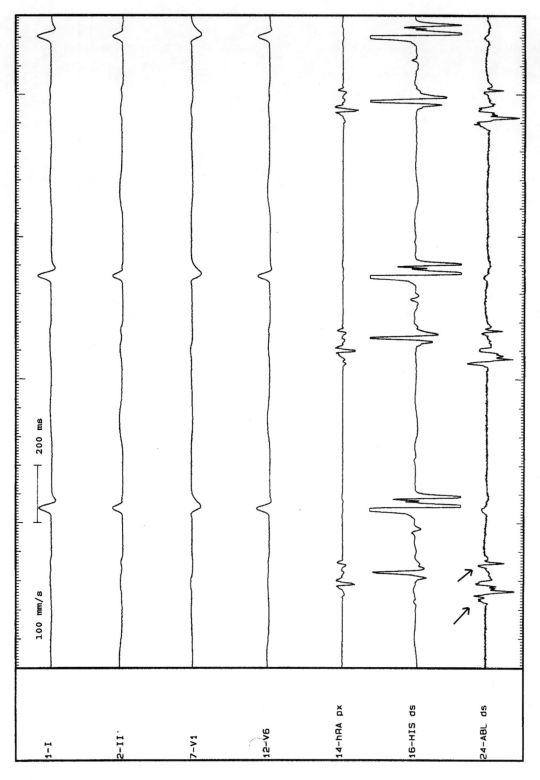

Figure 4. Intracardiac recordings from the high right atrium (100 mm/s). Here are represented four surface ECG leads (I, II, V_1, V_6), one bipolar recording from the high right atrium (hRA px), one bipolar recording from the His bundle region (HIS ds), and one bipolar recording from the distal poles of the ablation catheter (ABL ds). In that site, the local electrogram is prolonged (150 ms), and fragmented with a double potential (arrows).

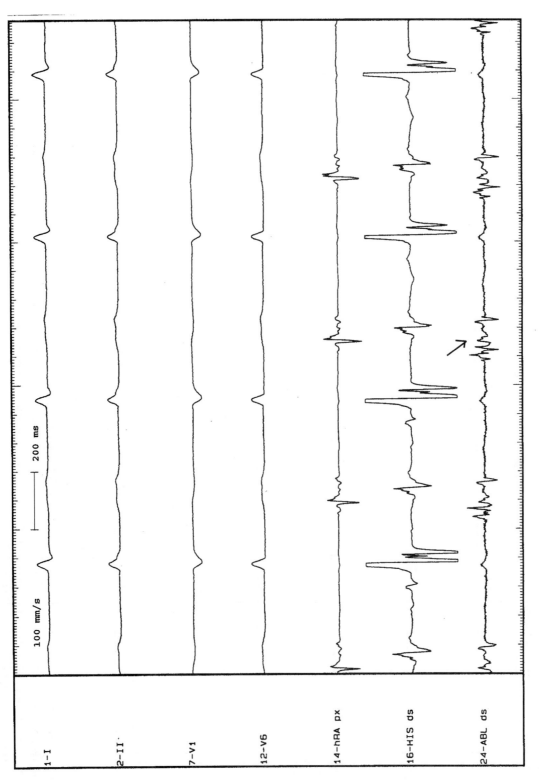

Figure 5. Intracardiac recordings at the successful ablation site (100 mm/s). Same display as Figure 4. In that site, the local electrogram is even more prolonged (160 ms), and more fragmented (arrow). The optimal site was found in the high right atrium in the region of the atriotomy scar.

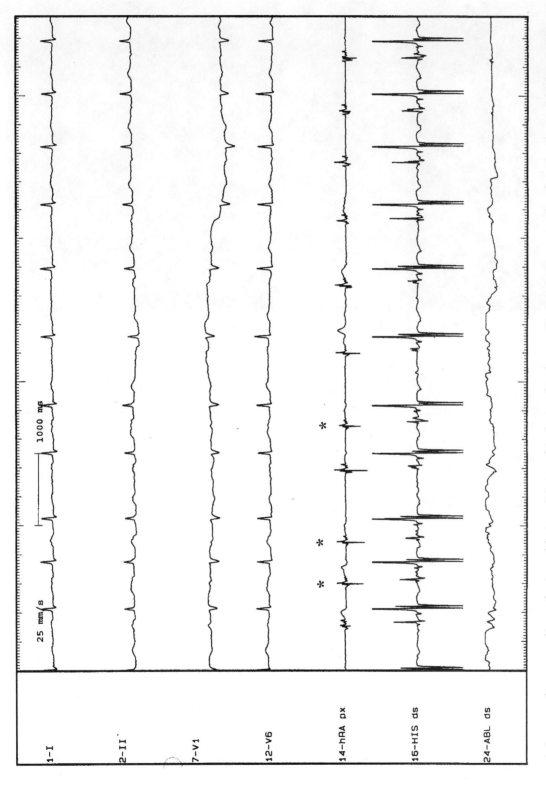

Figure 6. Intracardiac recordings during ablation (25 mm/s). Same display as Figure 5. Six seconds after the first radiofrequency current application, atrial tachycardia is interrupted and a few atrial premature beats are observed (*) before restauration of sinus rhythm. After the procedure, atrial tachycardia was no more inducible, even during isoproterenol infusion, and no recurrences have been observed after a follow-up of 8 months.

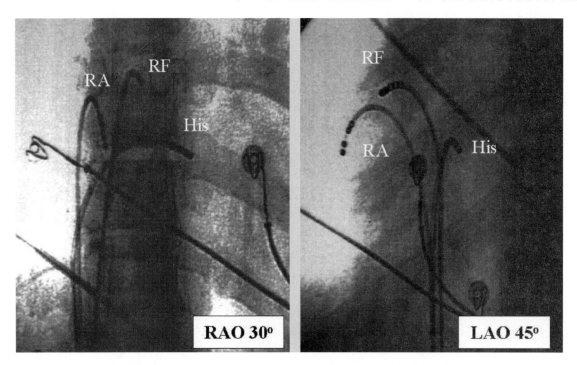

Figure 7. Chest X-ray showing catheter position.

successful, AV junction ablation with pacemaker implantation may be considered in patients with rapid ventricular rates despite pharmacological treatment.

In the present case, the ablation procedure was guided by local conduction delays and was easy, with termination of the arrhythmia during the first radiofrequency current application.

Suggested Reading

Coumel P, Flammang D, Attuel P, et al. Sustained intra-atrial reentrant tachycardia: Electrophysiologic study of 20 cases. *Clin Cardiol* 1979;2:167-178.

Haines DE, DiMarco JP. Sustained intra-atrial reentrant tachycardia: Clinical, electrocardiographic and electrophysiologic characteristics and long-term follow-up. *J Am Coll Cardiol* 1990;15:1345-1354.

Walsh EP, Saul P, Hulse E, et al. Transcatheter ablation of ectopic atrial tachycardia in young patients using radiofrequency current. *Circulation* 1992;86:1138-1146.

Chapter 5

Permanent Left Atrial Tachycardia

Medical History

This is a 46-year-old man with paroxysmal irregular palpitations for 12 years, most of the time induced by physical activity. Initially, palpitations lasted for only 5 to 15 minutes, but occurred several times per day. Over the years, the tachycardia became permanent with ventricular rates between 50 and 230 beats/min. The 12-lead ECG shows a tachycardia with narrow QRS complexes; Holter recording shows intermittent 2:1 or 3:1 atrioventricular (AV) block, confirming the diagnosis of atrial tachycardia. Antiarrhythmic drugs like ß-blockers, sotalol, flecainide or propafenone showed no effect. Echocardiography revealed a progressive diffuse decrease in left ventricular systolic function during follow-up.

Comments

Permanent left atrial tachycardias are rare in our experience. Normally, atrial tachycardias are paroxysmal and the mechanism can be reentry, enhanced automaticity or triggered activity. The differential diagnosis in the presence of a 1:1 AV conduction and a long R-P interval includes: 1) permanent junctional reciprocating tachycardia (PJRT); 2) atypical atrioventricular node reentrant tachycardia ("fast-slow"' AVNRT); and 3) atrial tachycardia. If no AV block can be induced by carotid sinus massage or adenosin, the diagnosis must be confirmed by pacing maneuvers during tachycardia. Radiofrequency catheter ablation is possible with a high success rate (>80 %), but the risks of the transseptal puncture and embolism must be mentioned. The mapping techniques generally use one fixed and stable intracardiac reference (either the His bundle or the coronary sinus atrial electrogram) and two steerable ablation catheters for mapping. The ablation is performed at the site where the earliest intracardiac atrial activation (in reference to the surface P-wave) is recorded.

From: RETAC: *Radiofrequency Catheter Ablation for the Treatment of Cardiac Arrhythmias: A Practical Atlas with Illustrative Cases.*
© Futura Publishing Company, Inc. Armonk, NY, 2002.

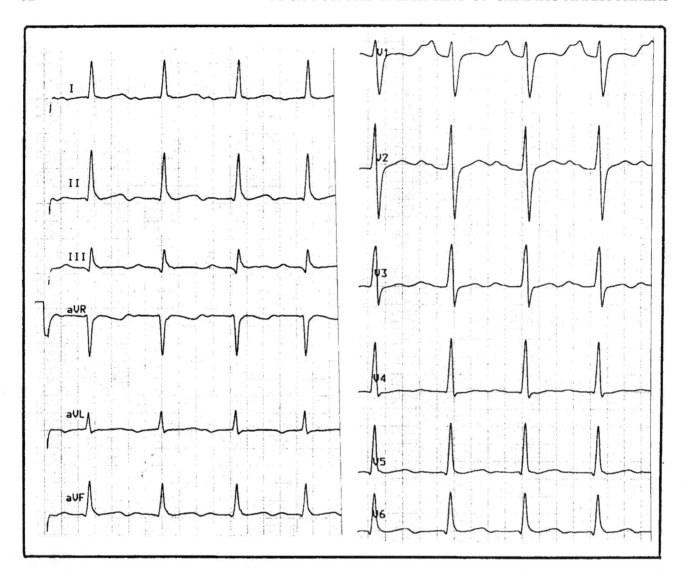

Figure 1. Twelve-lead resting ECG. Paper speed 50 mm/s. Atrial tachycardia at a rate of 140 beats/min with 1:1 AV-conduction. The P wave morphology (flat or negative in I and AVL, giant and positive in V_1) is in favor of a left atrial tachycardia.

Suggested Reading

Kay GN, Chong F, Epstein AE, et al. Radiofrequency ablation for treatment of primary atrial tachycardias. *J Am Coll Cardiol* 1993;21:901-909.

Lesh M, Van Hare GF, Epstein LM, et al. Radiofrequency catheter ablation of atrial arrhythmias. *Circulation* 1994;89:1074-1089.

Weiss C, Hatala R, Cappato R, et al. The encircling mapping technique: A simplified approach to ablation of ectopic atrial tachycardia. *J Am Coll Cardiol* 1994;23:82-89.

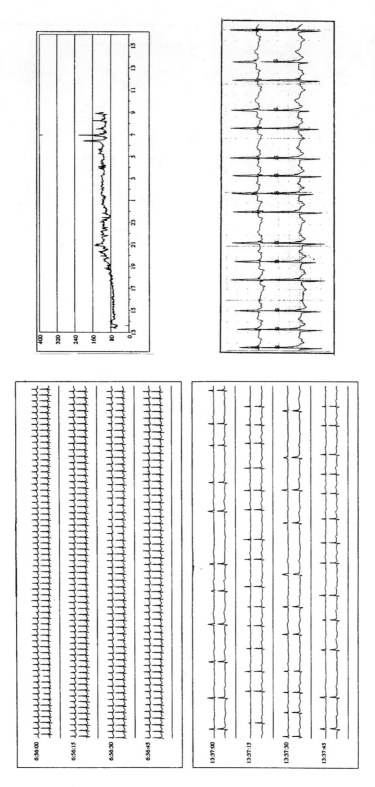

Figure 2. Holter recording showing permanent atrial tachycardia with a ventricular rate between 50 and 223 beats/min. The broad heart rate spectrum is first due to the variability of AV-conduction, but also to a variable atrial rate. This observation suggests that the rate of the atrial tachycardia depends on the autonomic status in the patient.

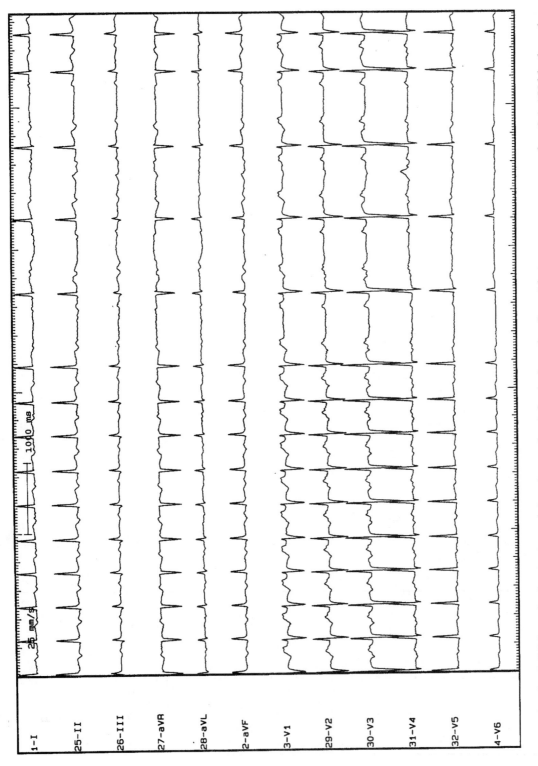

Figure 3. Twelve-lead ECG at the beginning of the electrophysiological study. Carotid sinus massage provokes 2:1 AV block and confirms the diagnosis of atrial tachycardia. If the carotid sinus massage is ineffective, intravenous adenosine can be used. The differential diagnosis of such a long RP tachycardia, with the P wave in the second half of the R-R interval, includes an atypical atrioventricular node reentrant tachycardia (AVNRT) using the slow pathway retrogradely, a permanent junctional reciprocating tachycardia (PJRT) and an atrial tachycardia.

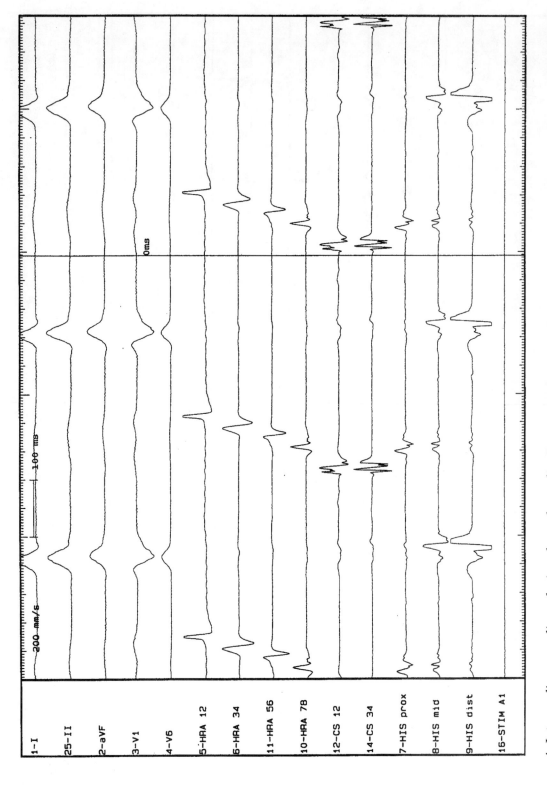

Figure 4. Intracardiac recordings during the tachycardia. Paper speed 200 mm/s. Here are represented five surface ECG leads (I, II, aVF, V₁, V₆), four bipolar recordings from the high right atrium (HRA 12, 34, 56, 78), two bipolar recordings from the coronary sinus (CS 12, 34), and three bipolar recordings from the His bundle region (HIS prox, mid, dist). The earliest atrial activation during tachycardia occurs inside the coronary sinus, in a posterolateral position, 30 ms before the beginning of the P wave on the surface ECG, confirming the diagnosis of a left atrial tachycardia.

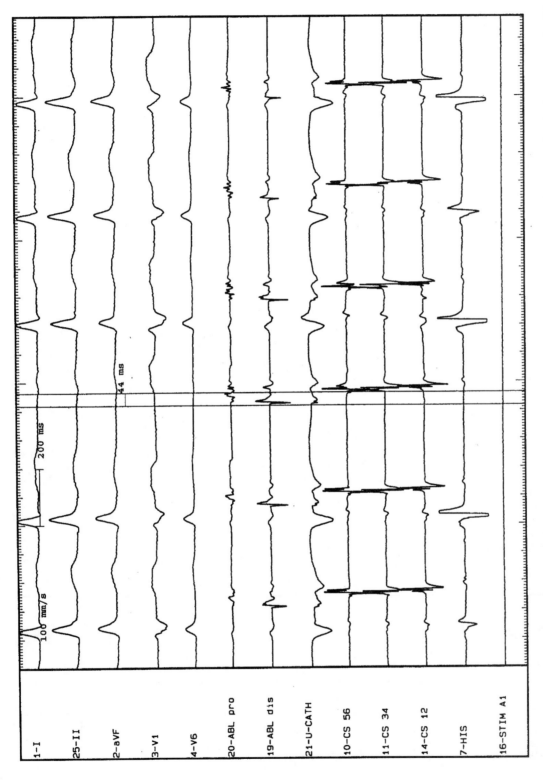

Figure 5. Intracardiac recordings before ablation. Paper speed 100 mm/s. Here are represented 5 surface ECG leads (I, II, aVF, V_1, V_6), two bipolar recordings from the ablation catheter (ABL pro, dis), one unipolar recording obtained from the tip of the ablation catheter (U-CATH), three bipolar recordings from the coronary sinus (CS 12, 34, 56) and one bipolar recording from the His bundle region (HIS). The ablation catheter was advanced into the left atrium through a transseptal sheath, and positioned in the posterolateral region. The earliest atrial activation occurs 44 ms before the beginning of the P wave on the surface ECG, and the unipolar electrogram (U-CATH) shows a QS complex, indicating that this site represents the origin of atrial ectopy.

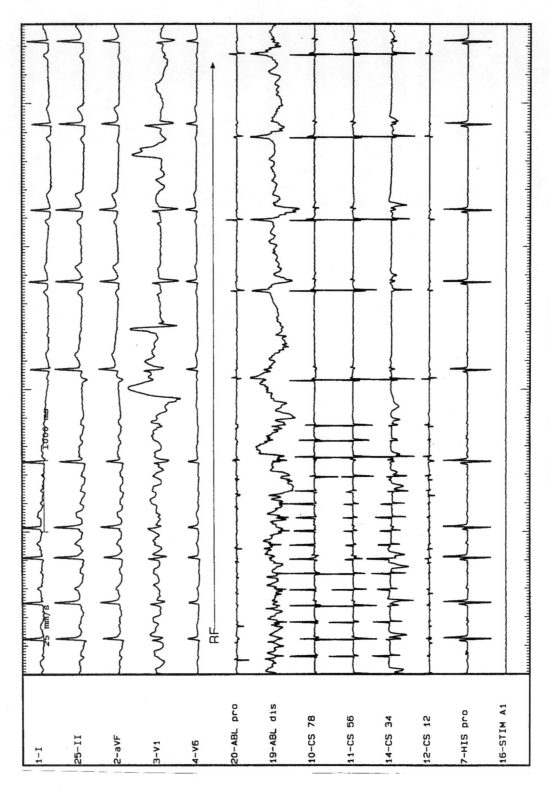

Figure 6. Intracardiac recordings during ablation (paper speed 25 mm/s). Radiofrequency current application at this location (with a maximal temperature of 55°C and a power limit of 50 Watts) terminates the tachycardia after 10 seconds.

Chapter 6

Catheter Ablation of Typical (Type I) Atrial Flutter

Medical History

A 66-year-old male patient presented with a history of typical atrial flutter for the last 4 years. He underwent coronary artery bypass grafting at the age of 60, and suffered from dilated cardiomyopathy with a left ventricular ejection fraction of 25%. Because dilated cardiomyopathy was possibly related to the chronic atrial arrhythmia, the patient was referred for radiofrequency catheter ablation.

Comments

Atrial flutter is often resistant to antiarrhythmic drugs, and carries a potential risk of thromboembolism and, as in the present case, of tachycardiomyopathy. Radiofrequency catheter ablation of the cavotricuspid isthmus is now considered to be the method of choice to treat atrial flutter, with a primary success rate of 90% if complete bidirectional isthmus conduction block is obtained. The ablation procedure is often performed during atrial flutter, and the catheter is positioned in the cavotricuspid isthmus in order to obtain electrograms coinciding with the plateau of the flutter wave on the surface ECG. An ablation line is drawn from the tricuspid annulus to the inferior vena cava using punctate lesions. A standard 4-mm tip ablation catheter may be used like for any other type of ablation but irrigated-tip or 8-mm tip catheters have been found more effective, with a more rapid achievement of bidirectional isthmus block. Bidirectional isthmus block should be demonstrated by activation mapping during pacing from the low lateral right atrium and proximal coronary sinus, and/or by recording double potentials all along the line of block.

From: RETAC: *Radiofrequency Catheter Ablation for the Treatment of Cardiac Arrhythmias: A Practical Atlas with Illustrative Cases.* © Futura Publishing Company, Inc. Armonk, NY, 2002.

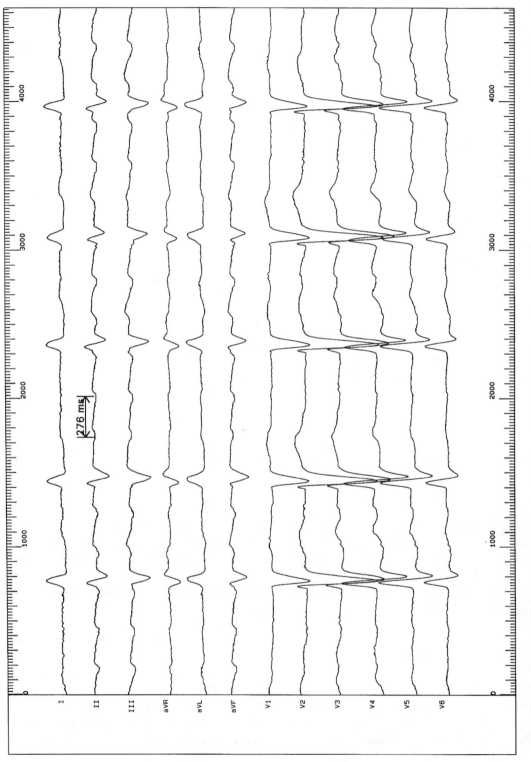

Figure 1. Twelve-lead ECG (50 mm/s) showing typical (type I) atrial flutter, with an atrial cycle length of 276 ms and 2:1 atrioventricular conduction.

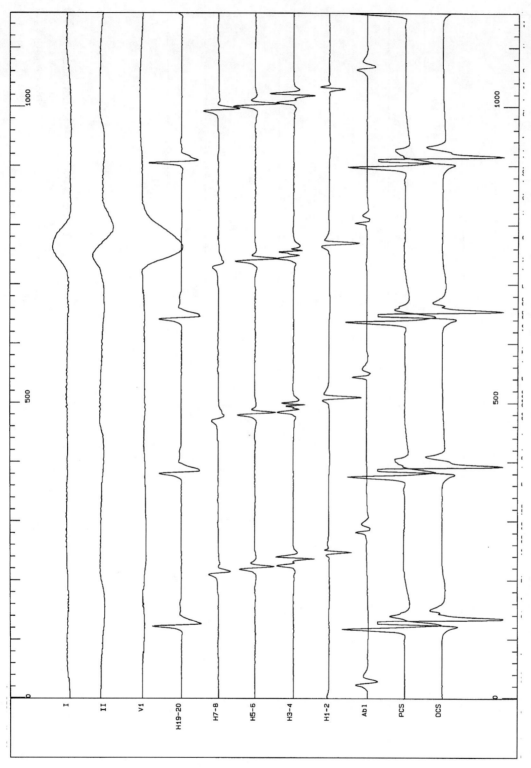

Figure 2. Intracardiac recordings during atrial flutter. On the figure are shown three surface ECG leads (I, II and V_1) together with eight bipolar intracardiac recordings (H19-20 to H1-2) = catheter positioned on the right lateral wall, from the high to low right atrium; Abl = bipolar recording from the tip of the ablation catheter positioned in the cavotricuspid isthmus; PCS = proximal coronary sinus; DCS = distal coronary sinus). The atrial activation sequence is counterclockwise. Paper speed 200 mm/s.

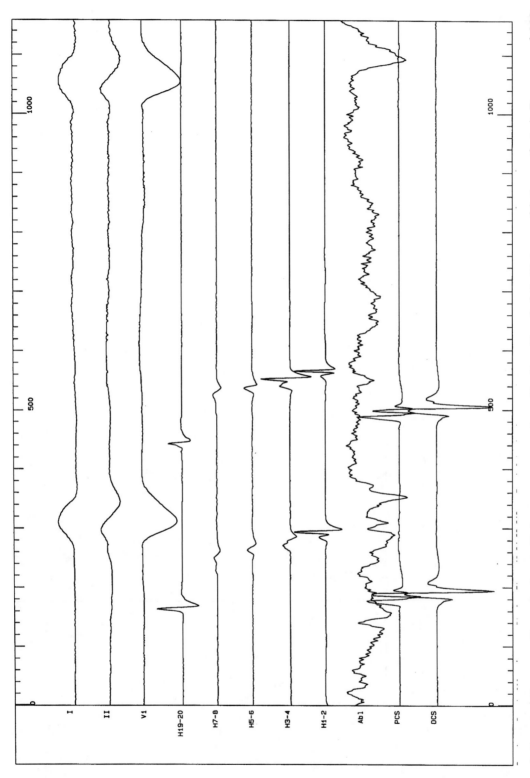

Figure 3. Intracardiac recordings during radiofrequency current application ("cooled-tip" 4-mm ablation catheter). Paper speed 200 mm/s. On the figure are shown three surface ECG leads (I, II, V_1) together with eight bipolar intracardiac recordings (same abbreviations as Figure 2). The atrial flutter is interrupted in the cavo-tricuspid isthmus during radiofrequency current application (in the present case, three radiofrequency current applications of 1 minute each were applied before successful interruption of the atrial arrhythmia).

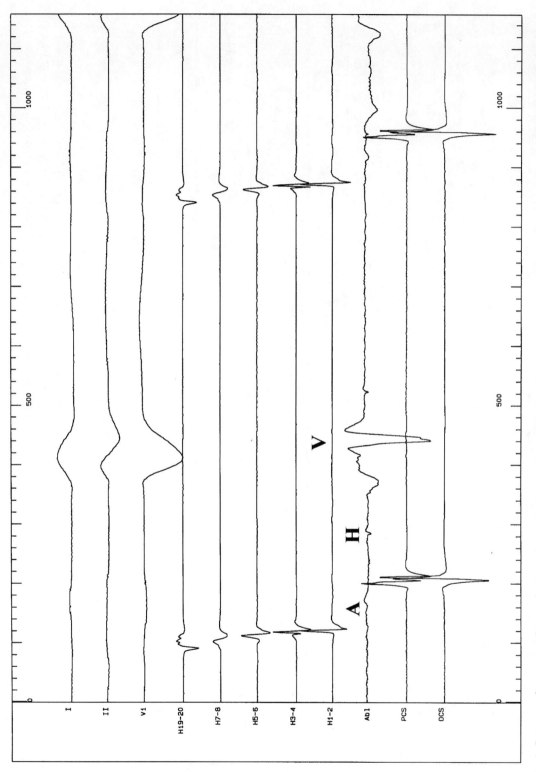

Figure 4. Intracardiac recordings during sinus rhythm after radiofrequency current application. Paper speed 200 mm/s. On the figure are shown three surface ECG leads (I, II, V$_1$) together with eight bipolar intracardiac recordings (same abbreviations as Figure 2). The ablation catheter is now in the His bundle region. AH interval = 120 ms; HV interval = 60 ms; interatrial conduction time (HRA-CS) = 90 ms.

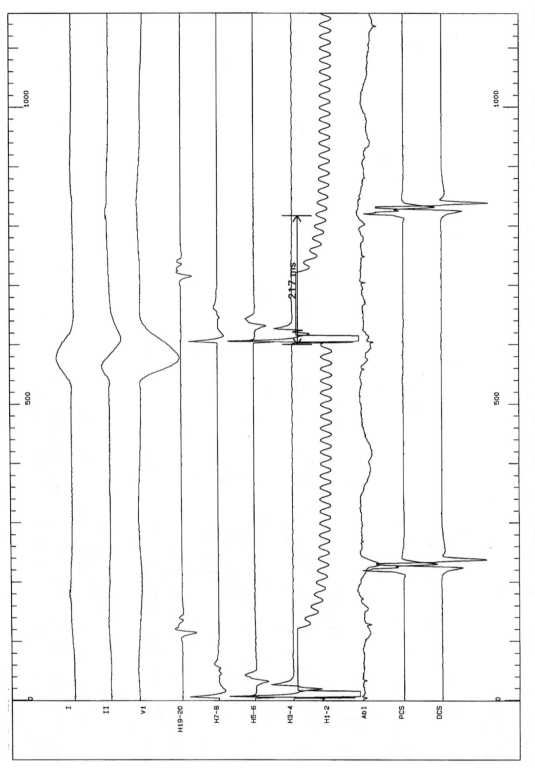

Figure 5. Intracardiac recordings after the ablation procedure, showing counterclockwise isthmus conduction block. Paper speed 200 mm/s. On the figure are shown three surface ECG leads (I, II and V_1) together with eight bipolar intracardiac recordings (same abbreviations as Figure 2). The low right atrium is paced through poles H1-2, and conduction time between the low right atrium and the proximal coronary sinus is prolonged to 217 ms.

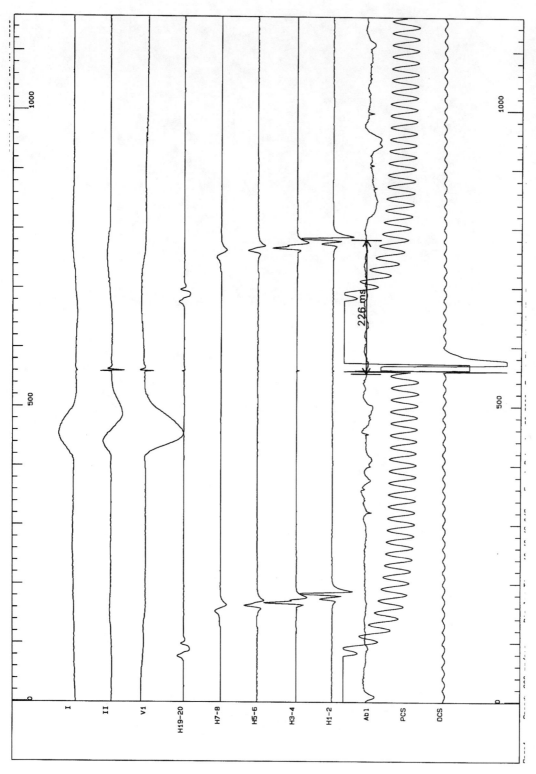

Figure 6. Intracardiac recordings after the ablation procedure, showing clockwise isthmus conduction block. Paper speed 200 mm/s. On the figure are shown three surface ECG leads (I, II, V$_1$) together with eight bipolar intracardiac recordings (same abbreviations as Figure 2). The proximal coronary sinus (PCS) is paced, and conduction time between the PCS and the low right atrium (H1-2) is prolonged to 226 ms.

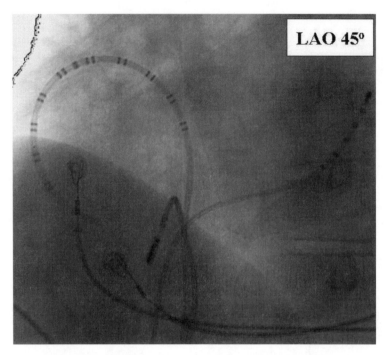

Figure 7. Chest X-ray showing catheter position

Suggested Reading

Luchsinger JA, Steinberg JS. Resolution of cardiomyopathy after ablation of atrial flutter. *J Am Coll Cardiol* 1998;32:205-210.

Fischer B, Jaïs P, Shah DC, et al. Radiofrequency catheter ablation of common atrial flutter in 200 patients. *J Cardiovasc Electrophysiol* 1996;7:1225-1233.

Poty H, Saoudi N, Aziz AA, et al. Radiofrequency catheter ablation of type I atrial flutter: Prediction of late success by electrophysiological criteria. *Circulation* 1995;92:1389-1392.

Jaïs P, Shah DC, Haïssaguerre M, et al. Prospective randomized comparison of irrigated-tip versus conventional-tip catheters for ablation of common flutter. *Circulation* 2000;101:772-776.

Chapter 7

Clockwise (Atypical) Atrial Flutter

Medical History

This 62-year-old patient had suffered an anterior wall myocardial infarction in 1992, treated with thrombolysis. He had three subsequent episodes of pulmonary edema related to an extensive myocardial scar (left ventricular ejection fraction 25%). A first episode of atrial flutter in October 2000 was treated by overdrive pacing and amiodarone, but over the next 3 months he presented with two additional episodes of symptomatic atrial flutter. Echocardiography confirmed the low ejection fraction and showed significant left and right atrial enlargement. The ECG showed clockwise atrial flutter, and radiofrequency catheter ablation was proposed.

Comments

Radiofrequency ablation of clockwise isthmus-dependent type II atrial flutter is feasible with a high rate of primary success. In fact, the rate of success and rate of recurrence are very similar to those of type I counterclockwise atrial flutter. The target for ablation is the same in both arrhythmias: the isthmus between the tricuspid valve annulus and the inferior vena cava. In the present case, a cineangiogram of the isthmus was performed before the ablation procedure in order to define anatomy. The radiofrequency catheter ablation was performed during atrial flutter using a long-curve 8-mm tip catheter introduced into a long 8-French sheath for better stabilization in the isthmus. The ablation catheter was positioned perpendicularly to 40° LAO fluoroscopic view, and each radiofrequency current application had a duration of 60 seconds, with a power setting of 60 Watts and a temperature limit of 55°C. After interruption of atrial flutter during radiofrequency current application, it is essential to confirm isthmus block by pacing maneuvers (pacing from the proximal coronary sinus to demonstrate clockwise isthmus block).

From: RETAC: *Radiofrequency Catheter Ablation for the Treatment of Cardiac Arrhythmias: A Practical Atlas with Illustrative Cases.*
© Futura Publishing Company, Inc. Armonk, NY, 2002.

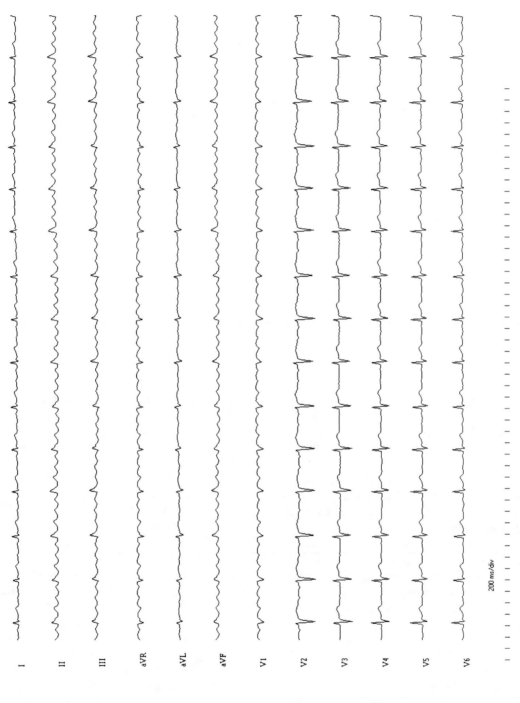

Figure 1. Twelve-lead ECG tracing showing a clockwise atrial flutter at 290 beats/min with a positive atrial deflection in lead II, III and aVF and a negative deflection in V₁ with a 4:1 ventricular response at 75 beats/min.

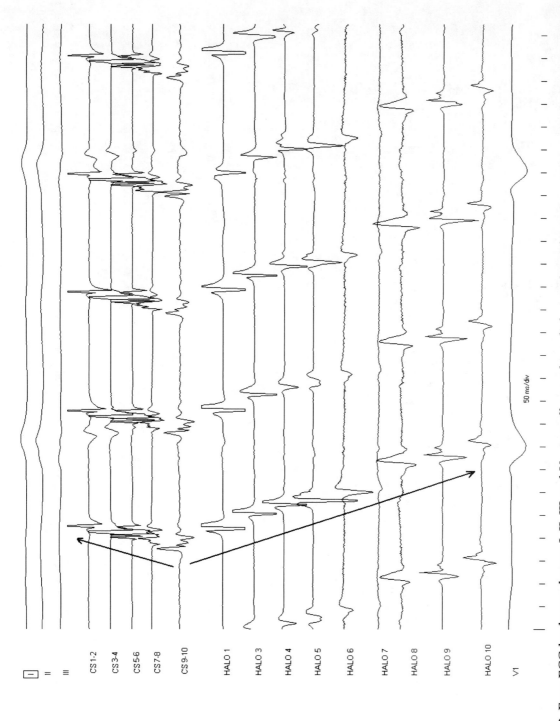

Figure 2. Four ECG leads are shown: I, II, III and V₁, as well as endocardial recordings from the coronary sinus (CS 1-2 to CS 9-10 from the distal part to the proximal one) and from a Halo catheter located in the right atrium at the level of the tricuspid annulus, crossing the cavo-tricuspid isthmus (Halo 1 to Halo 10 from the region of the coronary sinus os to the upper antero-lateral portion of the right atrium). We observe a clockwise progression of the electrical activation from Halo 1 to Halo 10. The coronary sinus is activated from the proximal portion (CS 9-10) to the distal one (CS 1-2).

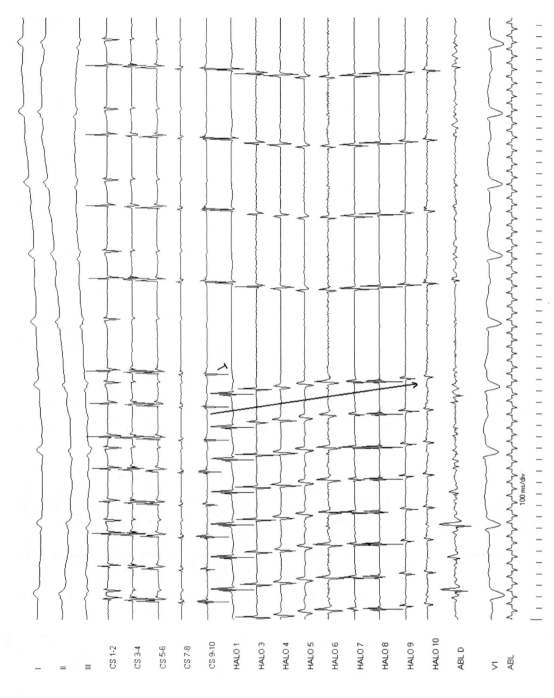

Figure 3. Same recordings as in Figure 2, during radiofrequency ablation. ABL is a reference marker of energy delivery during ablation. The Halo catheter has been pulled back towards the postero-lateral part of the tricuspid annulus. The flutter is interrupted at the isthmus, precluding depolarisation to conduct from the coronary sinus os region to Halo1. Sinus rhythm is restored.

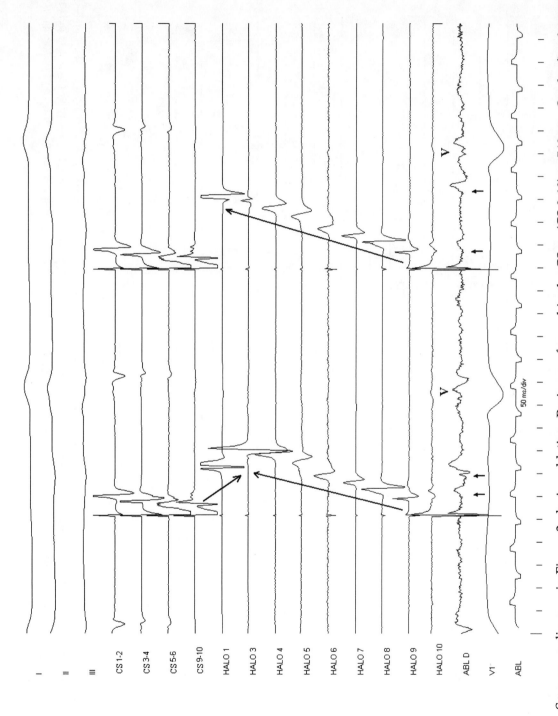

Figure 4. Same recordings as in Figure 3, during ablation. Pacing performed in the CS os (CS 9-10) at 540 ms. On the first beat, we observe a clear collision of two wave fronts, one coming from CS 9-10 to Halo 10 and one travelling towards Halo 1, colliding near Halo 3. This means that conduction through the isthmus is still possible. Atrial activity in ABLD has two components but closely spaced. The second beat shows, during ablation, a shift of Halo 1 and Halo 3 with the electrograms no more collided but depolarized sequentially form Halo 10 to Halo 1, indicating a conduction block between the region of the CS os and Halo 1. A clear separation of the potentials on ABLD can be observed.

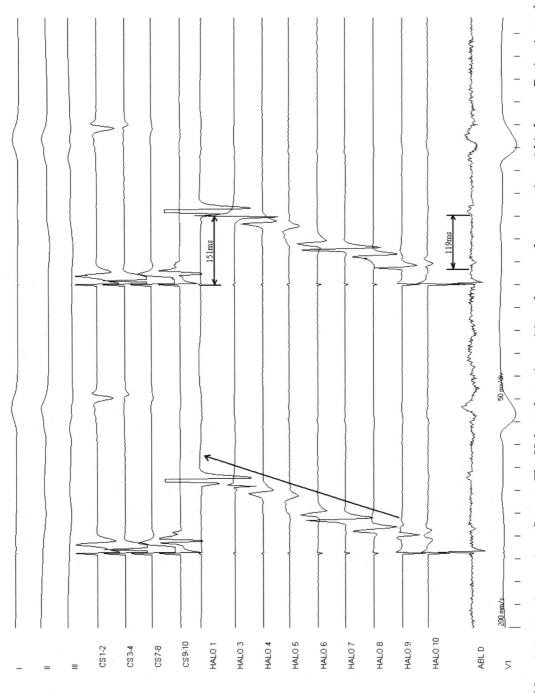

Figure 5. Abbreviations as in previous figures. The Halo catheter is positioned across the cavo-tricuspid isthmus. Pacing is performed at the CS os and confirms the conduction block with a delay of activation of 119 ms between the two potentials at the level of the isthmus (ABLD).

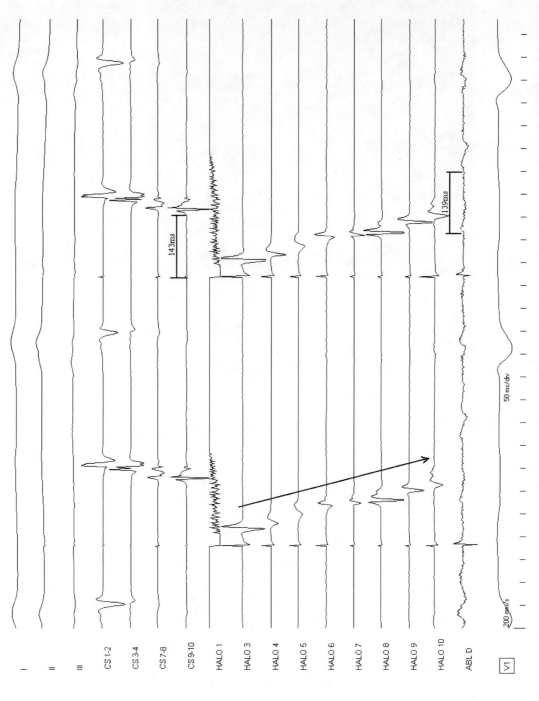

Figure 6. Pacing at the lateral part of the isthmus confirms the isthmus block in the other direction (counterclockwise) with a delay of activation at the level of the isthmus (ABLD) of 139 ms.

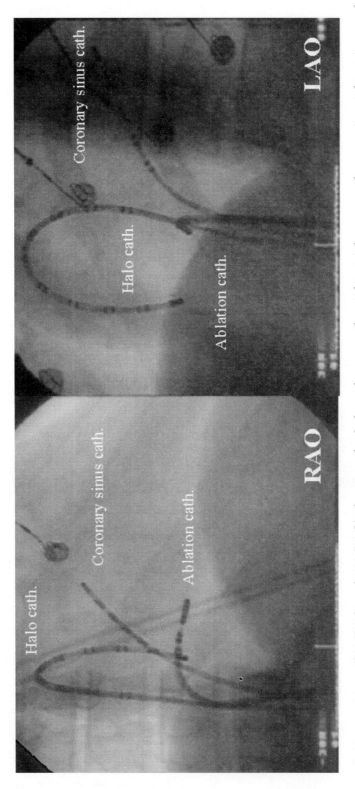

Figure 7. X-ray picture (30° RAO and 40° LAO) showing the halo catheter on the right atrial septum, the superior right atrium and the lateral wall during ablation. A decapolar catheter is positioned in the coronary sinus. An 8-mm tip catheter is placed on the cavo-tricuspid isthmus via an 8-French specific introducer for RF ablation.

Suggested Reading

Lesh M, Kalman J. To fumble flutter or tackle tach ? Toward updated classifiers for atrial tachyarrhythmias. *J Cardiovasc Electrophysiol* 1996;7:460-466.

Nakagawa H, Lazzara R, Khastgir T, et al. Role of the tricuspid annulus and the eustachian valve/ridge on atrial flutter: Relevance to catheter ablation of the septal isthmus and a new technique for rapid identification of ablation success. *Circulation* 1996;94:407-424.

Heidbüchel H, Willems R, Van Rensburg H, et al. Right atrial angiographic evaluation of the posterior isthmus. Relevance for ablation of typical atrial flutter. *Circulation* 2000;101: 2178-2184.

Schwartzman D, Callans DJ, Gottlieb CD, et al. Conduction block in the inferior vena caval-tricuspid valve isthmus: Association with outcome of radiofrequency ablation of Type I atrial flutter. *J Am Coll Cardiol* 1996;28:1519-1531.

Chapter 8

Counterclockwise (Typical) Atrial Flutter

Medical History

This 59-year-old patient presented with paroxysmal atrial arrhythmias of 6 months duration. The atrial arrhythmia was extremely symptomatic with severe impairment of quality of life. Atrial fibrillation had been diagnosed and amiodarone was prescribed. Echocardiography showed no structural heart disease, with borderline atrial enlargement. During amiodarone therapy, atrial fibrillation was transformed into typical (counterclockwise) atrial flutter and it was decided to perform an ablation of the cavo-tricuspid isthmus to prevent further recurrences. The ablation procedure in this case was performed during sinus rhythm.

Comments

Radiofrequency catheter ablation is considered today as the best curative therapy for typical (counter-clockwise) isthmus-dependent type I atrial flutter. In order to achieve the lowest recurrence rate, complete bidirectional cavotricuspid isthmus block has to be obtained (endpoint for the ablation procedure). The most widely used techniques to assess the presence of isthmus conduction block are detailed atrial activation mapping and identification of widely split double potentials along the ablation line. Prolongation of transisthmus interval by more than 50% in both directions is also associated with an excellent prognosis.

In patients with recurrent atrial arrhythmias, a combined approach using antiarrhythmic agents and ablation techniques can often be used, especially when atrial fibrillation is transformed into typical atrial flutter by drugs like in the present case, or when the predominant clinical arrhythmia is atrial flutter.

From: RETAC: *Radiofrequency Catheter Ablation for the Treatment of Cardiac Arrhythmias: A Practical Atlas with Illustrative Cases.* © Futura Publishing Company, Inc. Armonk, NY, 2002.

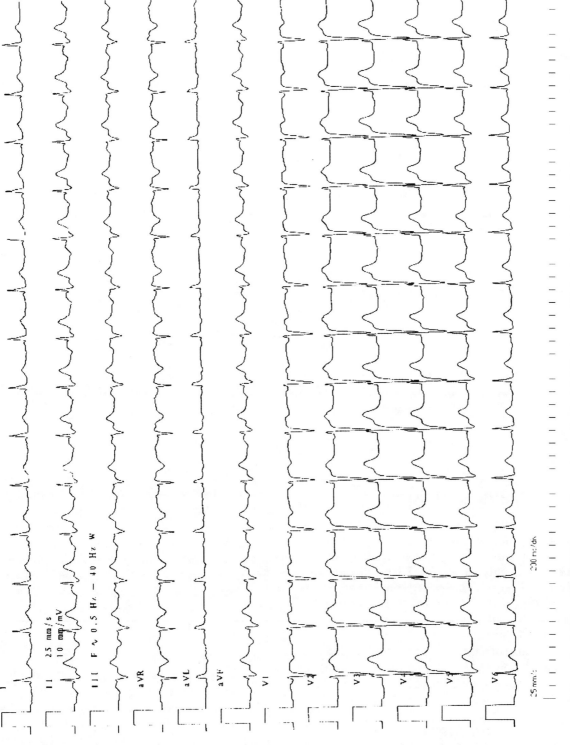

Figure 1. Twelve-lead ECG recording of a typical atrial flutter at 180 beats/min (slowed down by amiodarone).

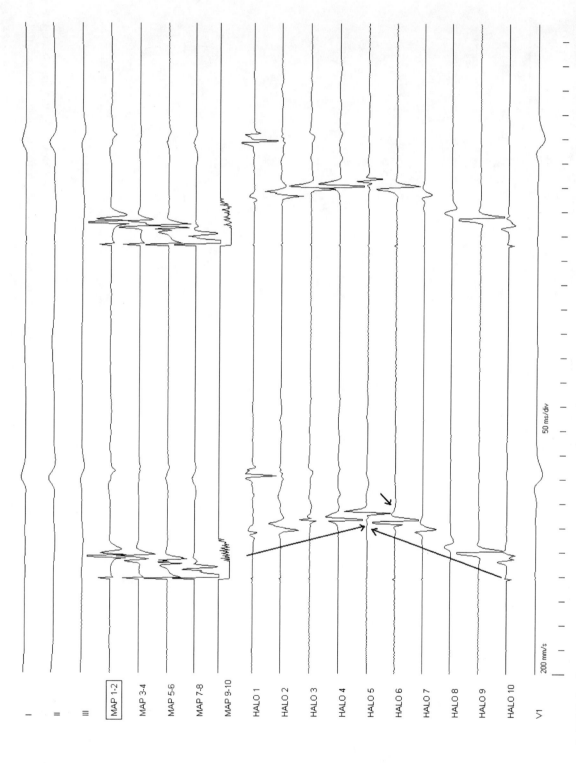

Figure 2. ECG leads I, II, III and V$_1$ are shown. MAP 1-2 to 9-10 represent recordings from the distal coronary sinus (CS) to the proximal part. A Halo catheter is positioned against the lateral wall of the right atrium, crossing the cavo-tricuspid isthmus. Pacing from the CS os reveals a collision of two wave fronts, one coming from the septum, descending along lateral wall and one passing through the isthmus and partially ascending the lateral wall. The collision occurs at Halo 5 (small arrow).

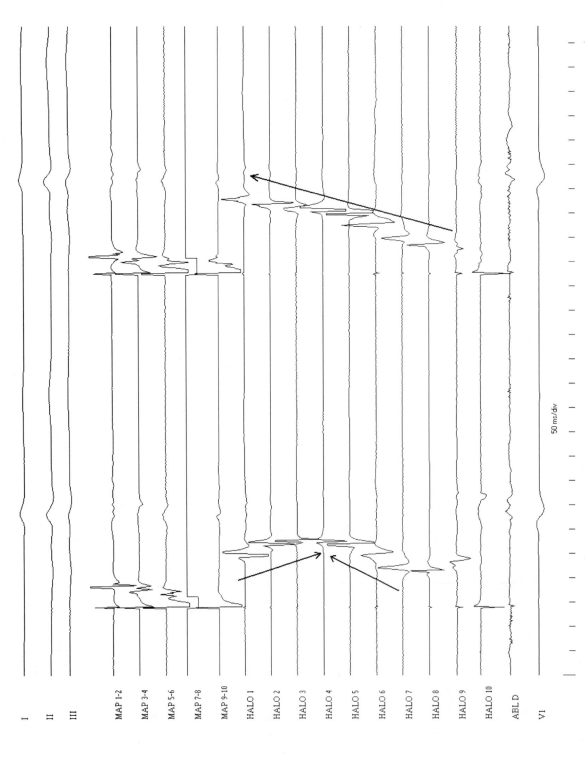

Figure 3. Same recordings as in Figure 2, during radiofrequency (RF) ablation while pacing from the CS os. On the first beat, the collision is still present. On the second beat, the collision disappears during RF application, because of the interruption of conduction in the isthmus. The wavefront has to travel all around the right atrium to the opposite side of the isthmus.

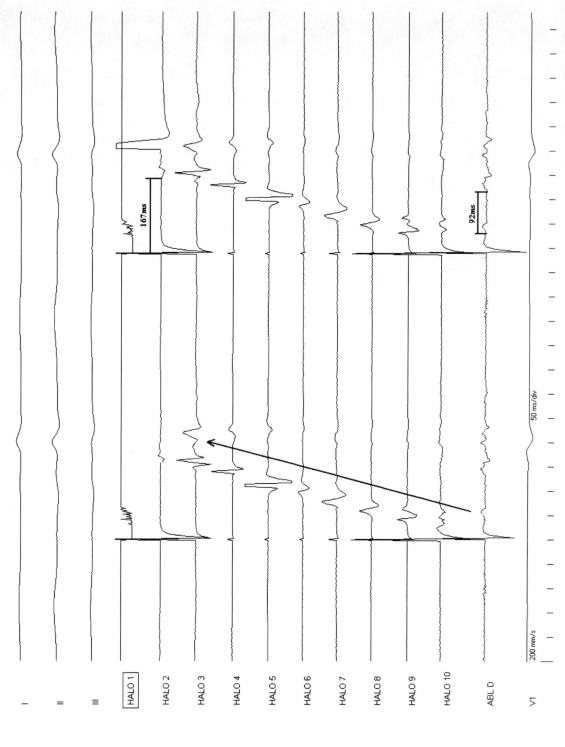

Figure 4. Abbreviations as in previous figures. After having interrupted the conduction through the isthmus, pacing from the CS os (Halo1) reveals a conduction block in the isthmus with a very late deflection on Halo 2 at the opposite side of the isthmus. On the ablation catheter, positioned on the isthmus, we observe a significant delay of 92 ms between the two components of the potentials at both parts of the isthmus.

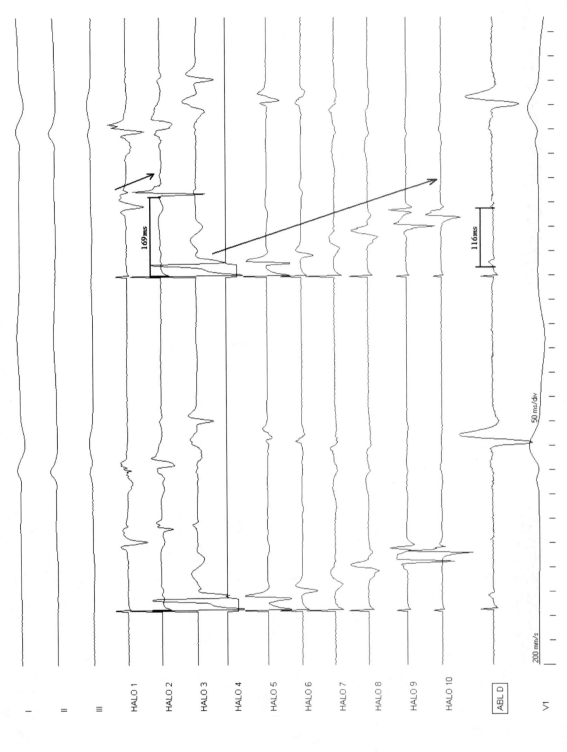

Figure 5. Same display as in Figure 4. Pacing from the lateral part of the isthmus (Halo 4) shows an upward depolarization along the lateral wall and a counterclockwise depolarization towards Halo 2 which is positioned on the isthmus. Halo 2 also records the potentials from the other side of the isthmus when the wavefront coming from the lateral wall has travelled downwards along the septum. The ablation catheter (ABLD), lying on the cavo-tricuspid annulus shows a marked delay between the two potentials (116 ms).

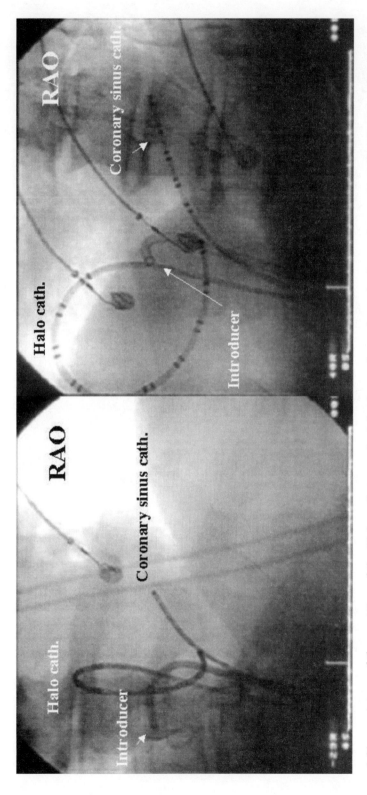

Figure 6. X-ray picture of the position of the Halo catheter and of the decapolar catheter in the coronary sinus (30° RAO and 40° LAO views). The Halo catheter encircles the tricuspid annulus, covering the upper, lateral and lower part during pacing before and during ablation. The decapolar catheter is located in the proximal and medial part of the coronary sinus.

Suggested Reading

Feld GK, Fleck RP, Chen PS, et al. Radiofrequency catheter ablation for the treatment of human type I atrial flutter: Identification of a critical zone in the reentrant circuit by endocardial mapping techniques. *Circulation* 1992;86:1233-1240.

Kalman J, Olgin J, Saxon L, et al. Electrocardiographic and electrophysiologic characterization of atypical atrial flutter in man: Use of activation and entrainment mapping and implications for catheter ablation. *J Cardiovasc Electrophysiol* 1997;8:121-144.

Takahashi R, Iesaka Y, Takahashi A, et al. Clinical significance of residual slow cavotricuspid isthmus conduction after ablation of typical atrial flutter. *Pacing Clin Electrophysiol* 2000;23:1902-1907.

Scheinman MM, Huang S. The 1998 NASPE prospective catheter ablation registry. *Pacing Clin Electrophysiol* 2000;23:1020-1028.

Waldo AL. Treatment of atrial flutter. *Heart* 2000;84:227-232.

Oral H, Sticherling C, Tada H, et al. Role of transisthmus conduction intervals in predicting bidirectional block after ablation of typical atrial flutter. *J Cardiovasc Electrophysiol* 2001;12:169-174.

Chapter 9

Incisional Tachycardia and Atrial Flutter after Orthotopic Heart Transplantation

Medical History

A 56-year-old male patient benefited from orthotopic heart transplant in 1993 because of idiopathic drug-resistant dilated cardiomyopathy. A first episode of atrial tachycardia was diagnosed in 1998, successfully treated with digoxine and β-blockers. Two years later, the arrhythmia recurred with shortness of breath, palpitations, and exercise intolerance. The arrhythmia proved to be resistant to digoxin, metoprololol and propafenone, and the patient was referred for electrophysiologic evaluation and radiofrequency catheter ablation.

Comments

Atrial arrhythmias are frequent after orthotopic cardiac transplantation; they include atrial fibrillation, atrial flutter and ectopic atrial tachycardias. Atrial fibrillation has been associated with an increased risk of subsequent death whereas atrial flutter has not, and most atrial arrhythmias occur in the absence of significant rejection. Atrial flutter in heart transplant patients is usually drug-resistant and radiofrequency catheter ablation should be considered in those patients. Double-spike electrograms are frequently recorded in the low posterior region of the donor heart, but mapping is frequently difficult due to the large circumference of the sutured right atrium. In the present case, two different atrial arrhythmias were observed: one ectopic atrial tachycardia in the recipient heart successfully ablated after careful mapping of the atrial suture line, and one typical atrial flutter in the donor heart successfully treated by conventional isthmus ablation.

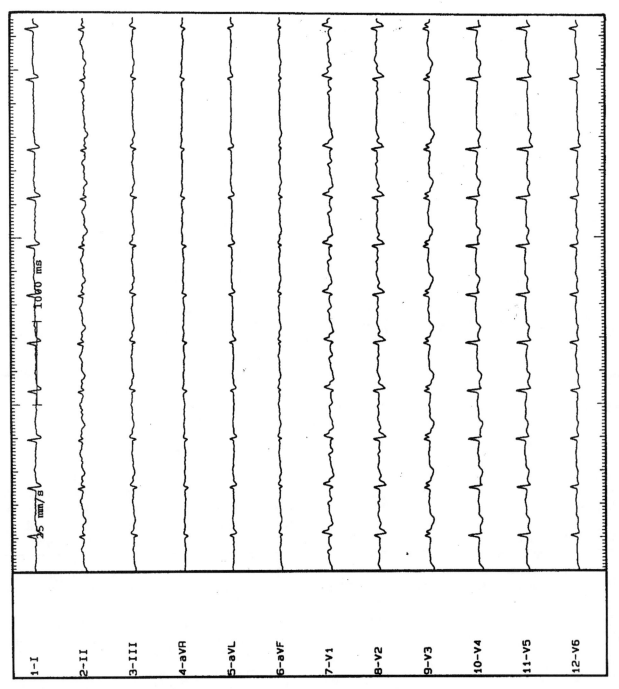

Figure 1. Twelve-lead resting ECG (25 mm/s) showing permanent supraventricular tachycardia at a rate of 210 beats/min with 2:1 atrioventricular block. P wave appears positive in inferior leads with a morphology almost identical to the one observed during sinus rhythm.

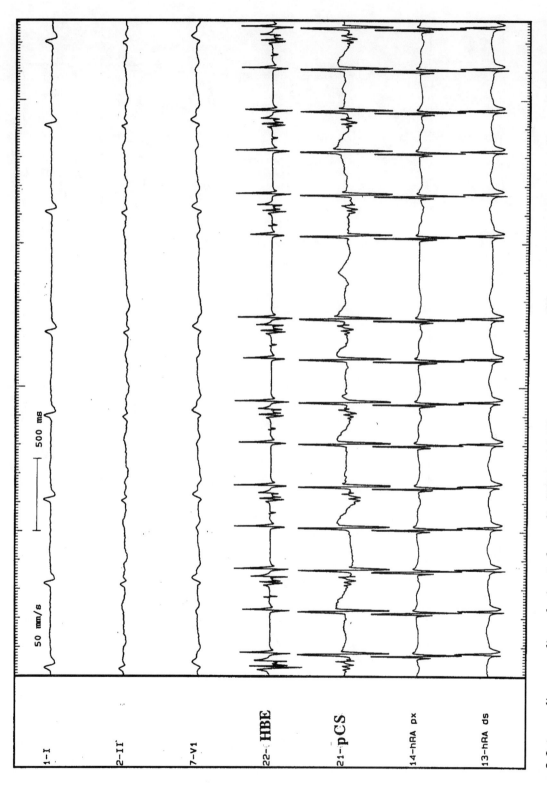

Figure 2. Intracardiac recordings during tachycardia (50 mm/s). Here are represented three surface ECG leads (I, II, V_1), one bipolar recording from the His bundle region (HBE), one bipolar recording from the proximal coronary sinus (pCS), and two bipolar recordings from the high right atrium (hRA px = proximal; hRA ds = distal). Atrial tachycardia is present with a cycle length of 290 ms. An apparent spontaneous termination is observed in the middle of the figure.

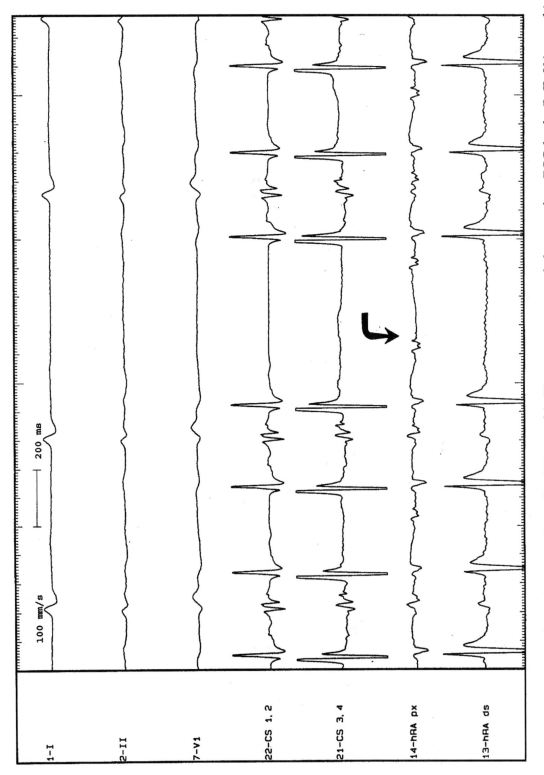

Figure 3. Intracardiac recordings during tachycardia (100 mm/s). Here are represented three surface ECG leads (I, II, V₁), two bipolar recordings from the coronary sinus (CS 1,2 = distal; CS 3,4 = proximal), one bipolar recording from the recipient right atrium (hRA px), and one bipolar recording from the donor right atrium (hRA ds). In the recipient right atrium (hRA px) marked fragmentation of the local electrogram is observed (total duration = 105 ms), with a double potential. During the apparent spontaneous termination of the tachycardia, the intracardiac recording reveals permanent atrial tachycardia in the recipient right atrium with conduction block to the donor right atrium (arrow).

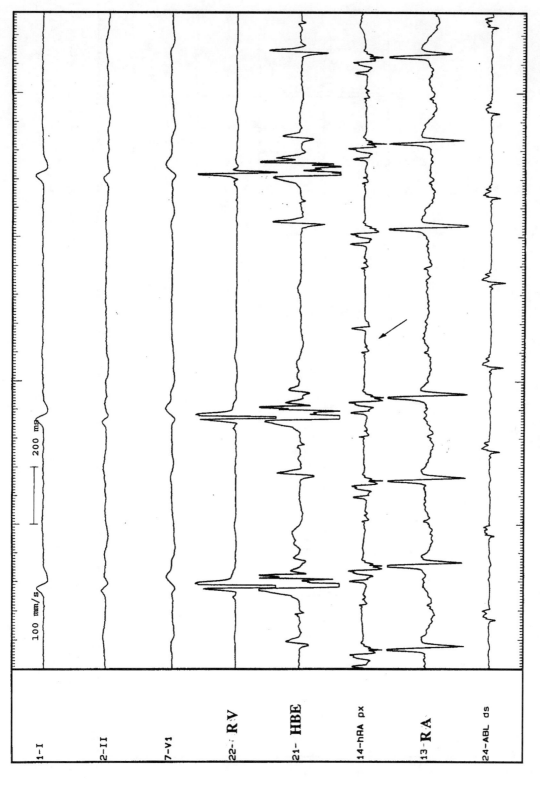

Figure 4. Intracardiac recordings during tachycardia (100 mm/s) at the successful site. Here are represented three surface ECG leads (I, II, V$_1$), one bipolar recording from the right ventricle (RV), one bipolar recording from the His bundle region (HBE), one bipolar recording from the region of the atrial scar (hRA px), one bipolar recording from the donor right atrium (RA), and one bipolar recording from the distal poles of the ablation catheter (ABL ds) positioned in the recipient right heart. The double potential is clearly identified in the recipient right atrium (hRA px, arrow) and dissociation between the recipient and the donor right atrium is present. The local electrogram in the recipient heart precedes the surface P wave by 133 ms. Radiofrequency current application at that site terminated the recipient atrial tachycardia.

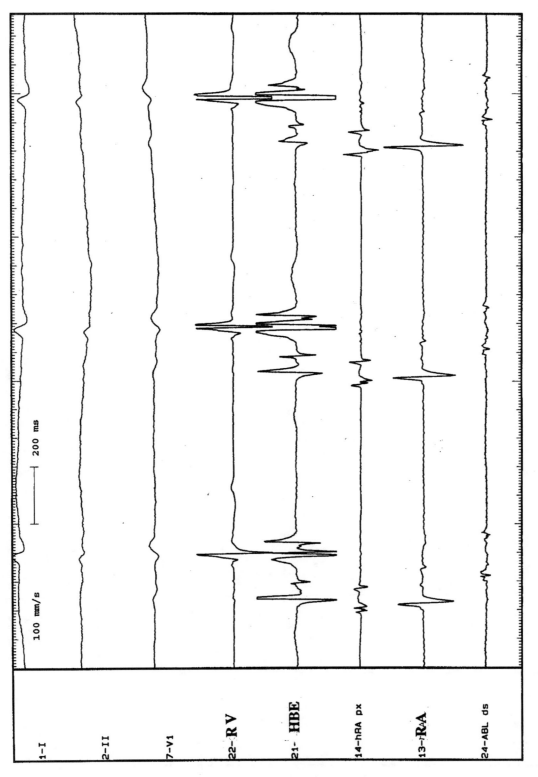

Figure 5 : Intracardiac recordings (100 mm/s) during sinus rhythm after successful catheter ablation. Same display as Figure 4. In the recipient right atrium (ABL ds) the double potential is still present, as well as in the region of the atrial scar (hRA px). A-H interval = 70 ms; H-V interval = 50 ms.

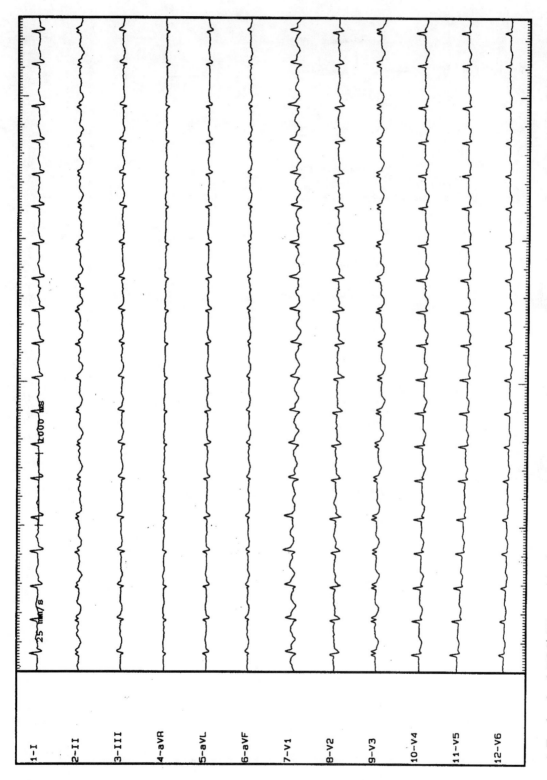

Figure 6. Twelve-lead ECG (25 mm/s) of type I atrial flutter induced after the ablation procedure during programmed atrial stimulation under isoproterenol infusion. The induced arrhythmia is clearly different from the one shown in Figure 1, with negative P waves in inferior leads, a cycle length of 210 ms, and 2:1 atrioventricular block (ventricular rate now 130 beats/min).

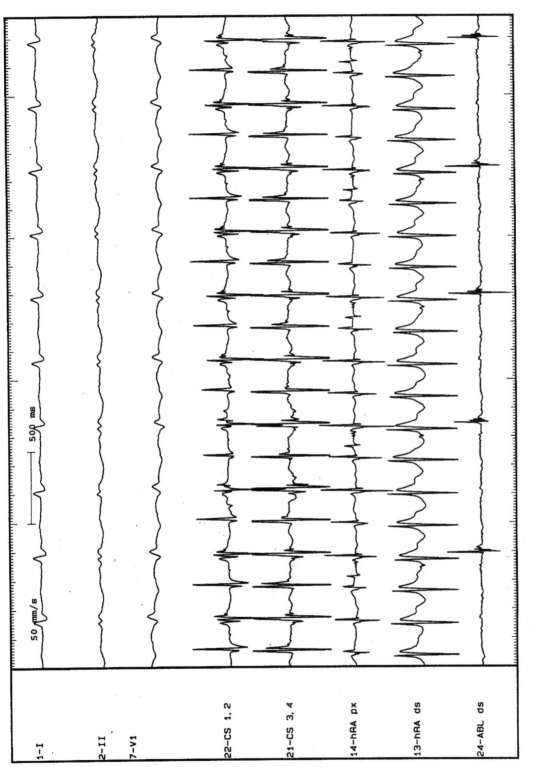

Figure 7. Intracardiac recordings during atrial flutter (50 mm/s). Here are represented three surface ECG leads (I, II, V$_1$), two bipolar recordings from the coronary sinus (CS 1,2 = distal; CS 3,4 = proximal), two bipolar recordings from the donor right atrium (hRA px = proximal; hRA ds = distal), and one bipolar recording from the distal poles of the ablation catheter positioned in the recipient right atrium (ABL ds). Counterclockwise atrial flutter is present in the donor heart, and sinus rhythm is present in the recipient heart (ABL ds) with complete dissociation between the two atria.

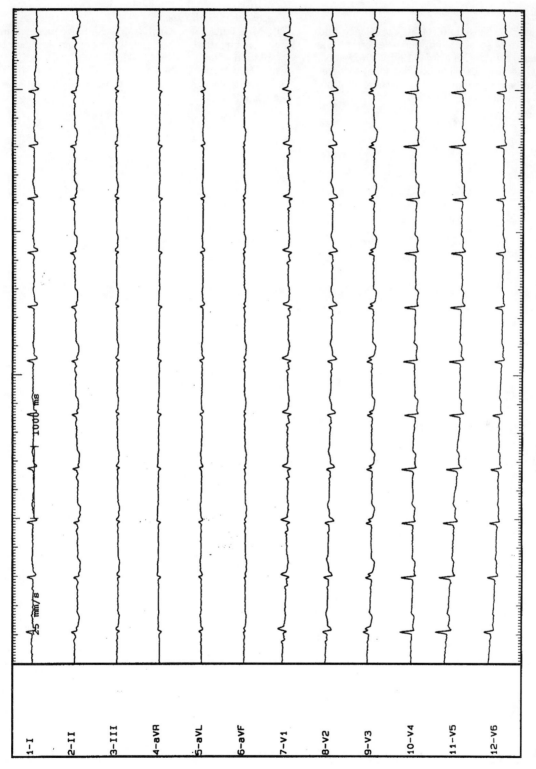

Figure 8. Twelve-lead ECG (25 mm/s) at the end of the ablation procedure showing normal sinus rhythm. Cavotricuspid isthmus ablation was performed as usual, with 10 successive punctiform radiofrequency applications in the anterior isthmus, and bidirectional isthmus block was confirmed by low right atrium and coronary sinus stimulation. No recurrences of atrial arrhythmias were observed during a follow-up of 8 months.

Suggested Reading

Pavri BB, O'Nunain SS, Newell JB, et al. Prevalence and prognostic significance of atrial arrhythmias after orthotopic cardiac transplantation. *J Am Coll Cardiol* 1995;25:1673-1680.

Li YG, Gronefeld G, Hohnloser SH. Radiofrequency catheter ablation of atrial flutter after orthotopic heart transplantation. *J Cardiovasc Electrophysiol* 1996;7:1986-1990.

Pinski SL, Bredikis AJ, Winkel E, et al. Radiofrequency catheter ablation of atrial flutter after orthotopic heart transplantation: Insights into the redefined critical isthmus. *J Heart Lung Transplant* 1999;18:292-296.

Pitt MP, Bonser RS, Griffith MJ. Radiofrequency catheter ablation for atrial flutter following orthotopic heart transplantation. *Heart* 1998;79:412-413.

Cosio FG, Pastor A, Nunez A, et al. How to map and ablate atrial scar macroreentrant tachycardia of the right atrium. *Europace* 2000;2:193-200.

Chapter 10

Atrial Flutter Ablation in a Heart Transplant Patient

Introduction

A 48-year-old patient had an orthotopic heart transplant performed in 1987. He was admitted on August 8, 1998 for acute congestive heart failure. No evidence for acute rejection was found. The ECG on admission revealed supraventricular tachycardia without any definite atrial activity but with a constant atrioventricular conduction pattern. The ventricular rate was 140 beats/min. Symptomatic treatment of heart failure and preventive anticoagulation were initiated. Amiodarone (at a dose of 1 g/day) and digoxin (0.25 mg/day) were added in order to decrease the ventricular rate and to try to restore sinus rhythm. Five days later the patient was still short of breath with a NYHA class III dyspnea. It was then decided to perform an electrophysiologic study to determine the mechanism of the arrhythmia and eventually to perform radiofrequency catheter ablation.

Comments

The clinical and electrocardiographic follow-up at 2, 6, and 12 months did not show any recurrence of supraventricular arrhythmias, and this result was obtained without any preventive antiarrhythmic therapy. This experience confirms that radiofrequency catheter ablation can be used safely and effectively in heart transplant patients and that the results may be comparable to those obtained in normal patients, because the reentrant circuit of the flutter (as in this case) may involve the isthmus between the tricuspid valve annulus and the inferior vena cava.

From: RETAC: *Radiofrequency Catheter Ablation for the Treatment of Cardiac Arrhythmias: A Practical Atlas with Illustrative Cases.*
© Futura Publishing Company, Inc. Armonk, NY, 2002.

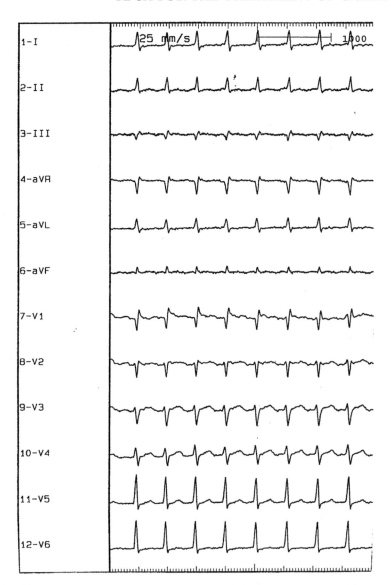

Figure 1. Twelve-lead ECG (25 mm/s) at baseline. Observe the supraventricular arrhythmia without any precise atrial activity while a fixed conduction to ventricles is present. Ventricular rate was 140 beats/min.

Suggested Reading

Pavri BB, O'Nunain SS, Newell JB, et al. Prevalence and prognostic significance of atrial arrhythmias after orthotopic cardiac transplantation. *J Am Coll Cardiol* 1995;25:1673-1680.

Li YG, Gronefeld G, Hohnloser SH. Radiofrequency catheter ablation of atrial flutter after orthotopic heart transplantation. *J Cardiovasc Electrophysiol* 1996;7:1086-1090.

Arenal A, Almendral J, Munoz R, et al. Mechanism and location of atrial flutter in transplanted hearts: Observations during transient entrainment from distant sites. *J Am Coll Cardiol* 1997;30:539-546.

Pitt MP, Bonser RS, Griffith MJ. Radiofrequency catheter ablation for atrial flutter following orthotopic heart transplantation. *Heart* 1998;79:412-413.

Pinski SL, Bredikis AJ, Winkel E, et al. Radiofrequency catheter ablation of atrial flutter after orthotopic heart transplantation: Insights into the redefined critical isthmus. *J Heart Lung Transplant* 1999;18:292-296.

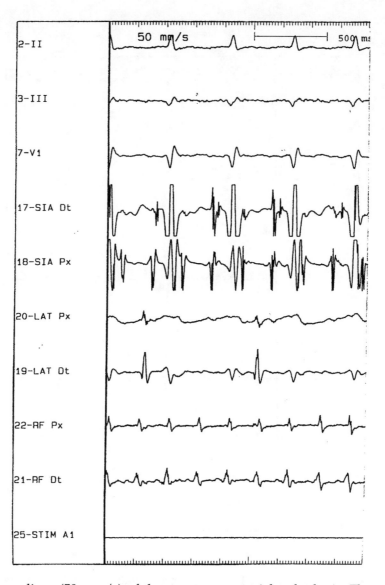

Figure 2. Intracardiac recordings (50 mm/s) of the spontaneous atrial arrhythmia. Three quadripolar catheters were inserted through the right femoral vein and used to map the right atrium. One catheter was positioned in the septal region close to the His bundle (SIA Dt and SIA Px), one in the high part of the lateral wall of the donor's right atrium, and one steerable catheter (RF Dt and RF Px) was used to explore successively the lower part of the lateral wall of the donor's right atrium, the recipient right atrium, the junction between the two atria, and the isthmus between the tricuspid valve and the inferior vena cava. Mapping of these different regions showed that the arrhythmia was located in the donor atrium (21-RF Dt and 22-RF Px), whereas the native atrium was in sinus rhythm (19-LAT Dt and 20-LAT Px).

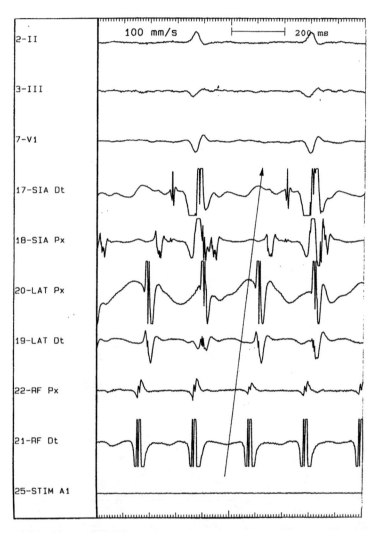

Figure 3. Intracardiac recordings (100 mm/s) showing the activation sequence of the atrial arrhythmia in the donor's right atrium corresponding to a clockwise atrial flutter (type II). The right lateral wall shows a caudo-cranial activation whereas the septum has a cranio-caudal activation. Mapping and resetting with the steerable catheter confirmed that the isthmus was part of the circuit. SIA Dt and Px = interatrial septum of the donor's right atrium; LAT Dt and Px = high lateral wall of the donor's right atrium; RF Dt and Px = steerable radiofrequency catheter located on low lateral wall of the donor's right atrium.

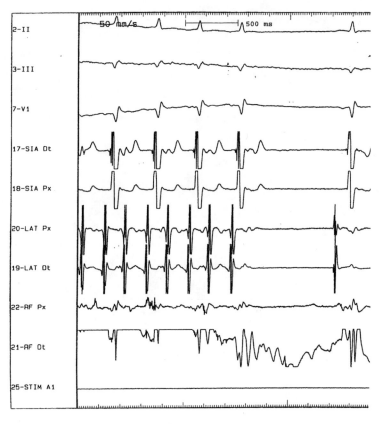

Figure 4. Intracardiac recordings (50 mm/s) at the successful site. Radiofrequency was delivered during 60 seconds at a maximal temperature of 65°C through a steerable catheter with a 4-mm tip and a thermocouple temperature control. The first site was in the tricuspid region of the isthmus. The catheter was then slightly pulled back towards the inferior vena cava and several other radiofrequency current applications were made until the arrhythmia stopped. The atrial flutter was interrupted during the 15th radiofrequency application applied close to the inferior vena cava. SIA Dt and Px = quadripolar catheter located in the right ventricle; LAT Dt and Px = catheter positioned in the high lateral wall of the donor's right atrium; RF Dt and Px = radiofrequency catheter located in the isthmus between the tricuspid valve and the inferior vena cava.

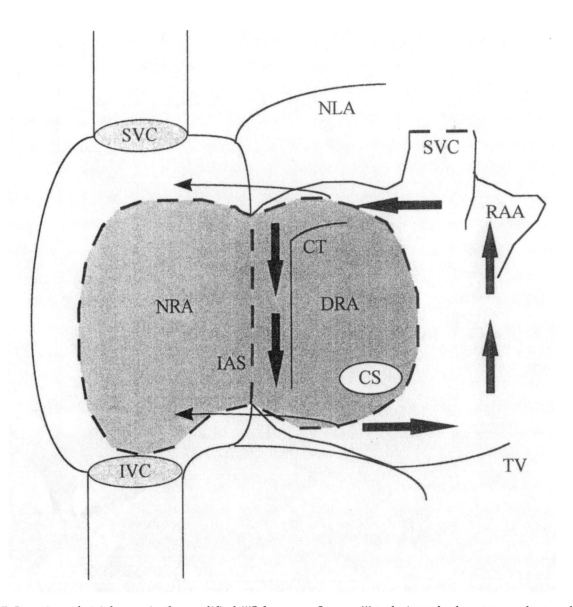

Figure 5. Location of atrial scars in the modified '"Schumway-Lowers'" technique for heart transplant and atrial flutter circuits. Anterior view of opened right atrium. The interatrial suture is circumferential and goes from the interatrial septum to the lateral wall. Note that the suture crosses perpendicularly the isthmus between the inferior vena cava and the tricuspid valve. Large arrows indicate the circuit of the flutter, dotted lines indicate the location of the right atrial scar, thin arrows indicate side-by-side suture. SVC = superior vena cava; IVC = inferior vena cava; NRA = native right atrium; NLA = native left atrium; DRA = donor's right atrium; IAS = interatrial septum; CT = crista terminalis; RAA = right atrial appendage; CS = coronary sinus; TV = tricuspid valve.

Chapter 11

Catheter Ablation of Focal Atrial Fibrillation Originating from the Pulmonary Veins

Medical History

A 34-year-old female patient suffered from recurrent episodes of paroxysmal atrial fibrillation (ventricular rate 160-200 beats/min) for more than 10 years. Her major complaint was palpitation with dizziness, but she never experienced syncope. Clinical examination, resting 12-lead ECG during sinus rhythm and echocardiography were all within normal limits. Atrial fibrillation recurred on a daily basis despite treatment with β-blockers, propafenone, sotalol, quinidine, digoxin, amiodarone, or flecainide.

Comments

The pulmonary veins are an important source of ectopic beats initiating frequent paroxysms of atrial fibrillation, especially in patients with so-called "'lone'" atrial fibrillation. These arrhythmogenic foci are amenable to radiofrequency catheter ablation, which can suppress the trigger and reduce the propensity to develop atrial fibrillation. This type of catheter ablation is curative but requires a transseptal approach and a careful mapping of all pulmonary veins to identify the focus. The procedure is usually long and difficult, and early recurrences are frequently observed, necessitating in many cases two or three successive ablation sessions. Complications include thromboembolic events during or after the procedure, and pulmonary vein stenosis.

Suggested Reading

Haïsaguerre M, Jaïs P, Shah DC, et al. Spontaneous initiation of atrial fibrillation by ectopic beats originating in the pulmonary veins. *N Engl J Med* 1998;339:659-666.

From: RETAC: *Radiofrequency Catheter Ablation for the Treatment of Cardiac Arrhythmias: A Practical Atlas with Illustrative Cases.* © Futura Publishing Company, Inc. Armonk, NY, 2002.

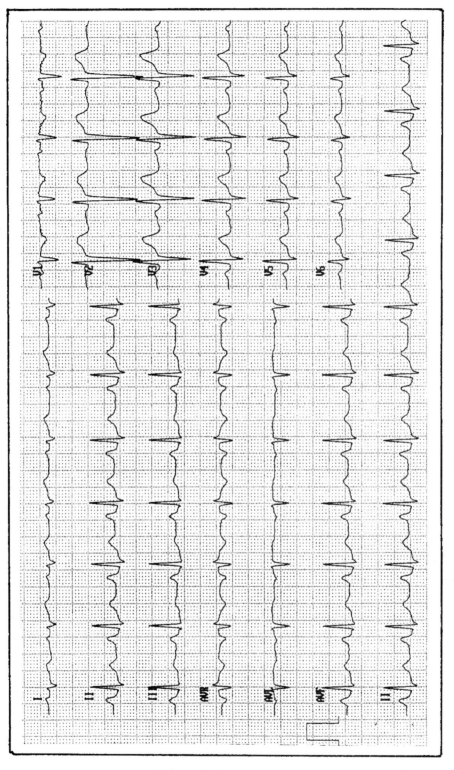

Figure 1. Twelve-lead ECG (25 mm/s) during sinus rhythm showing tall P waves in inferior leads without any other abnormality.

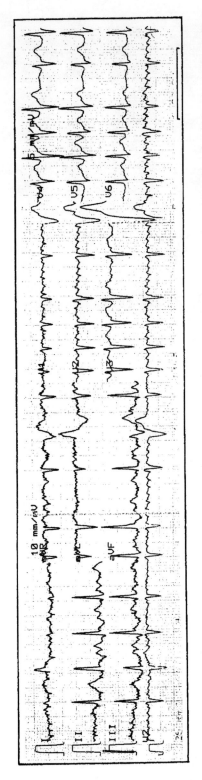

Figure 2. Twelve-lead ECG (25 mm/s) recorded during an episode of severe palpitations. Atrial fibrillation is present, with a ventricular rate of 130 to 190 beats/min and several ventricular ectopic beats.

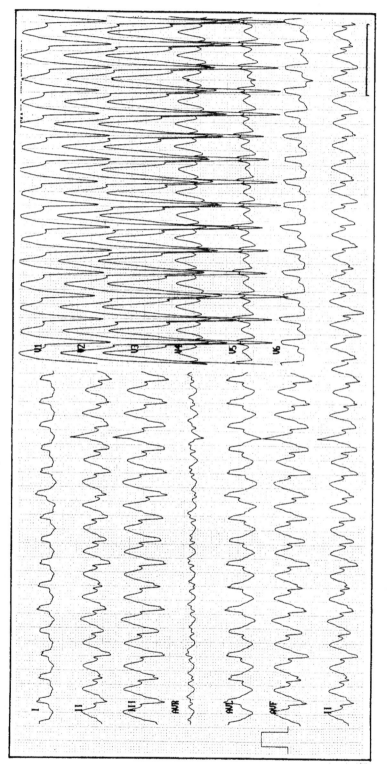

Figure 3. Twelve-lead ECG (25 mm/s) recorded during an episode of severe dizziness during treatment with flecainide showing a regular wide QRS complex tachycardia at a rate of 185 beats/min (atrial tachycardia with 1:1 AV conduction).

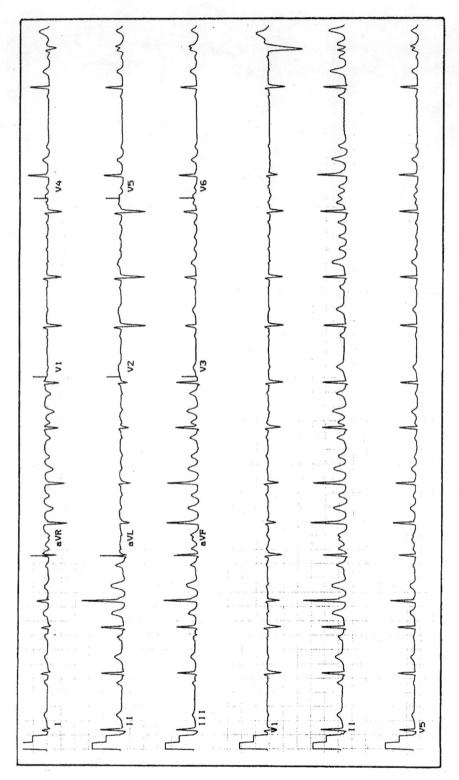

Figure 4. Twelve-lead ECG recording (25 mm/s) without any antiarrhythmic drug treatment showing incessant bursts of atrial tachycardia. The atrial arrhythmia is relatively well organized, at least during the first few seconds, and the initiating premature atrial beat exhibits a classical "P on T'" phenomenon. The same aspect was observed during 24-hour Holter monitoring.

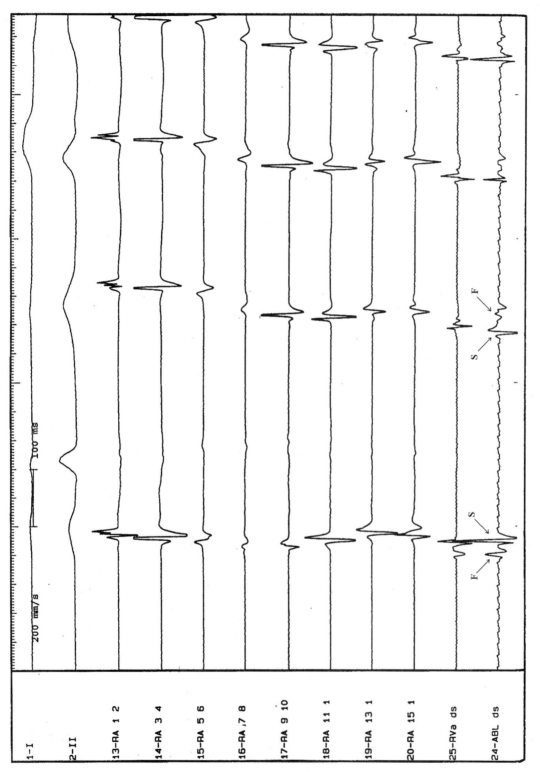

Figure 5. Intracardiac recording (200 mm/s) during spontaneous initiation of atrial fibrillation. A halo catheter was positioned in the right atrium (RA 1 to RA 15) and the ablation catheter (ABL ds and ABL pr) was positioned in the right upper pulmonary vein (RUPV). Note that during sinus rhythm a double potential was identified in the RUPV: the first deflection (arrow-F) was a far-field potential and the second deflection (arrow-S) a spike representing the arrhythmogenic activity originating from the pulmonary vein. During initiation of the atrial arrhythmia there was an inversion of the activation sequence, the spike from the RUPV preceded the onset of P wave by 30 ms and ABL ds preceded ABL px indicating that the arrhythmogenic activity was coming from the pulmonary vein to the left atrium.

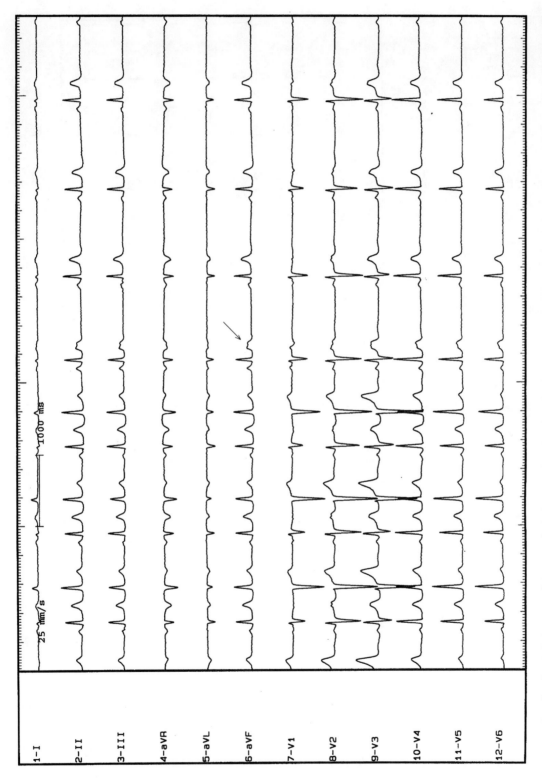

Figure 6. Twelve-lead ECG (25 mm/s) recorded during the third radiofrequency current application at the os of the right upper pulmonary vein. Overt atrial bigeminy was present, and transition to concealed atrial bigeminy (arrow) is observed during radiofrequency current application. No salvoes of atrial tachycardia were observed at that time.

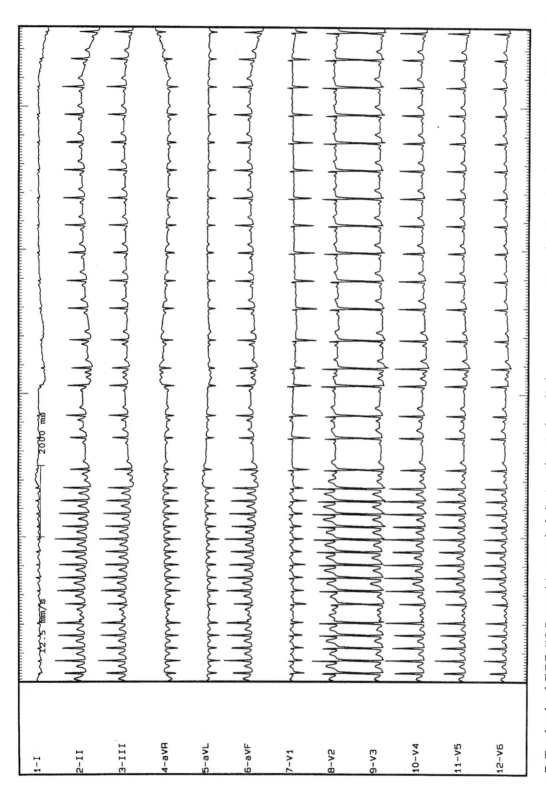

Figure 7. Twelve-lead ECG (12.5 mm/s) recorded during the sixth radiofrequency current application showing progressive interruption of atrial ectopic activity and return to normal sinus rhythm.

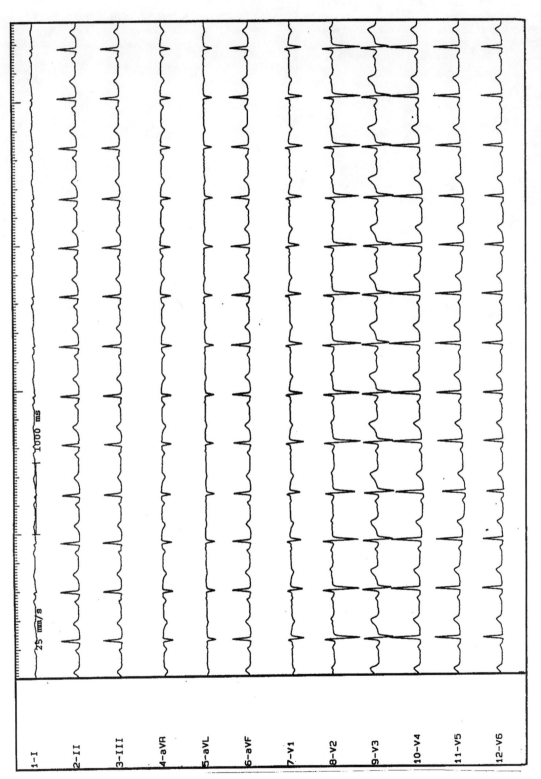

Figure 8. Twelve-lead ECG (25 mm/s) recorded after the ablation procedure showing normal sinus rhythm without any atrial ectopic beat. During a 10-month follow-up without any antiarrhythmic drugs, the patient showed no recurrences of atrial arrhythmia.

Jaïs P, Haïssaguerre M, Shah DC, et al. A focal source of atrial fibrillation treated by discrete radiofrequency ablation. *Circulation* 1997;95:572-576.

Chen SA, Hsieh MH, Tai CT, et al. Initiation of atrial fibrillation by ectopic beats originating from the pulmonary veins. Electrophysiological characteristics, pharmacological re-sponses, and effects of radiofrequency ablation. *Circulation* 1999;100:1879-1886.

Tse HF, Lau CP, Kou W, et al. Comparison of endocardial activation times at effective and ineffective ablation sites within the pulmonary veins. *J Cardiovasc Electrophysiol* 2000;11:155-159.

Chapter 12

Focal Paroxysmal Atrial Fibrillation

Medical History

This is a 45-year-old woman with a 4-year history of daily episodes of irregular rapid palpitations lasting from seconds up to 3 hours. Holter monitoring showed frequent short-coupled atrial premature beats initiating atrial fibrillation. Multiple antiarrhythmic drugs including β-blockers, verapamil, quinidine, sotalol, and propafenone had been tried, but without any beneficial effect on the arrhythmia. Physical examination, echocardiography, and exercise stress testing were normal. An electrophysiologic study was performed with the aim to localize the origin of the atrial premature beats and to try to eliminate the premature ectopic beats by radiofrequency ablation.

Comments

Atrial fibrillation can be initiated by focal triggers located in the pulmonary veins in more than 85% of the cases. Haïssaguerre and coworkers were the first to show that these patients can be cured from atrial fibrillation by ablating the focal triggers. In the present case, the focal source was mapped and ablated like an atrial arrhythmia. The limitations of this kind of approach are multiple:

- Long procedure time (3-4 hours) due to inconstant focal activity and/or long lasting episodes of atrial fibrillation during the ablation procedure.

- High recurrence rate (up to 60 %) after an initial successful ablation of pulmonary vein foci, either because of recovery of the same focus (occurring in more than 70% of the cases) or because of the presence of a second focus (up to 30% of the cases).

- Risk of a pulmonary vein stenosis if the ablation is performed deep inside the pulmonary vein.

From: RETAC: *Radiofrequency Catheter Ablation for the Treatment of Cardiac Arrhythmias: A Practical Atlas with Illustrative Cases.* © Futura Publishing Company, Inc. Armonk, NY, 2002.

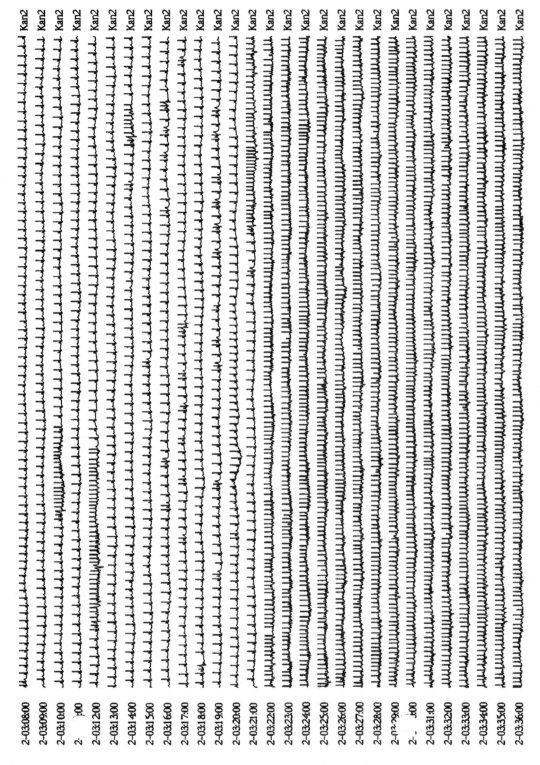

Figure 1. Holter monitoring disclosing frequent atrial premature beats and short episodes of atrial fibrillation.

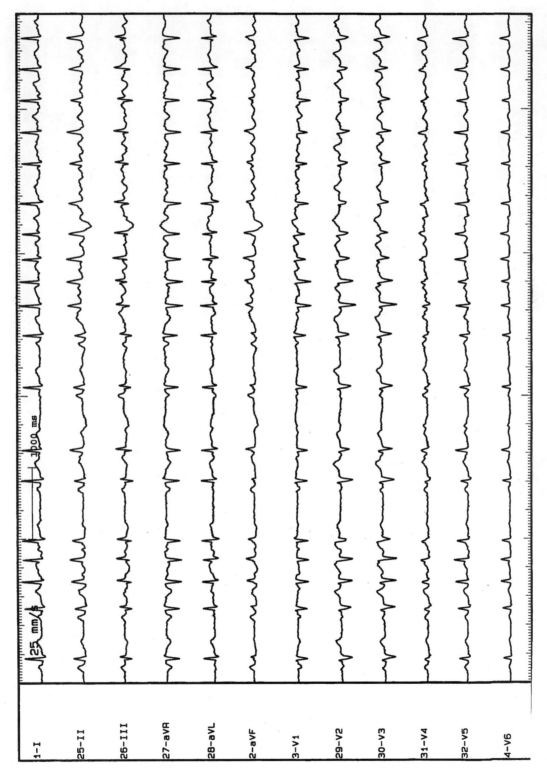

Figure 2. Twelve-lead surface ECG at the beginning of the electrophysiological study with frequent short-coupled atrial premature beats with P on T phenomenon and short runs of atrial tachycardia degenerating into atrial fibrillation. Paper speed 25 mm/s.

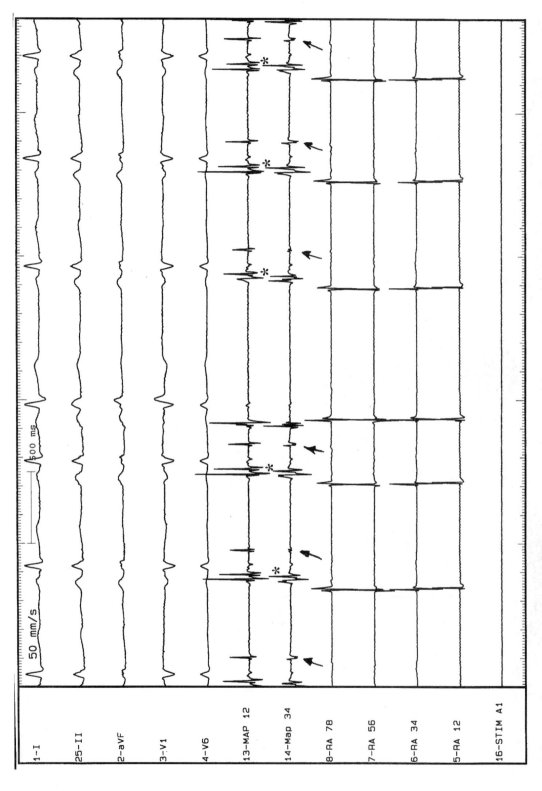

Figure 3. Intracardiac recordings at the baseline. Paper speed 50 mm/s. Five surface ECG leads (I, II, aVF, V_1, V_6) are represented together with two bipolar recordings from the quadripolar ablation catheter (MAP 12 and MAP 34) placed transseptally into the left lower pulmonary vein, and four bipolar recordings from an octopolar catheter in the right atrium (RA12, 34, 56, 78). The ablation catheter (MAP) located in the pulmonary vein records a very sharp potential (arrow) after each sinus beat. After the third sinus beat this pulmonary-vein activity is conducted to the atrium, giving rise to an ectopic P-wave on the surface ECG. After sinus beat 1, 2, 4, 5, and 6, the focal discharge is blocked inside the pulmonary vein (concealed ectopic activity) without any change in the surface ECG. Because during sinus rhythm the pulmonary vein is activated passively from the left atrium, the same sharp spike-like potential can be observed just after the left atrial potential (*).

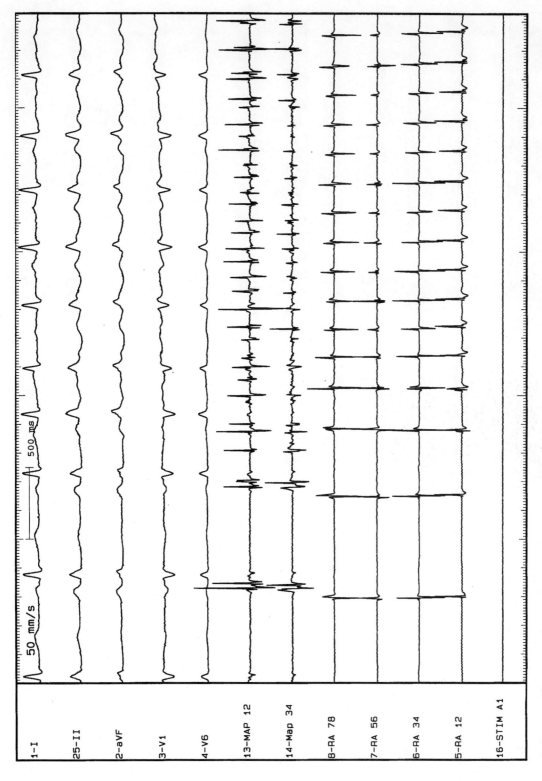

Figure 4. Intracardiac recordings during the spontaneous initiation of a sustained episode of atrial flutter. Paper speed 50 mm/s. Same display as in Figure 3. Rapid discharge from the pulmonary vein focus with a cycle length of 150 ms is observed, giving rise to atrial flutter in the surface ECG.

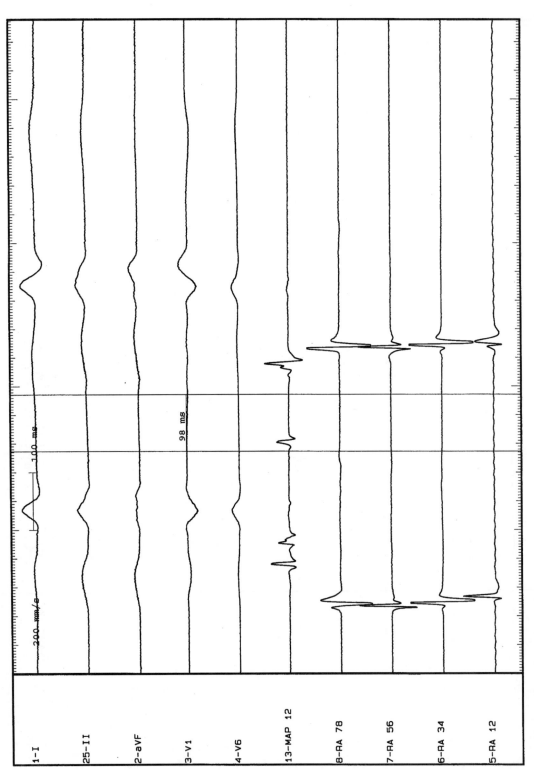

Figure 5. Intracardiac recordings (200 mm/s) showing the earliest activation during ectopy relative to the P wave. Mapping position (MAP 12) is 2 cm inside the pulmonary vein. Radiofrequency ablation at this site (60 seconds, with a temperature of 55°C and a power limit of 30 Watts) eliminated all focal activities and atrial fibrillation.

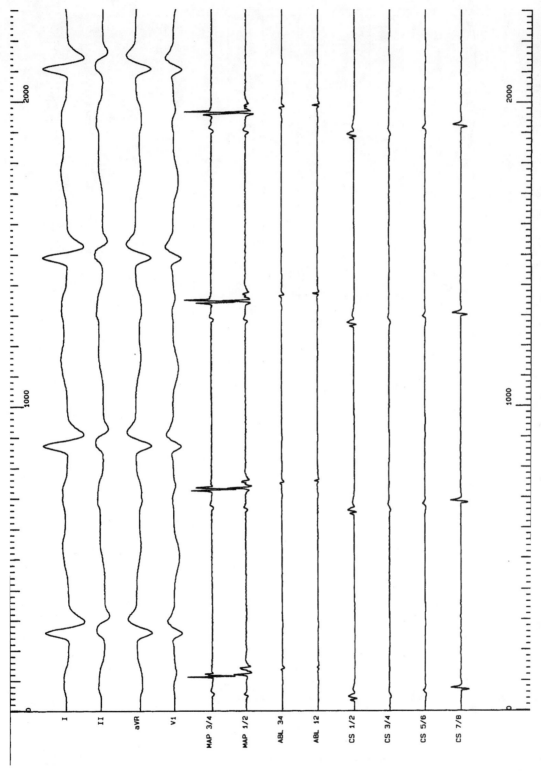

Figure 6. Intracardiac recordings of pulmonary-vein potentials in another patient. Paper speed 100 mm/s. Here are represented four surface ECG leads (I, II, aVR, V_1), two bipolar recordings from the right upper pulmonary vein (MAP 1/2 and MAP {{frac34}}), two bipolar recordings from the left upper pulmonary vein (ABL 12 and ABL 34), and four bipolar recordings from the coronary sinus (CS 12, 34, 56, 78). The mapping catheter at the exit of the right upper pulmonary vein shows a relatively late pulmonary-vein potential at the roof of the vein during sinus rhythm.

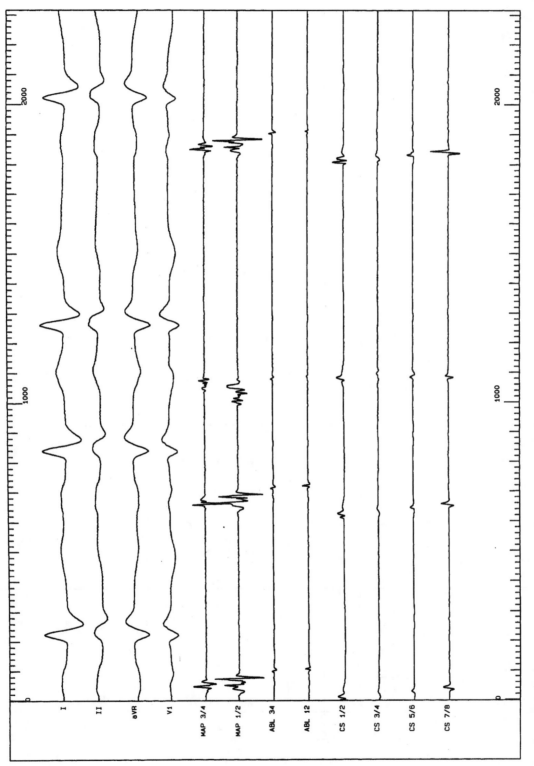

Figure 7. Intracardiac recordings during spontaneous ectopy. Paper speed 100 mm/s. Same display as in Figure 6. The mapping catheter (MAP 12 and MAP 34) has now been turned down to the bottom of the same vein. There is fusion between the pulmonary-vein potential and the atrial potential, indicating the entrance site into the vein.

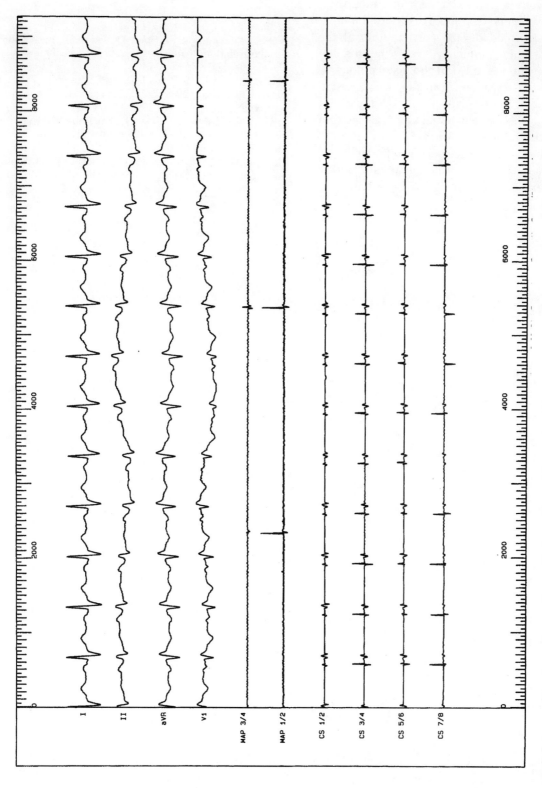

Figure 8. Intracardiac recordings after radiofrequency ablation at the site shown in Figure 7. Paper speed 25 mm/s. Same display as Figure 7. Sixty seconds of radiofrequency current application resulted in dissociation between sinus rhythm and a slow automatic activity recorded inside the pulmonary vein, demonstrating its successful pulmonary vein isolation.

As a result of these limitations, the mapping and ablation strategies were recently changed: after identification of an arrhythmogenic pulmonary vein, the ablation is now performed during sinus rhythm at the
junction between the pulmonary vein and the left
atrium in order to abolish all local and distal pulonary-
vein potentials (PV-isolation). If this endpoint is successfully achieved, the recurrence rate is only about
35%, and 70% of the patients remain in sinus rhythm
without antiarrhythmic drugs during follow up.

In our opinion, pulmonary vein isolation will certainly become an efficient and safe therapeutic option
for the treatment of paroxysmal atrial fibrillation in
the near future.

Suggested Reading

Jaïs P, Haïssaguerre M, Shad DC, et al. A focal source of
atrial fibrillation treated by discrete radiofrequency ablation.
Circulation 1997;95:572-576.

Haïssaguerre M, Jaïs P, Shah D, et al. Spontaneous initiating
of atrial fibrillation by ectopic beats originating in the pulmonary veins. *N Engl J Med* 1998;339:659-666.

Robbins IM, Colvin EV, Doyle T, et al. Pulmonary vein stenosis after catheter ablation of atrial fibrillation. *Circulation*
1998;98:1769-1775.

Haïssaguerre M, Jaïs P, Shah D, et al. Electrophysiological
endpoint for catheter ablation of atrial fibrillation initiated
from multiple pulmonary vein foci. *Circulation* 2000;
101:1409-1417.

Chapter 13

Atrial Flutter Ablation During Sinus Rhythm

Introduction

Isthmus-dependent atrial flutter ablation is currently a well recognized and accepted curative therapy with success rates of 85% to 95%. This is the case of a 57-year-old female patient presenting with paroxysmal type I atrial flutter degenerating into atrial fibrillation. Class Ic and III antiarrhythmic drugs were ineffective and an isthmus ablation was proposed to avoid further recurrences. In that particular case, the ablation procedure was performed during sinus rhythm using anatomic criteria.

Comments

Radiofrequency catheter ablation of atrial flutter may be performed during sinus rhythm. Change in activation time (here from 80 to 180 ms) and activation sequence before and after ablation as well as modification of P wave morphology on the surface ECG and presence of double potentials all along the line of ablation confirm the isthmus block. In the present case, because the patient had also sustained episodes of atrial fibrillation, anticoagulant therapy was continued together with a class Ic antiarrhythmic drug. Such a hybrid therapy may be proposed in patients with both atrial flutter and atrial fibrillation, either when atrial flutter is the predominant clinical arrhythmia or when atrial fibrillation is transformed into atrial flutter by antiarrhythmic drug therapy (mainly class Ic drugs).

Suggested Reading

Calkins H, Leon AR, Deam AG, et al. Catheter ablation of atrial flutter using radiofrequency energy. *Am J Cardiol* 1994;73:353-356.

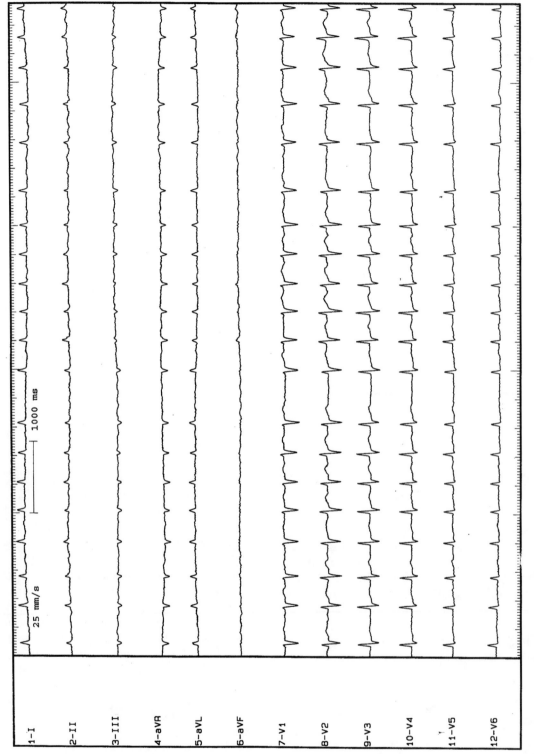

Figure 1. Twelve-lead ECG (25 mm/s) before ablation showing persistent atrial fibrillation with a rapid ventricular response.

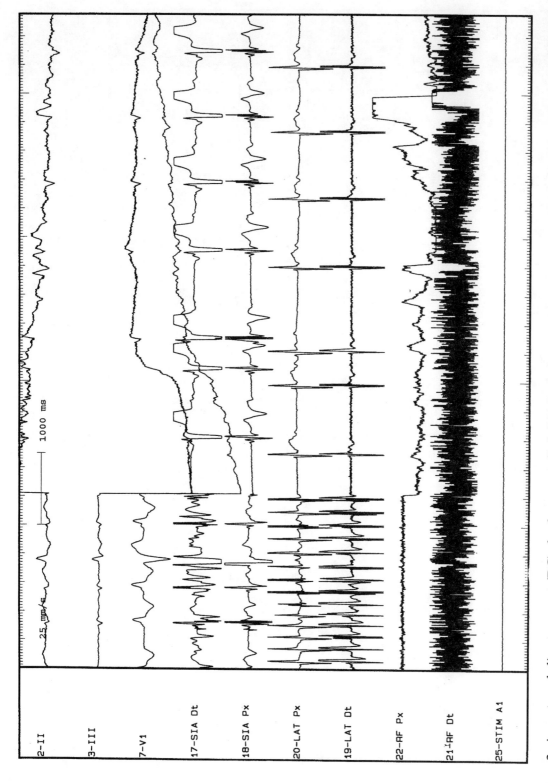

Figure 2. An external direct current (DC) shock was applied (320 Joules) to restore sinus rhythm. Here are displayed three surface ECG leads (II, III, V_1) and six intracardiac recordings: two bipolar recordings from the right ventricle (SIA Dt and SIA Px), two bipolar recordings from the low lateral right atrium (LAT Px and LAT Dt), and two bipolar recordings from the ablation catheter located in the inferior vena cava and not connected (RF Px and RF Dt). A channel for stimulation (STIM A1) is also displayed. Paper speed 25 mm/s. Sinus rhythm is restored immediately with a normal sinus node recovery time.

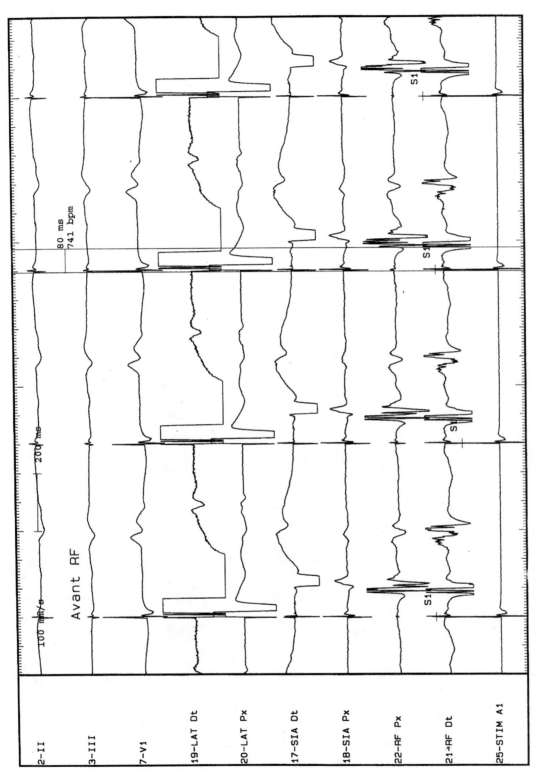

Figure 3. Intracardiac recordings (100 mm/s) during low lateral right atrial pacing (S1-S1 600 ms) before ablation. Same configuration as Figure 2, except that the right ventricular catheter has now been pulled back in the septal region of the right atrium (SIA Dt and SIA Px) and the ablation catheter is now in the proximal coronary sinus (RF Px and RF Dt). The conduction time between the low lateral right atrium and the proximal coronary sinus is short (80 ms), and the activation of the proximal coronary sinus occurs before the activation of the septal area, proving the absence of conduction block in the isthmus.

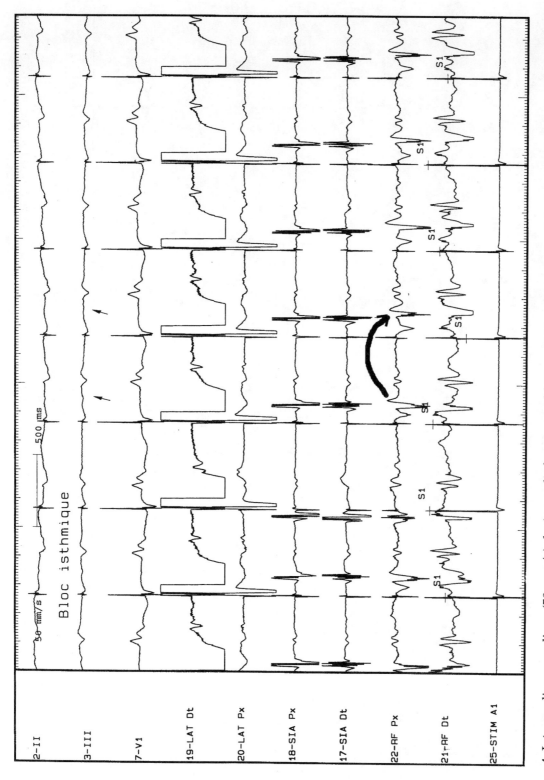

Figure 4. Intracardiac recordings (50 mm/s) during radiofrequency ablation which was performed during continuous low lateral right atrial pacing (S1-S1 600 ms). An internally irrigated-tip catheter was used for this procedure. Same configuration as Figure 3. Conduction block across the isthmus was achieved during the eighth radiofrequency current application. Note the instantaneous modification of P wave morphology in lead III (thin arrows) and the sudden apparition of a clearly separated double potential at the site of ablation (large arrow).

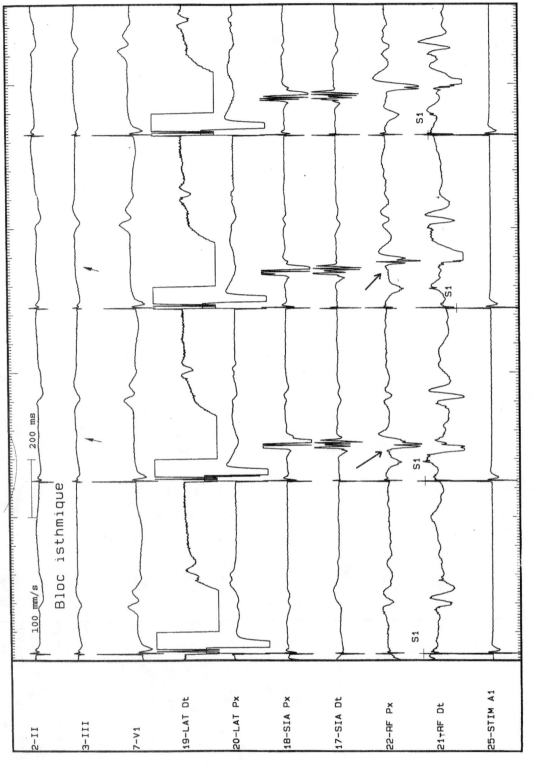

Figure 5. Same as Figure 4, but at a paper speed of 100 mm/s.

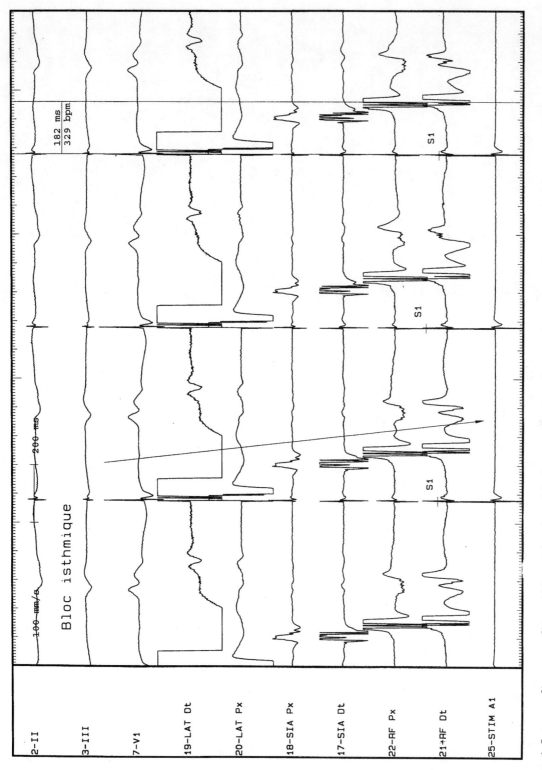

Figure 6. Intracardiac recordings 100 mm/s after ablation confirming counterclockwise isthmus block. Same display as Figure 3. Pacing is performed from the low lateral right atrium wall (S1-S1 600 ms). The activation time between the low lateral right atrium and the proximal coronary sinus is now 180 ms, and the proximal coronary sinus (RF Px and RF Dt) is activated late compared to the septal region of the right atrium (SIA Px and SIA Dt).

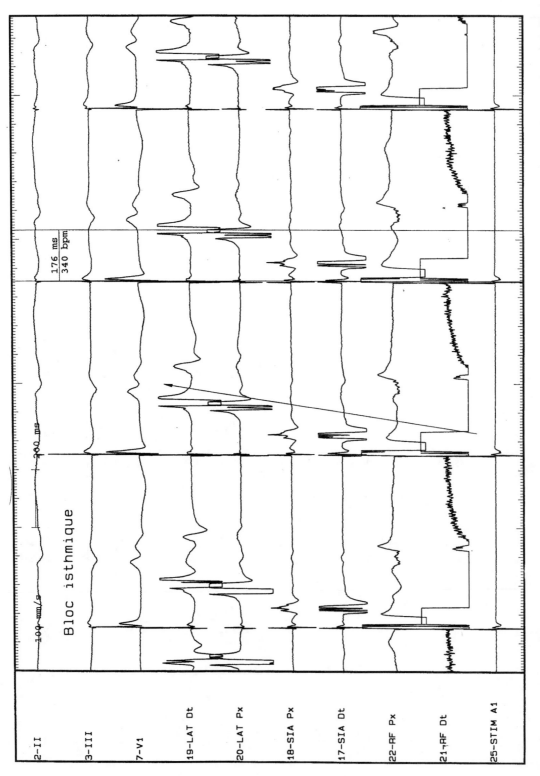

Figure 7. Intracardiac recordings 100 mm/s after ablation confirming clockwise isthmus block. Same display as Figures 3 and 6. Pacing is now performed from the proximal coronary sinus (S1-S1 600 ms). The activation time between the proximal coronary sinus (RF Dt) and the low lateral right atrium is 176 ms and the low lateral right atrium is activated late compared to the septal region of the right atrium (SIA Px and SIA Dt).

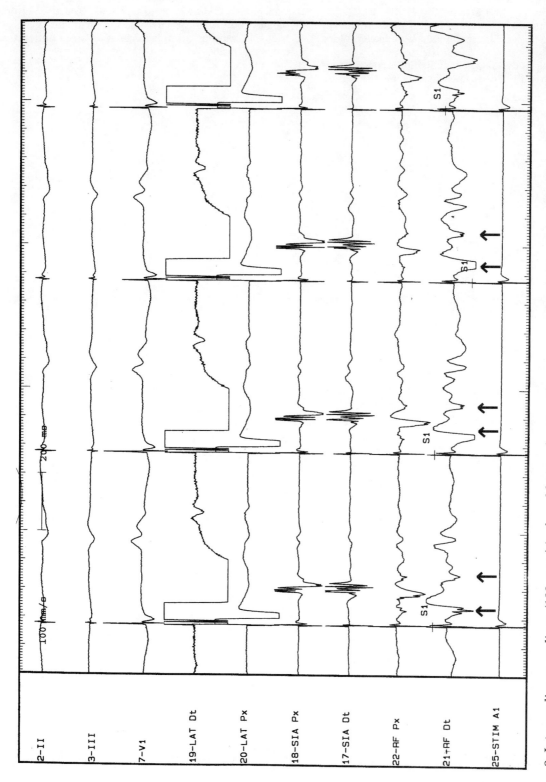

Figure 8. Intracardiac recordings (100 mm/s) after ablation showing the presence of double potentials (arrows) in the inferior vena cava – tricuspid valve isthmus. Same display as Figure 3, with pacing (S1-S1 600 ms) from the low lateral right atrial wall. The presence of double potentials all along the cavo-tricuspid isthmus confirms conduction block.

Cosio FG, Lopez GM, Goicolea A, et al. Radiofrequency ablation of the inferior vena cava – tricuspid valve isthmus in
common atrial flutter. *Am J Cardiol* 1993;71:705-709.

Kirkorian G, Moncada E, Chevalier P, et al. Radiofrequency
ablation of atrial flutter: Efficacy of an anatomically guided
approach. *Circulation* 1994;90:2804-2814.

Poty H, Saoudi N, Abdel Aziz A, et al. Radiofrequency catheter ablation of atrial flutter – further insights into the various

types of isthmus block: Application to ablation during sinus
rhythm. *Circulation* 1996;94:3204-3213.

Cauchemez B, Haïssaguerre M, Fischer B, et al. Electrophysiological effects of catheter ablation of inferior vena cava –
tricuspid annulus isthmus in common atrial flutter. *Circulation* 1996;93:284-294.

Chapter 14

Catheter Ablation of a Parahisian Accessory Pathway

Medical History

A 22-year-old male patient presented with drug resistant paroxysmal supraventricular tachycardia (rate 200 beats/min) for many years. He never experienced syncope, but tachycardia episodes recurred on a monthly basis despite β-blockers and flecainide. Ventricular preexcitation was present on the 12-lead resting ECG with a delta-wave polarity suggesting an antero-septal location of the accessory pathway. Atrial vulnerability with rapid ventricular response has been documented on several occasions. An ablation procedure was proposed.

Comments

Radiofrequency catheter ablation of anteroseptal and parahisian accessory pathways is always a stressful experience because of the risk of complete atrioventricular (AV) block. In order to minimize the risk of AV block, several rules should be strictly respected: use of a catheter with temperature control, low cut-off point (50-55°C), low initial energy (5 to 15 Watts), catheter position more on the ventricular side, immediate interruption of radiofrequency current application in case of junctional rhythm, demand atrial pacing to avoid catheter dislodgement in case of abrupt changes in sinus rate. In the present case, we used a femoral approach, which offers a good catheter stability, but in selected cases a subclavian or a jugular approach may be preferable.

Suggested Reading

Schluter M, et al. Catheter ablation from right atrium of anteroseptal accessory pathways using radiofrequency current. *J Am Coll Cardiol* 1992;19:663-670.

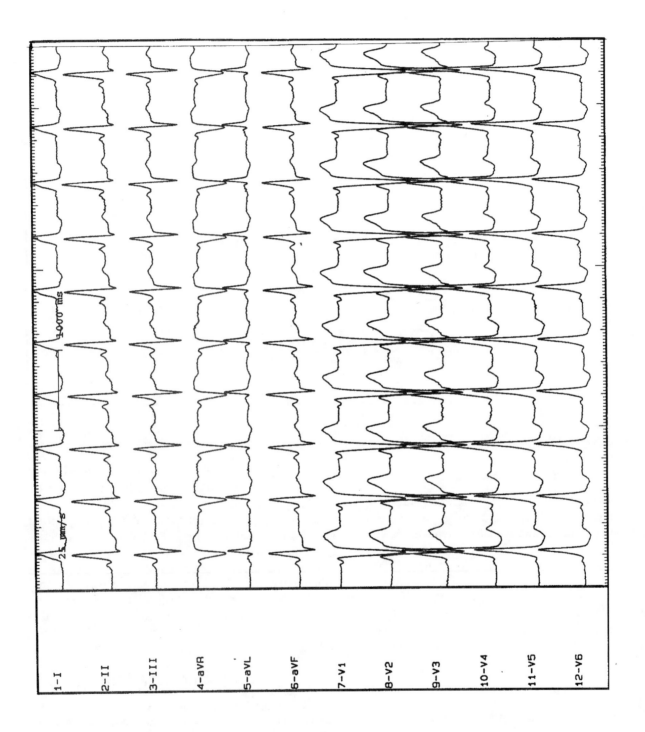

Figure 1. Twelve-lead ECG (25 mm/s) showing positive delta wave in DII, DIII, aVF. Of note is the aspect in V_1 with a discrete initial positive deflection.

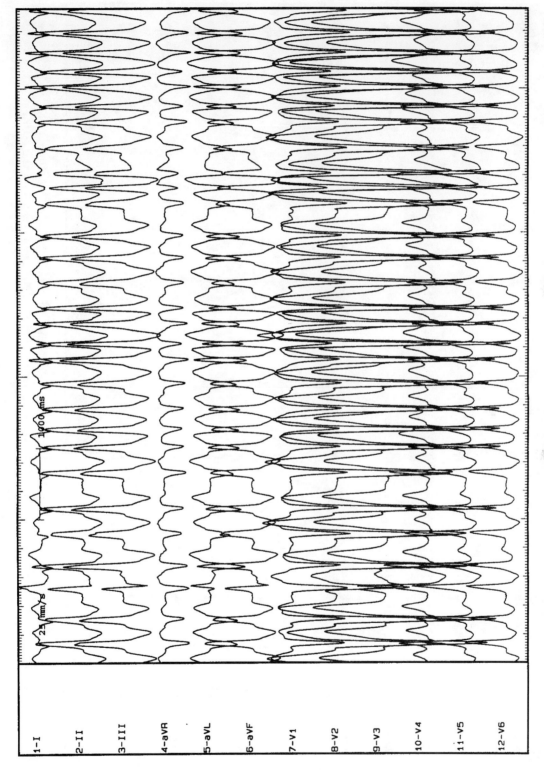

Figure 2. Twelve-lead ECG (25 mm/s) recorded during an episode of severe palpitations. Preexcited atrial fibrillation is present, with a ventricular rate of 190 to 280 beats/min (minimal RR interval = 210 ms).

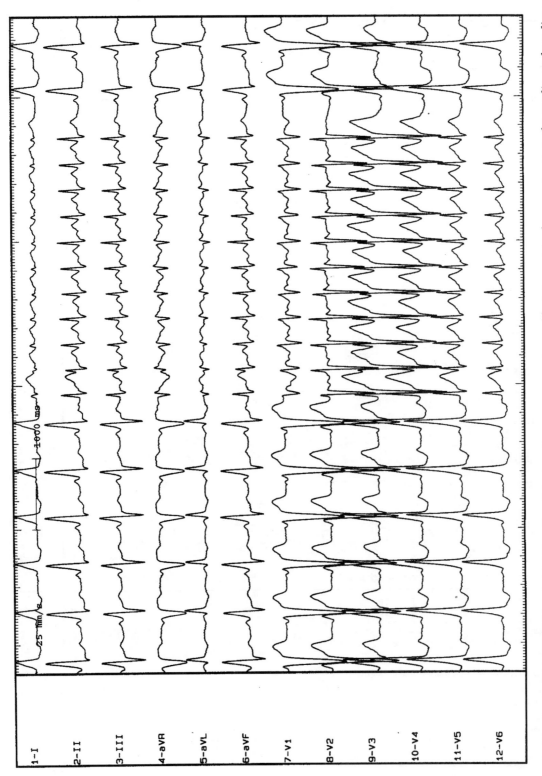

Figure 3. Twelve-lead ECG (25 mm/s) showing the spontaneous occurrence of atrioventricular reentrant tachycardia at baseline. The tachycardia episode is here nonsustained, at a rate of 175 beats/min, with narrow QRS complexes, and the retrograde P waves are visible just after the QRS complex, mainly in the inferior leads and in V_1-V_2.

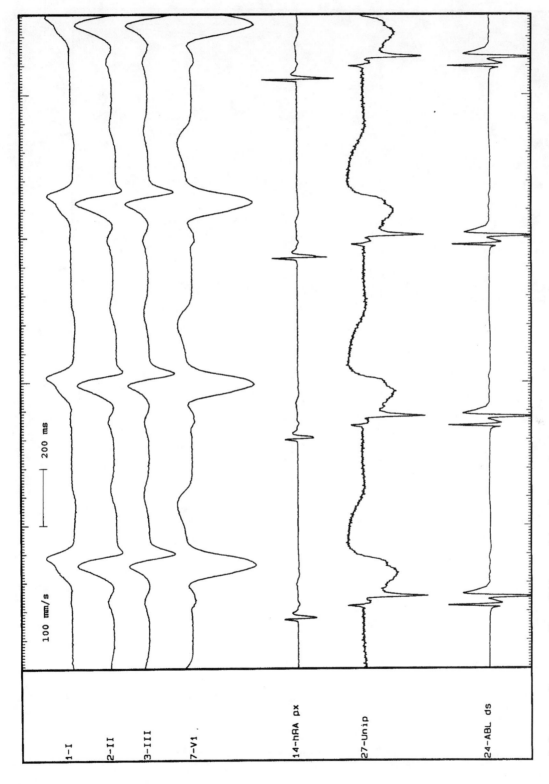

Figure 4. Intracardiac recording (100 mm/s) at the successful site despite a nonoptimal unipolar recording (no QS pattern but a slight notching between the atrial and the ventricular deflection) and a nonoptimal bipolar recording (no complete fusion between A and V). hRA px : high right atrium; Unip: unipolar recording on the distal tip of the ablation catheter; ABL ds: bipolar recording on the ablation catheter.

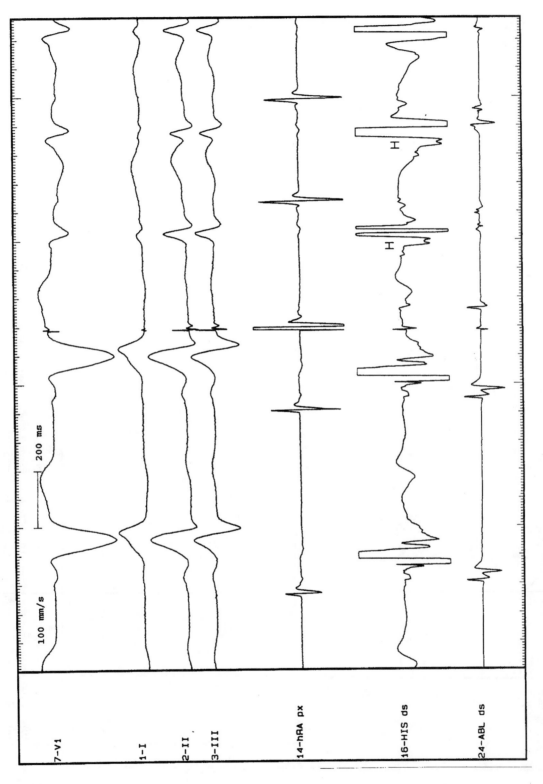

Figure 5. Intracardiac recording (100 mm/s) during initiation of atrioventricular reentrant tachycardia by atrial premature stimulation (A-S1: 280 ms). His ds: catheter positioned in the His bundle region.

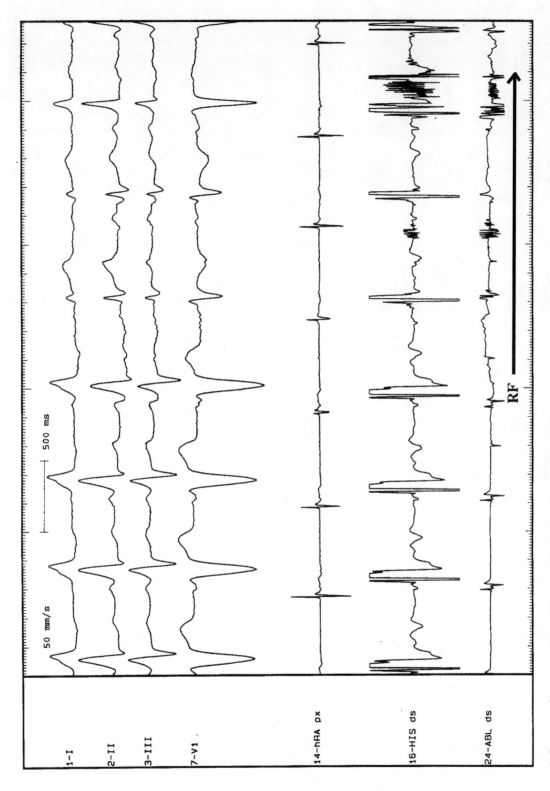

Figure 6. Intracardiac recording (50 mm/s) during the first radiofrequency (RF) current application. Energy was applied very carefully (10 Watts; 50°) and preexcitation disappeared immediately. Application of energy was maintained during 90 seconds. After the ablation procedure, conduction intervals were normal (H-V interval = 38 ms; A-H interval 85 ms).

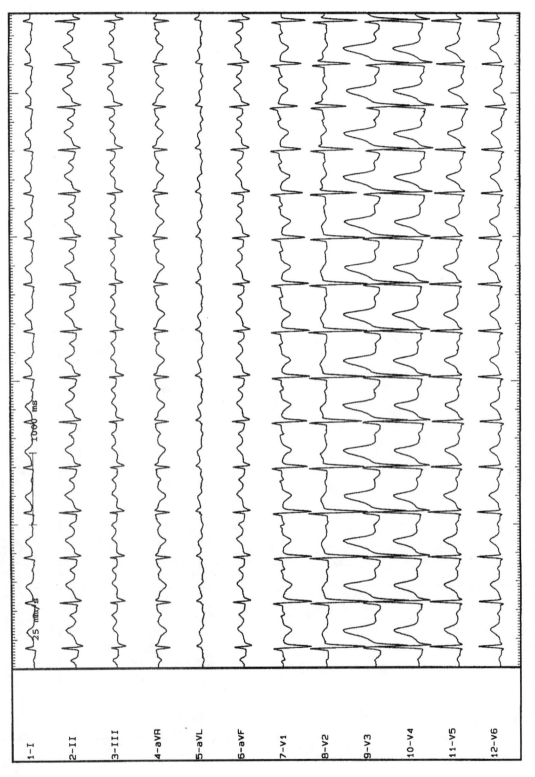

Figure 7. Twelve-lead ECG (25 mm/s) recorded after the ablation procedure. There is no ventricular preexcitation and the PR interval is normal.

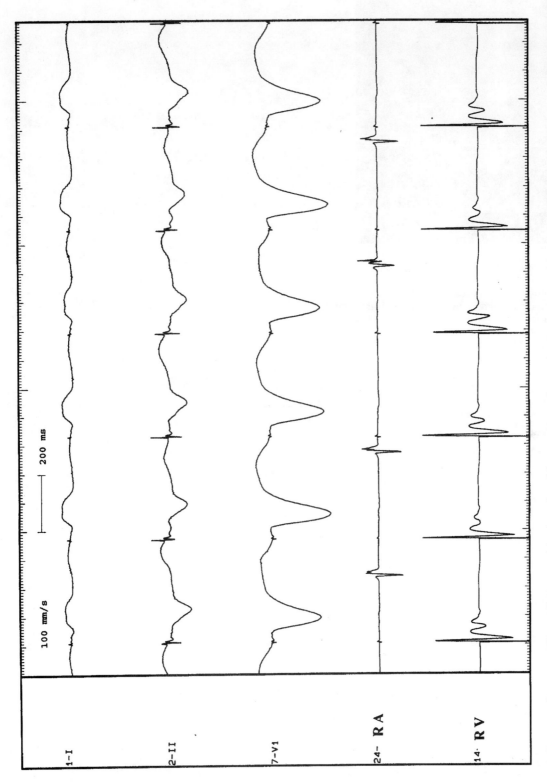

Figure 8. Intracardiac recordings (100 mm/s) after the ablation procedure. During ventricular pacing (S1-S1 : 350 ms) retrograde conduction occurs over the atrioventricular node with a Wenckebach phenomenon. RA: right atrium; RV: right ventricle.

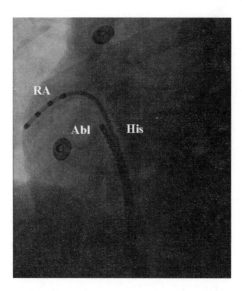

Figure 9. Chest X-ray of catheter position.

Kuck KH, Schlüter M, Gürsoy S, et al. Preservation of atrioventricular nodal conduction during radiofrequency current catheter ablation of midseptal accessory pathways. *Circulation* 1992;86:1743-1752.

Haïssaguerre M, Marcus F, Poquet F, et al. Electrocardiographic characteristics and catheter ablation of parahisian accessory pathways. *Circulation* 1994;90:1124-1128.

Brugada J, Puigfel M, Mont L, et al. Radiofrequency ablation of anteroseptal, para-hisian and mid-septal accessory pathways using a simplified femoral approach. *Pacing Clin Electrophysiol* 1998;21(Part I):735-741.

Chapter 15

Catheter Ablation Of An Accessory Pathway With Anterograde Decremental Conduction Properties

Medical History

An 80-year-old male patient presented with paroxysmal wide QRS complex tachycardia. The arrhythmia was badly tolerated with dyspnea and a diagnosis of possible ventricular tachycardia was made. Biatrial dilatation was present on echocardiography, but the left ventricular function appeared normal. Class Ic drugs and amiodarone were ineffective and the patient was referred for an electrophysiologic study.

Comments

Accessory pathways are frequently associated with the occurrence of atrial arrhythmias and not only in the elderly. Atrial fibrillation in Wolff-Parkinson-White (WPW) patients is correlated with the presence of concomitant reciprocating tachycardia. The mechanism of atrial fibrillation in WPW patients in unclear, but there are some arguments to support microreentry close to the atrial insertion of the accessory pathway.

From: RETAC: *Radiofrequency Catheter Ablation for the Treatment of Cardiac Arrhythmias: A Practical Atlas with Illustrative Cases.* © Futura Publishing Company, Inc. Armonk, NY, 2002.

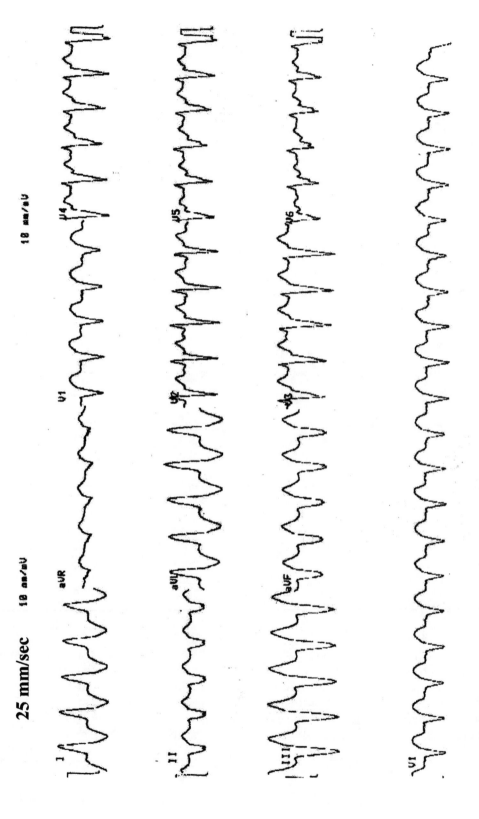

Figure 1. Twelve-lead ECG (25 mm/s) showing regular wide QRS complex tachycardia at a rate of 130 beats/min (cycle length 460 ms).

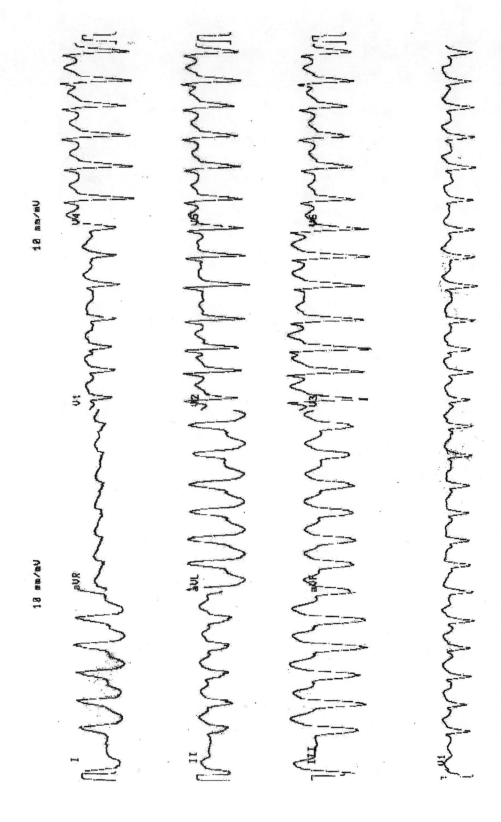

Figure 2. Twelve-lead resting ECG (25 mm/s) showing an irregular wide QRS complex tachycardia with the same morphological aspect, at a rate of 140 to 170 beats/min. On the basis of these two ECGs, the supposed diagnosis was atrial arrhythmia (atrial flutter and fibrillation) with a right posterolateral accessory pathway.

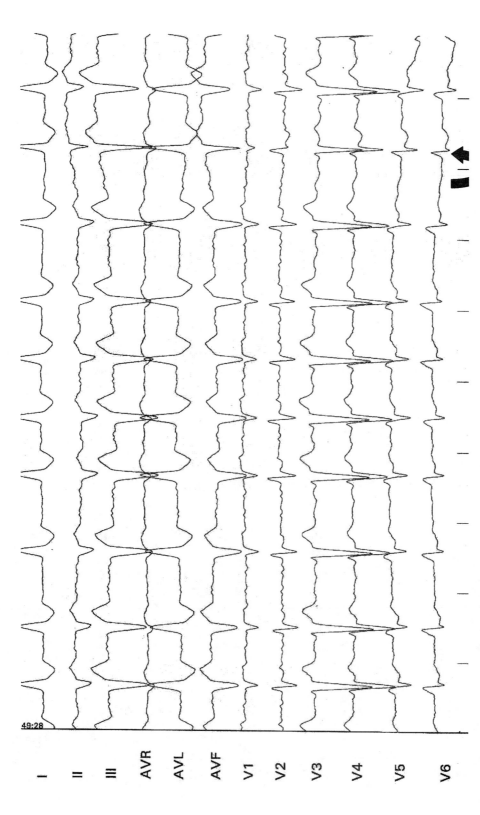

Figure 3. After 10 mg of intravenous ajmalin, a slow ventricular response (55 to 75 beats/min) was observed, with a left bundle branch pattern. One fusion beat is present (arrow).

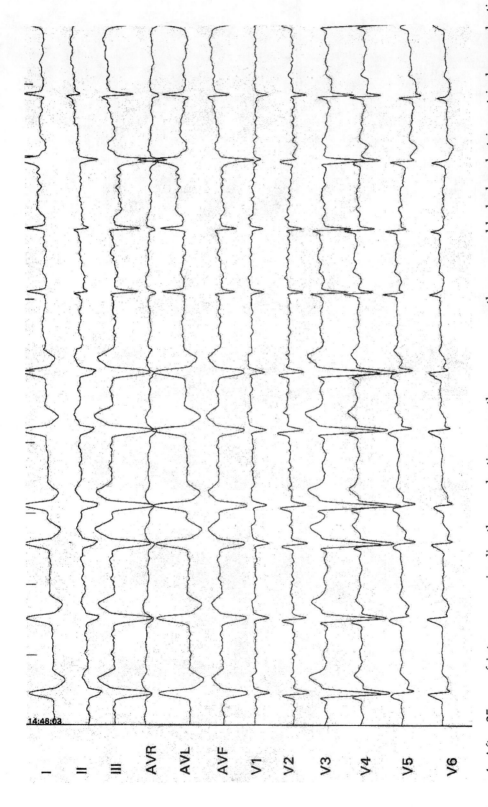

Figure 4. After 25 mg of intravenous ajmalin, the conduction over the accessory pathway was blocked and atrioventricular conduction occurred over the normal nodohisian conduction system with a narrow QRS complex. This response to ajmalin strongly suggests the presence of an accessory pathway.

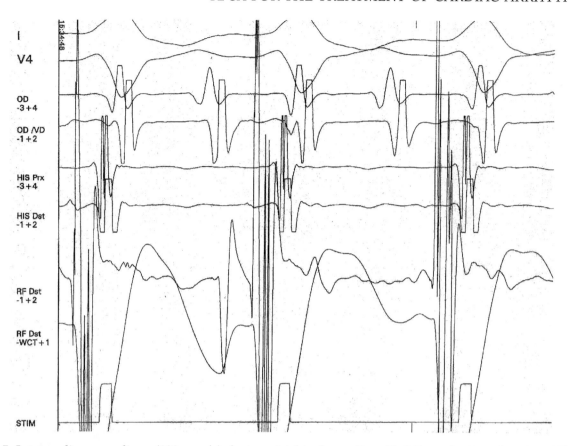

Figure 5. Intracardiac recordings (100 mm/s) during atrial tachycardia with 2:1 conduction showing AV fusion on the bipolar recording and a QS aspect on the unipolar recording. However, no success was obtained at this site. OD = right atrium; OD/VD = right atrium then right ventricle; His Prx = proximal His bundle region; His Dst = distal His bundle region; RF Dst = distal radiofrequency ablation catheter; RF Dst − WCT = unipolar recording on the distal tip of the ablation catheter.

Atrial flutter is quite rare in WPW patients, except in older individuals. In the present case, preexcited atrial arrhythmias were the first manifestations of the presence of an accessory pathway. The patient never experienced atrioventricular (AV) reentrant tachycardia, probably because of an impaired anterograde AV nodal conduction. The decremental conduction properties of the accessory pathway suggest the presence of Mahaim-like fibers. Finally, the occurrence of first- and second-degree AV block during radiofrequency current application implies that the accessory pathway was located quite close to the lower compact AV node with a relatively high risk of permanent AV block during ablation.

Suggested Reading

Campbell RF, Smith RA, Gallagher JJ, et al. Atrial fibrillation in the preexcitation syndrome. *Am J Cardiol* 1977;40:514-519.

Wathen M, Natale A, Wolfe K, et al. Initiation of atrial fibrillation in the Wolff-Parkinson-White syndrome: The importance of the accessory pathway. *Am Heart J* 1993;125:753-758.

Klein LS, Hacket FK, Zipes DP, et al. Radiofrequency catheter ablation of Mahaim fibers at the tricuspid annulus. *Circulation* 1993;87:738-747.

Sarter BH, Schwartzman D, Movsowitz C, et al. Atrial arrhythmias following successful ablation of atrial flutter associated with conduction block in the inferior vena caval-tricuspid valve isthmus (abstract). *Pacing Clin Electrophysiol* 1996;19:635.

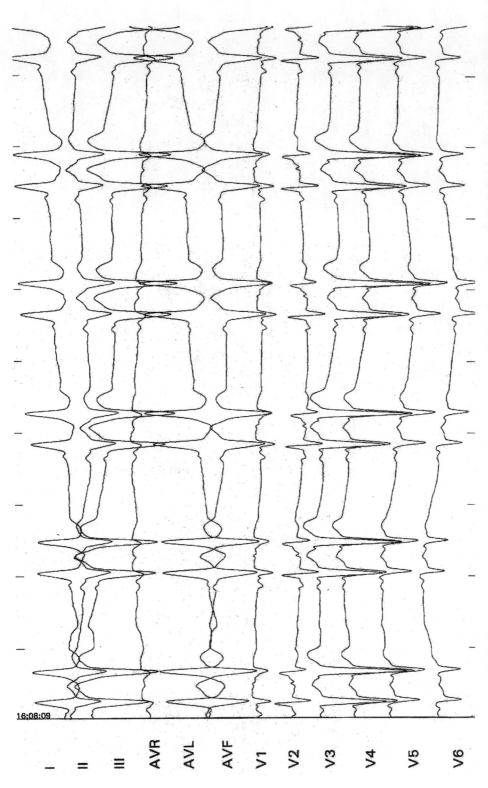

Figure 6. Twelve-lead ECG (25 mm/s) obtained after external direct current (DC) shock (200 Joules). Sinus rhythm has been restored and atrial bigeminy is observed. Ventricular preexcitation is present during sinus rhythm and on the atrial premature beats.

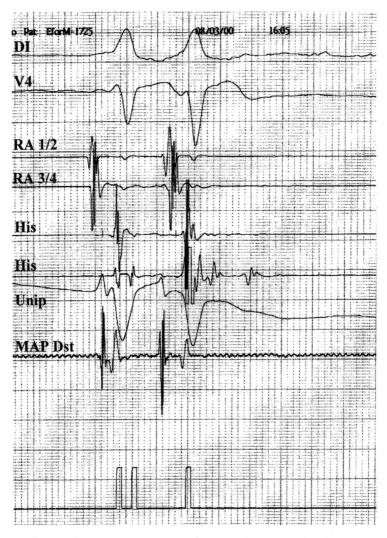

Figure 7. Intracardiac recordings (100 mm/s) with the mapping catheter in the close vicinity of the atrial insertion of the accessory pathway. Decremental conduction over the accessory pathway was present (AV 30 ms during sinus rhythm and 80 ms on the atrial premature beat), and the effective refractory period of the accessory pathway was 320 ms.

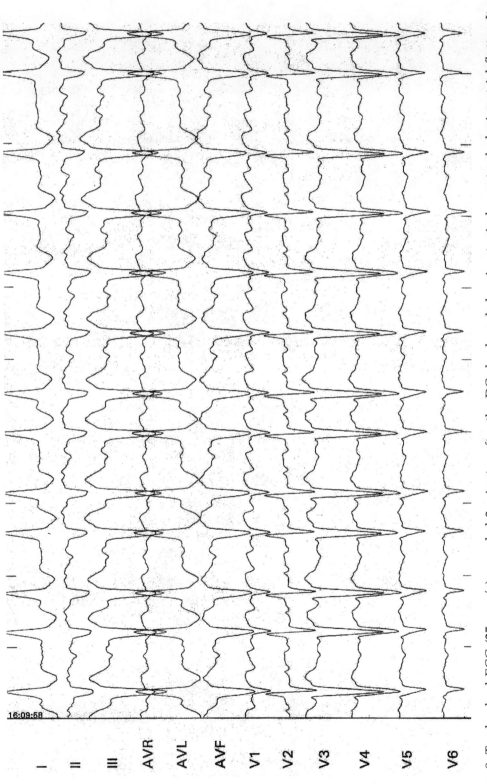

Figure 8. Twelve-lead ECG (25 mm/s) recorded 3 minutes after the DC shock and showing typical counterclockwise atrial flutter. It was then decided to perform an isthmus ablation to avoid recurrences of atrial flutter.

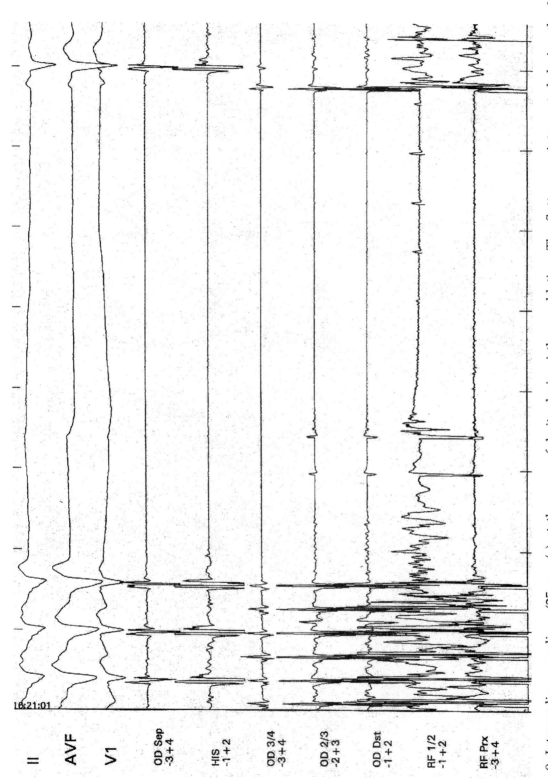

Figure 9. Intracardiac recordings (25 mm/s) at the successful site during isthmus ablation. The flutter was interrupted during the 10th radiofrequency current application. A long sinus node recovery time was observed. It was then decided to continue the ablation procedure and to target the accessory pathway.

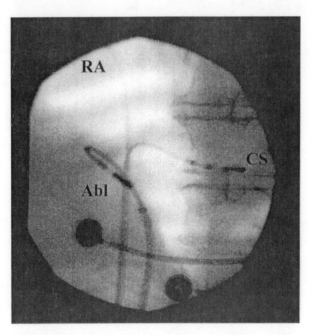

Figure 10. Forty-five degree LAO projection showing catheter position at the successful site. One catheter is positioned in the coronary sinus (CS), one catheter is positioned in the right atrium and the ablation catheter (Abl) in the posterior (inferior) region.

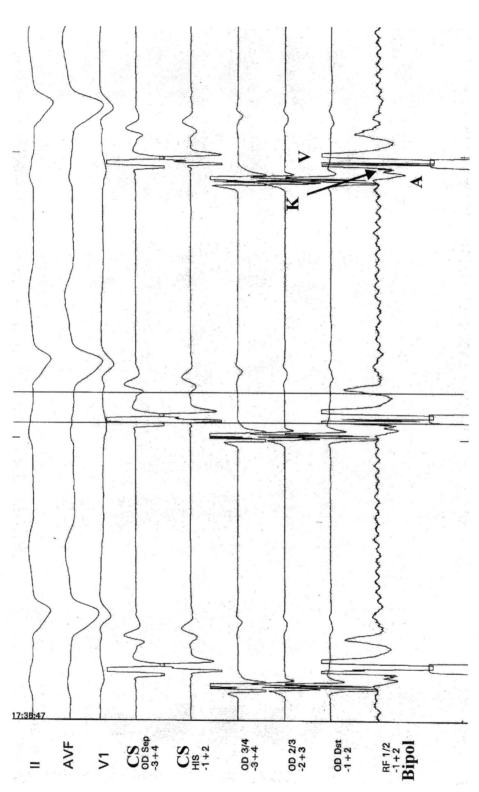

Figure 11. Intracardiac recordings (100 mm/s) at the successful site. The bipolar recording from the ablation catheter (RF ½ Bipol) disclosed atrioventricular fusion and the presence of a discrete Kent (K) potential. The interval between V and onset of delta wave is 60 ms. V : ventricle; A : atrium; CS : coronary sinus; OD : right atrium.

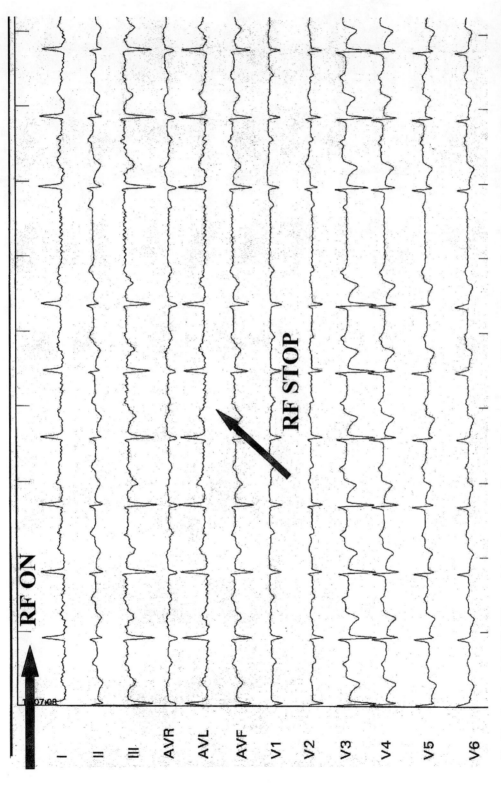

Figure 12. Twelve-lead ECG (25 mm/s) during the first radiofrequency (RF) current application. Preexcitation disappeared immediately but second-degree atrioventricular block type 1 (Wenckebach phenomenon) was observed. The RF current application was immediately interrupted.

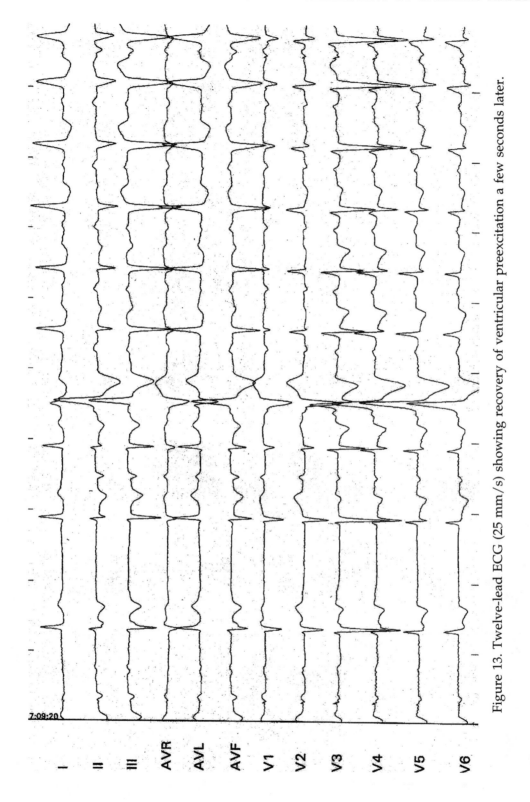

Figure 13. Twelve-lead ECG (25 mm/s) showing recovery of ventricular preexcitation a few seconds later.

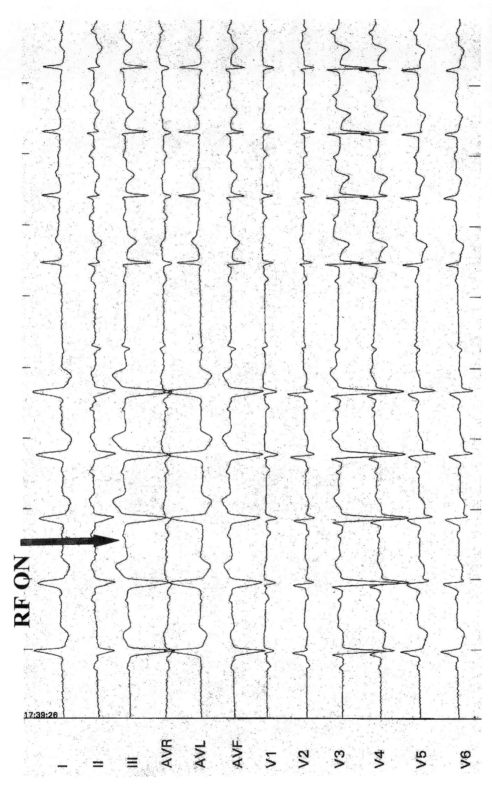

Figure 14. Twelve-lead ECG (25 mm/s) recorded during the second radiofrequency current application, and showing immediate disappearance of ventricular preexcitation. Note that there is a progressive prolongation of the PR interval during radiofrequency current application. During follow-up the patient showed no recurrence of preexcitation, no recurrence of atrial flutter, asymptomatic first degree AV block, and finally recurrence of atrial fibrillation with a ventricular rate of 60 to 70 beats/min without symptoms.

Chapter 16

Right Posteroseptal Accessory PathwayAblation

Introduction

It is well known that posteroseptal accessory pathways are sometimes difficult to ablate because of their location. In some cases it is necessary to ablate using a retrograde approach or inside the coronary sinus. Bipolar ablation between both sides of the septum is exceptionally needed. This is the case of a 35-year-old female with many episodes of atrioventricular reentrant tachycardia resistant to flecainide and β-blockers. Ablation was then performed. The mapping procedure was made difficult by the absence of optimal potentials during anterograde or retrograde conduction over the accessory pathway in the entire right posteroseptal region or even inside the coronary sinus and the mid-cardiac vein.

Comments

Posteroseptal accessory pathways are sometimes difficult to ablate. In this case, the nonoptimal local potential at the successful site of ablation may be explained by the poor anterograde conduction over the accessory pathway and by the prolonged A-H interval. In such a situation, mapping must be extremely careful and the ablation site must be targeted to the shortest A-V and V-A intervals, as well as to the best V-Delta wave precocity.

Suggested Reading

Schlüter M, Kuck KH. Radiofrequency current therapy of supraventricular tachycardia: Accessory atrioventricular pathways. *Pacing Clin Electrophysiol* 1993;16(part II):643-648.

Warin J, Haïssaguerre M, D'Ivernois C, et al. Catheter ablation of accessory pathways: Technique and results in 248 patients. *Pacing Clin Electrophysiol* 1990;13:1609-1616.

Dhala AA, Deshpande SS, Bremner S, et al. Transcatheter ablation of posteroseptal accessory pathways using a venous approach and radiofrequency energy. *Circulation* 1994; 90:1799-1810.

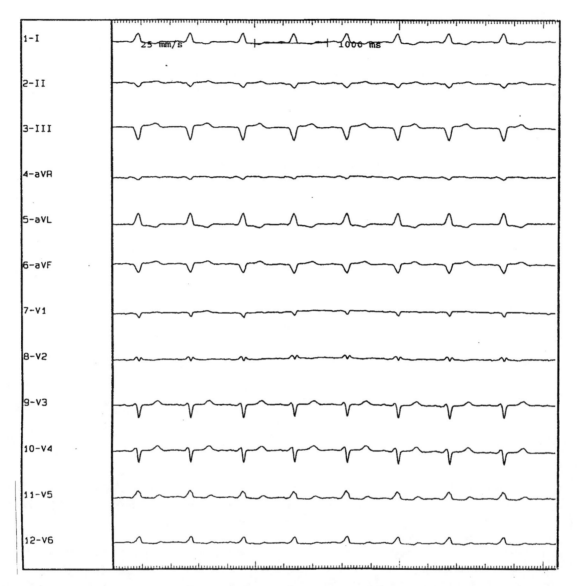

Figure 1. Twelve-lead ECG (25 mm/s) showing negative delta wave in DII, DIII, aVF and V$_1$. This pattern is quite typical of a right posteroseptal accessory pathway.

Calkins H, Kim YN, Schmaltz S, et al. Electrogram criteria for identification of appropriate target sites for radiofrequency catheter ablation of accessory atrioventricular connections. *Circulation* 1992;85:565-573.

Fitzpatrick AP, Gonzales RP, Lesh MD, et al. New algorithm for the localization of accessory atrioventricular connections using a baseline electrocardiogram. *J Am Coll Cardiol* 1994;23:107-116.

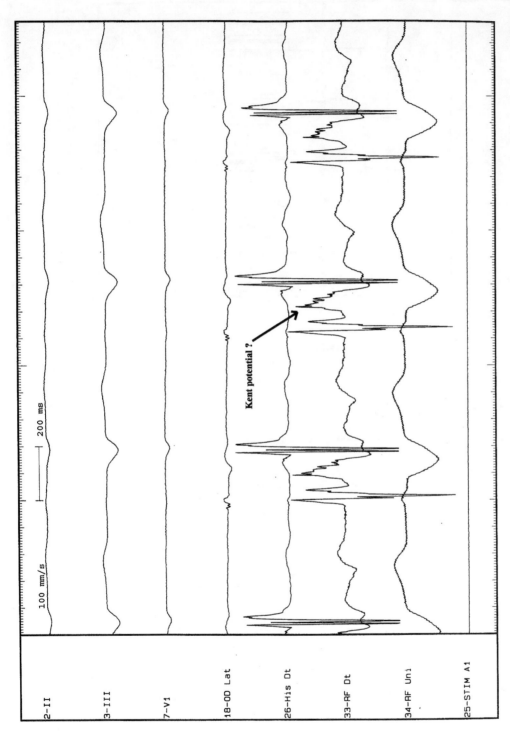

Figure 2. Intracardiac recording (100 mm/s) of the shortest atrioventricular (AV) interval. Mapping was initiated around the tricuspid annulus, towards the septum, around the coronary sinus os and to the posterior zone. No potential with AV fusion during bipolar recording or a QS pattern during unipolar recording was found. Then, the ablation catheter was moved inside the coronary sinus and the mid-cardiac vein, but the recorded potentials were worse than in the right septal region. We thought that the absence of fusion could be due to a poor anterograde conduction and then we looked for the shortest AV interval. The optimal potential was recorded in the posteroseptal zone in the close vicinity of the coronary sinus os, with a possible Kent potential (arrow). The ventricular potential was 50 ms before the delta wave at this site (RF Dt). Retrograde conduction showed a short ventriculo-atrial (V-A) interval but without fusion at that site. Of note is the absence of fusion and the poor unipolar tracing on the distal pole of the ablation catheter (RF Uni). OD lat = catheter in the lateral wall of the right atrium. His Dt = catheter in the distal His bundle region.

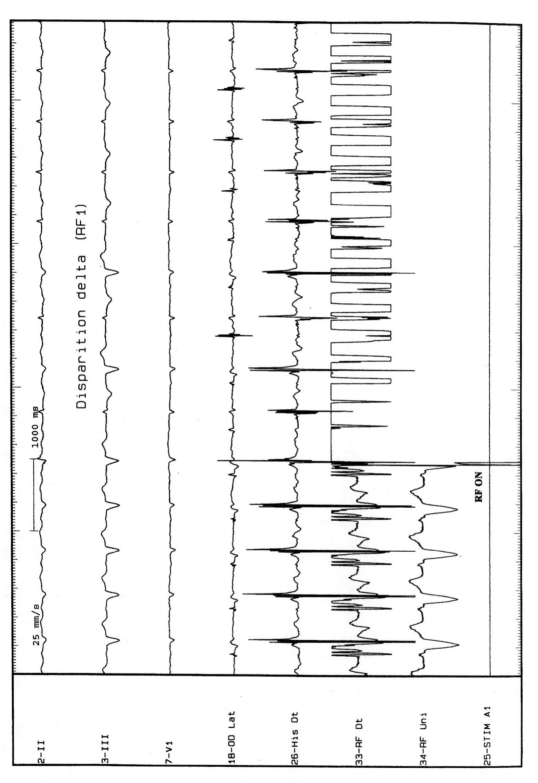

Figure 3. Intracardiac recording (25 mm/s) at the successful site. Delta wave disappeared within the first second of radiofrequency current application (arrow). No early recurrence was observed. Same abbreviations as Figure 2.

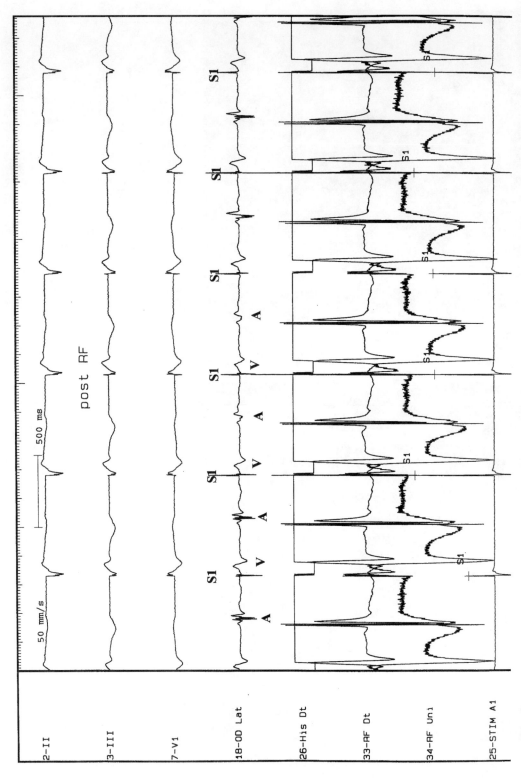

Figure 4. Intracardiac recording (50 mm/s) during ventricular pacing (S1-S1 700 ms) after the ablation procedure, showing 1 to 1 retrograde conduction over the atrioventricular node (V-A interval = 360 ms; retrograde Wenckebach period = 580 ms). Same abbreviations as Figure 2.

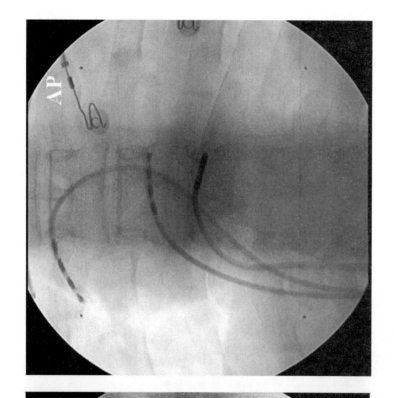

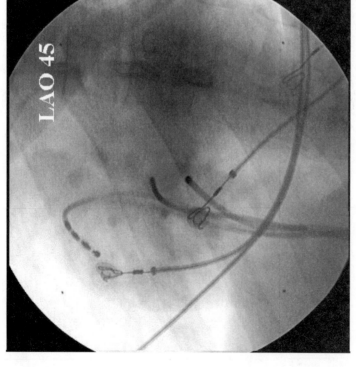

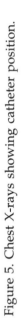

Figure 5. Chest X-rays showing catheter position.

Chapter 17

Accessory Atrioventricular Pathway in Ebstein's Anomaly

Medical History

A 17-year-old male patient had Ebstein's anomaly diagnosed at the age of 5. A 12-lead resting ECG revealed permanent ventricular preexcitation with a probable posterior accessory pathway. The clinical course was uneventful until the age of 14 when the patient began to experience sustained episodes of palpitations. A diagnosis of orthodromic atrioventricular reentrant tachycardia (AVRT) was made on the basis of the 12-lead ECG recorded during tachycardia. The tachycardia episodes were resistant to vagal maneuvers and sotalol was prescribed at a dosage of 80 mg twice a day, with partial success. Finally, on the basis

of the medical history, of the patient's age, and of the patient's desire, a radiofrequency catheter ablation procedure was scheduled.

Comments

Ventricular preexcitation is frequently present in Ebstein's anomaly (5% to 25%), and in up to 50% of the patients the accessory connections are multiple. Radiofrequency catheter ablation is the method of choice to cure patients with AVRT and is frequently proposed as a primary therapeutic option in young patients. However, radiofrequency catheter ablation of

From: RETAC: *Radiofrequency Catheter Ablation for the Treatment of Cardiac Arrhythmias: A Practical Atlas with Illustrative Cases.* © Futura Publishing Company, Inc. Armonk, NY, 2002.

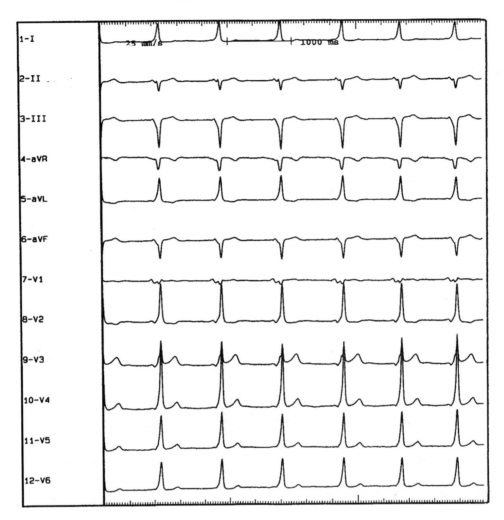

Figure 1. Twelve-lead resting ECG showing sinus rhythm with permanent ventricular preexcitation (posterior accessory pathway). Paper speed 25 mm/s.

AV connection in patients with Ebstein's anomaly is not easy because of the unusual location of the tricuspid valve leaflets, because of the multiplicity of accessory pathways, and because of abnormal morphology of endocardial potentials especially the atrialized right ventricle.

All these difficulties were encountered in the present case: presence of two different but closely related accessory pathways, difficulties in locating the site of the accessory pathway (two sessions were necessary to ablate successfully the two accessory pathways), misinterpretation of endocardial signals related to fragmentation of endocardial potentials in the atrialized right ventricle, necessity of using atrial extrastimuli to validate atrial components in multi-fragmented potentials, and complex geometry of the right ventricle making positioning of the ablation

catheter difficult. Similar experience was reported by Cappato et al. in 1996 in a series of 21 patients with AV connections in the setting of Ebstein's anomaly. These authors used right coronary artery mapping to improve localization of the accessory pathways and this technique apparently proved to be a useful tool in some patients. The use of long guiding sheaths may also be of some help when catheter position is difficult to maintain, or when tissue-contact is insufficient.

Despite all these technical difficulties, radiofrequency catheter ablation is feasible, safe, and efficient in patients with Ebstein's anomaly and this approach should be considered as a first choice therapy when Ebstein's anomaly is associated with episodes of supraventricular tachycardia related to the presence of an accessory pathway.

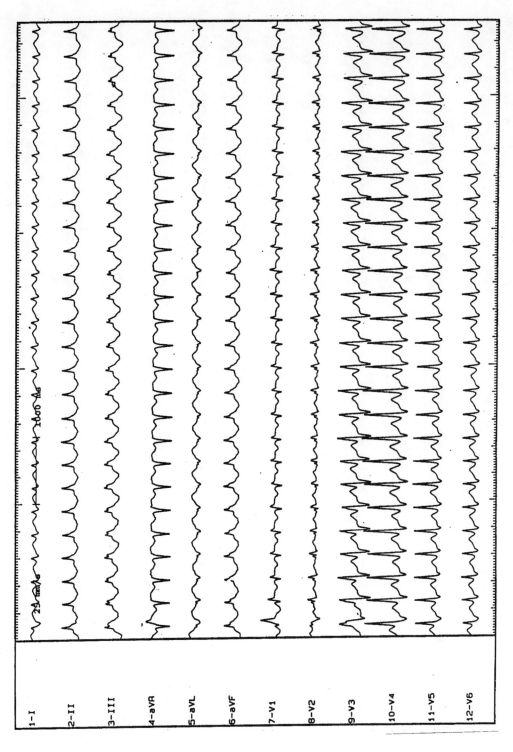

Figure 2. Twelve-lead ECG recorded during tachycardia, showing atrioventricular reentrant tachycardia (AVRT) at a rate of 180 beats/min (cycle length 330 ms) with right bundle branch morphology compatible with Ebstein's anomaly. Paper speed 25 mm/s.

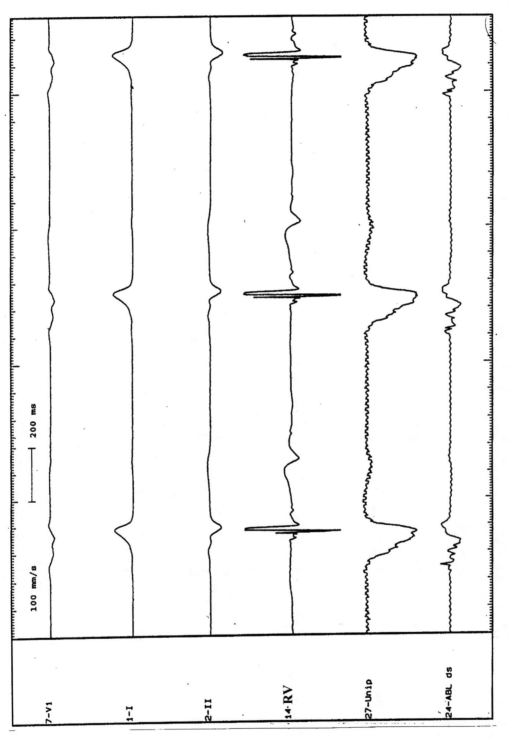

Figure 3. Here are represented three surface ECG leads (V₁, DI, DII), one bipolar intracardiac electrogram from the right ventricle (RV), one unipolar intracardiac electrogram from the tip of the ablation catheter (Unip) and one bipolar intracardiac electrogram from the distal poles of the ablation catheter (ABL ds). The ablation catheter is positioned in the posterior region, in the atrialized ventricle as shown by the marked electrogram fragmentation in ABL ds. Radiofrequency current application in that site was not successful despite an apparently optimal unipolar recording (QS pattern). Paper speed 100 mm/s.

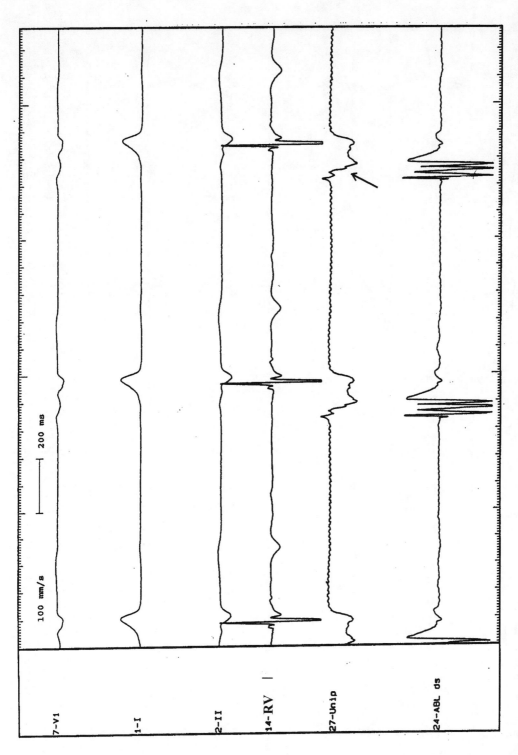

Figure 4. Same display as Figure 3. Paper speed 100 mm/s. The ablation catheter is positioned in the posterior region, on the annulus. The unipolar electrogram is slightly fragmented and an accessory potential is possibly present in the descending limb of the QS potential (arrow). The bipolar electrogram from the ablation catheter shows continuous electrical activity between atrium and ventricle. Radiofrequency current application in that site was successful but unmasked the presence of a second accessory pathway (see Figure 5).

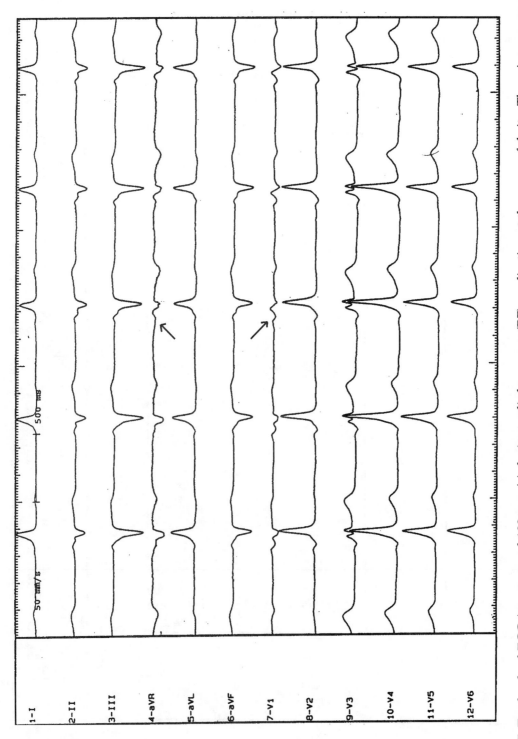

Figure 5. Twelve-lead ECG (paper speed 100 mm/s) during radiofrequency (RF) application at the successful site. There is no normalization of the surface ECG, but a distinctive change in lead aVR (from QR to RS) and in lead V_1 (from QS to RS) is present, attesting that RF application was successful to eliminate the first accessory pathway, but revealing the presence of another accessory pathway certainly located in the close vicinity.

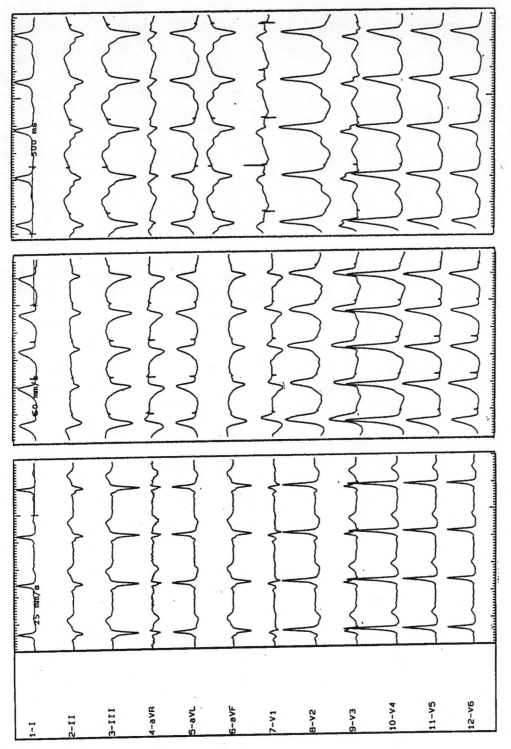

Figure 6. Different aspects of the preexcitation on the 12-lead ECG, essentially in leads aVR and V_1. **Left:** 12-lead ECG (paper speed 25 mm/s) showing the aspect of the preexcitation after the successful radiofrequency application. **Center:** 12-lead ECG (paper speed 50 mm/s) showing maximal preexcitation of the first accessory pathway during atrial stimulation. **Right:** 12-lead ECG (paper speed 50 mm/s) showing maximal preexcitation of the second accessory pathway during atrial stimulation.

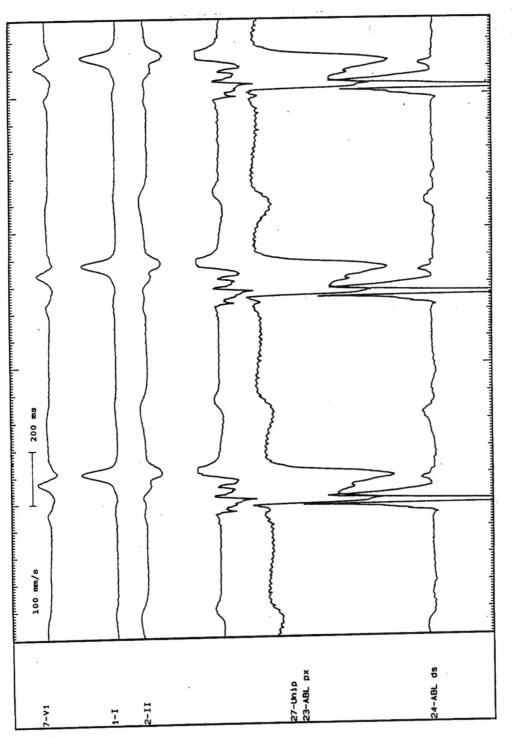

Figure 7. Here are represented three surface ECG leads (V₁, DI, DII), one bipolar intracardiac electrogram from the proximal poles of the ablation catheter (ABL px), one unipolar intracardiac electrogram from the tip of the ablation catheter (Unip), and one bipolar intracardiac electrogram from the distal poles of the ablation catheter (ABL ds). The ablation catheter is positioned in the posterior region, with fragmentation on the proximal poles of the ablation catheter and complete fusion between atrium and ventricle on the distal poles of the ablation catheter. Radiofrequency current application in that site was successful (see Figure 8). Paper speed 100 mm/s.

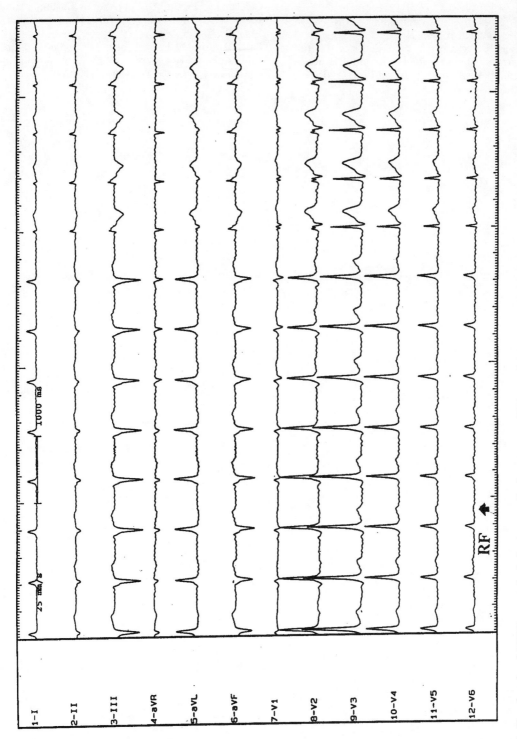

Figure 8. Twelve-lead ECG recorded during radiofrequency (RF) application in the site shown on Figure 7. Two seconds (arrow) after RF application, the preexcitation disappeared and the ECG returned to the aspect of Ebstein's anomaly. Paper speed 25 mm/s.

Suggested Reading

Cappato R, Schlüter M, Weiss C, et al. Radiofrequency current ablation of accessory atrioventricular pathways in Ebstein's anomaly. *Circulation* 1996;94:376-383.

Colavita PG, Packer DL, Pressley JC, et al. Frequency, diagnosis and clinical characteristics of patients with multiple accessory atrioventricular pathways. *Am J Cardiol* 1987;59:601-606.

Van Hare GF. Radiofrequency ablation of accessory pathways associated with congenital heart disease. *Pacing Clin Electrophysiol* 1997;20(part II):2077-2081.

Celermajer DS, Bull C, Till JA, et al. Ebstein's anomaly: Presentation and outcome from fetus to adult. *J Am Coll Cardiol* 1994;23:170-176.

Reich JD, Auld D, Hulse E, et al. The pediatric radiofrequency ablation registry's experience with Ebstein's anomaly. *J Cardiovasc Electrophysiol* 1998;9:1370-1377.

Chapter 18

Right Free Wall Accessory Pathway

Medical History

A 64-year-old female patient without any structural heart disease presented with frequent episodes of paroxysmal tachycardia. The 12-lead ECG showed a typical aspect of preexcitation with a delta wave polarity suggesting the presence of a posterolateral accessory pathway. After informed consent, it was decided to map the accessory pathway and to ablate it.

Comments

Lateral and postero-lateral accessory pathways are not frequent (6% of all accessory pathways) and they are sometimes very difficult to ablate because of unstable catheter position, poor tissue contact, and/or inadequate temperature. Precise location of the accessory pathway can be facilitated by the introduction of a mapping catheter into the right coronary artery. Stabilization of the catheter position (and hence better tissue contact) can be obtained by specially designed sheaths. In selected cases, a subclavian or a jugular approach can be used in order to improve tissue contact. The recurrence rate after successful ablation is significantly higher in patients with right lateral or right anteroseptal accesory pathways (10% to 20%) compared to patients with posteroseptal or left lateral accessory pathways (<5%).

Suggested Reading

Milstein S, Sharma AD, Guiraudon GM, et al. An algorithm for the electrocardiographic localization of accessory path-

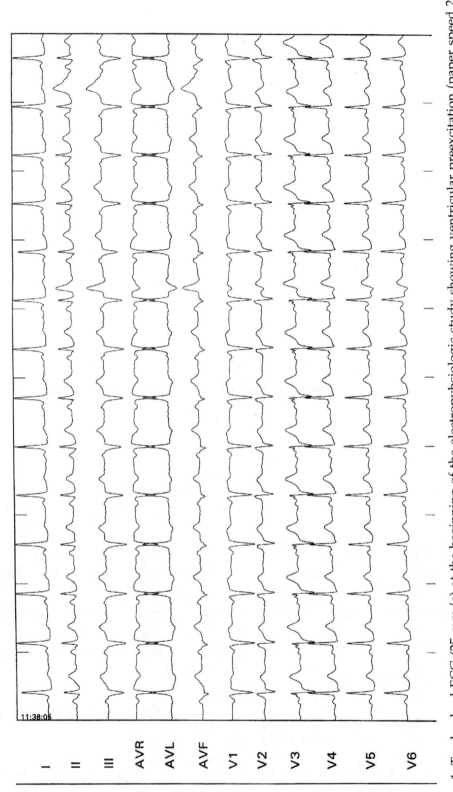

Figure 1. Twelve-lead ECG (25 mm/s) at the beginning of the electropyhsiologic study showing ventricular preexcitation (paper speed 25 mm/s)

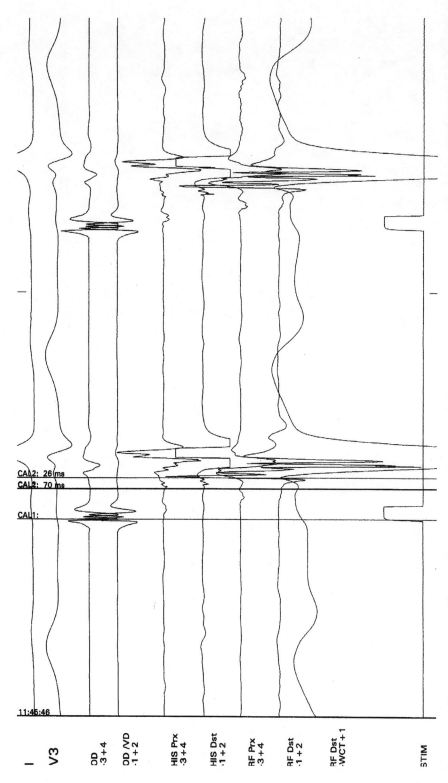

Figure 2. Intracardiac recordings (150 mm/s) during sinus rhythm before the ablation procedure. Here are displayed two surface ECG leads (I, V₃), two bipolar recordings from the high right atrium (OD 3+4 and OD 1+2), two bipolar recordings from the His bundle region (HIS Prx 3+4 and His Dst 1+2), two bipolar recordings obtained from the tip of the ablation catheter (RF Prx 3+4 and RF Dst 1+2), one unipolar recording obtained from the distal pole of the ablation catheter (RF Dst WCT+1), and the stimulation channel. During sinus rhythm A-H interval is 70 ms and H-V interval 26 ms.

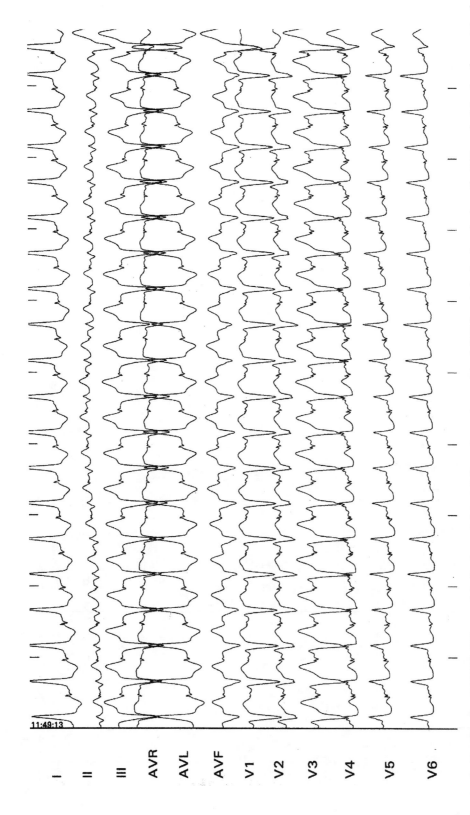

Figure 3. Twelve-lead ECG (25 mm/s) during right atrial pacing at a rate of 120 beats/min (cycle length 500 ms). Maximal ventricular preexcitation is present and the polarity of the delta wave suggests a right posterior location of the accessory pathway. In this case, the antegrade effective refractory period of the accessory pathway was 290 ms (not shown).

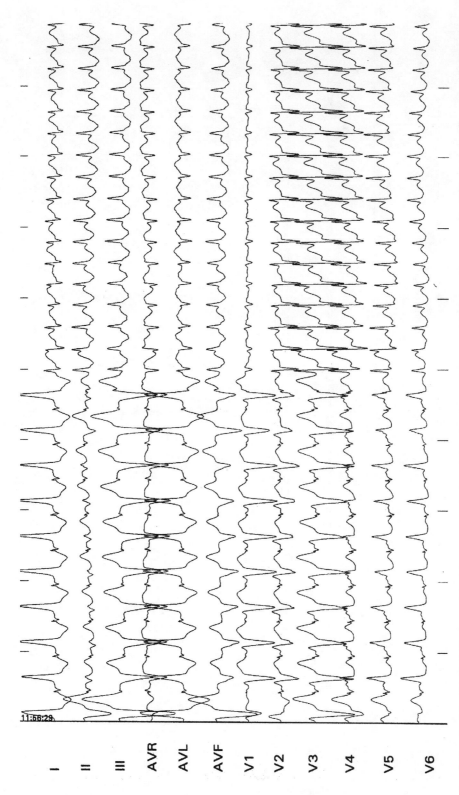

Figure 4. Twelve-lead ECG (25 mm/s) showing induction of orthodromic atrioventricular reentrant tachycardia during right atrial pacing.

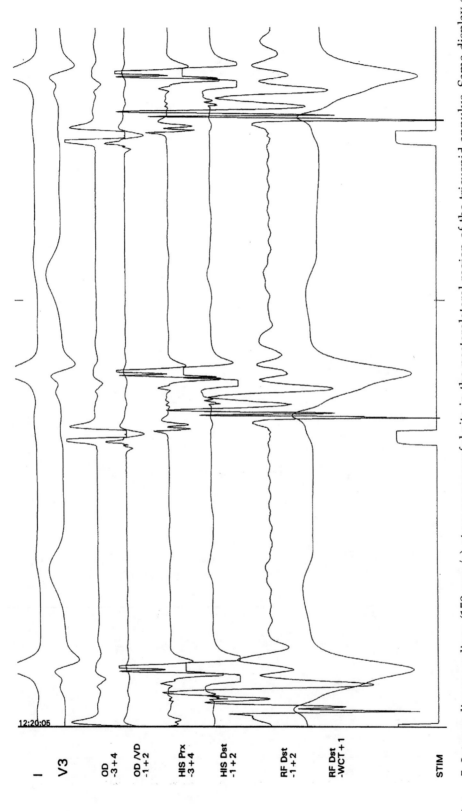

Figure 5. Intracardiac recordings (150 mm/s) at an unsuccessful site in the posterolateral region of the tricuspid annulus. Same display as Figure 2. The ablation catheter is located more on the atrial side (A > V).

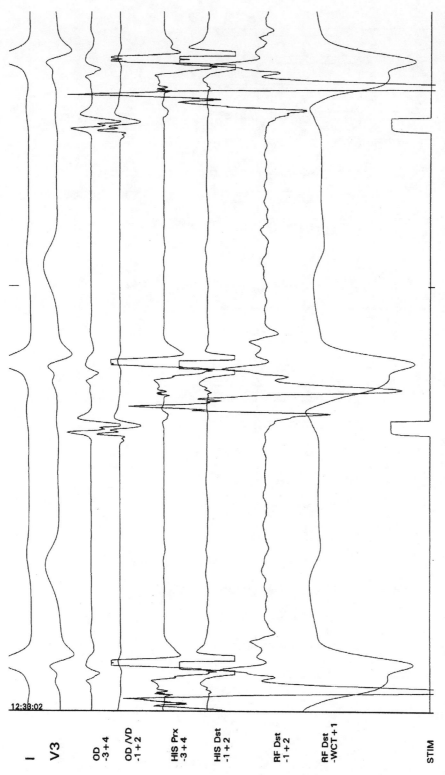

Figure 6. Intracardiac recordings (150 mm/s) at the successful site in the posterolateral region of the tricuspid annulus. Same display as Figure 2. Compared to the position shown on Figure 5, the ablation catheter was moved more laterally and more on the ventricular side.

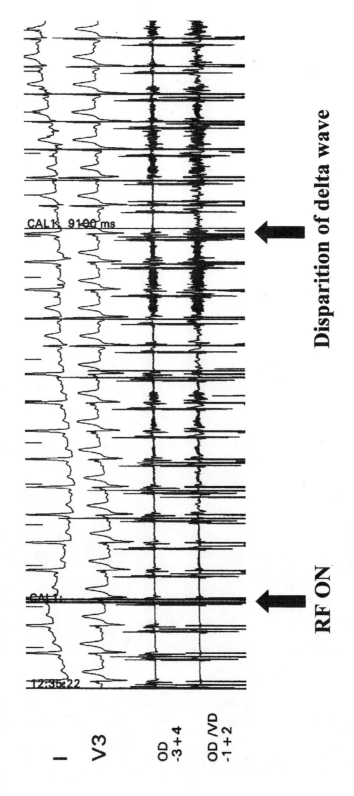

Figure 7. Intracardiac recordings (25 mm/s) during radiofrequency current application at the successful site (60°C, 50 Watts). Here are displayed two surface ECG leads (I, V₃) and two bipolar recordings from the high right atrium (OD 3+4, OD 1+2). Nine seconds after radiofrequency current application (RF ON) disparition of delta wave is observed.

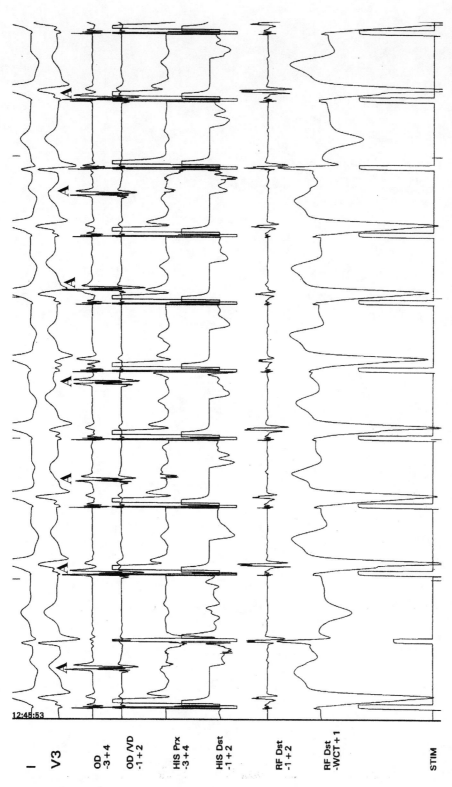

Figure 8. Intracardiac recordings (50 mm/s) during ventricular pacing after the ablation procedure, showing ventriculo-atrial dissociation. Same display as Figure 2.

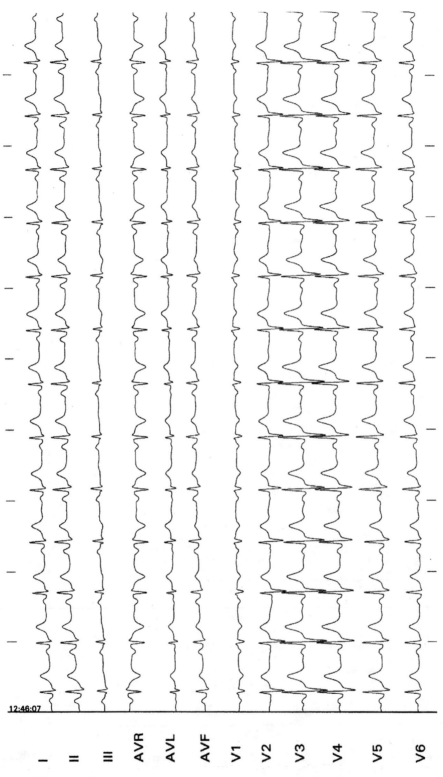

Figure 9. Twelve-lead ECG (25 mm/s) after the ablation procedure showing disparition of delta wave and normalization of the ECG.

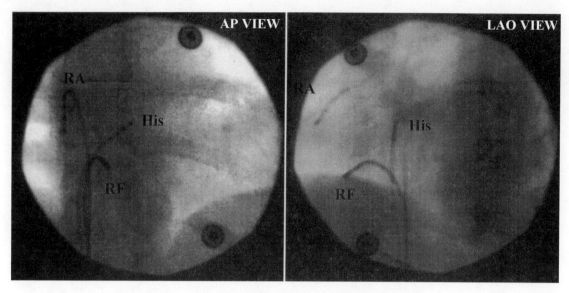

Figure 10. Chest X-ray showing catheter position.

ways in the Wolff-Parkinson-White syndrome. *Pacing Clin Electrophysiol* 1987;10:555-563.

Swartz JF, Tracy CM, Fletcher RD, et al. Radiofrequency endocardial catheter ablation of accessory atrioventricular pathway atrial insertion sites. *Circulation* 1993;87:487-499.

Kay GN, Epstein AE, Dailey SM, et al. Role of radiofrequency ablation in the management of supraventricular arrhythmias: Experience in 760 consecutive patients. *J Cardiovasc Electrophysiol* 1993;4:371-389.

Haissaguerre M, Fischer B, Warin JF, et al. Electrogram patterns predictive of successful radiofrequency catheter ablation of accessory pathways. *Pacing Clin Electrophysiol* 1992;15(suppl II):2138-2145.

Swartz JF, Cohen AI, Fletcher RD, et al. Right coronary epicardial mapping improves accessory pathway catheter ablation success (abstract). *Circulation* 1989;80:432.

Chapter 19

Catheter Ablation of a Right Posteroseptal Accessory Pathway During Atrial Fibrillation

Medical History

A 66-year-old female patient presented with paroxysmal episodes of regular narrow QRS complex tachycardia (rate 170 beats/min) alternating from time to time with episodes of atrial fibrillation for more than 10 years. She had no underlying heart disease and never experienced syncope. Arrhythmias proved to be resistant to all antiarrhythmics including sotalol, propafenone, and amiodarone. Ventricular preexcitation was present on the 12-lead resting ECG with a delta wave polarity suggesting a posteroseptal location of the accessory pathway. An ablation procedure was proposed.

Comments

Atrial fibrillation may occur in up to one third of patients with Wolff-Parkinson-White (WPW) syndrome. Transformation of atrioventricular reentrant tachycardia (AVRT) into atrial fibrillation is not uncommon, and some authors have suggested a direct

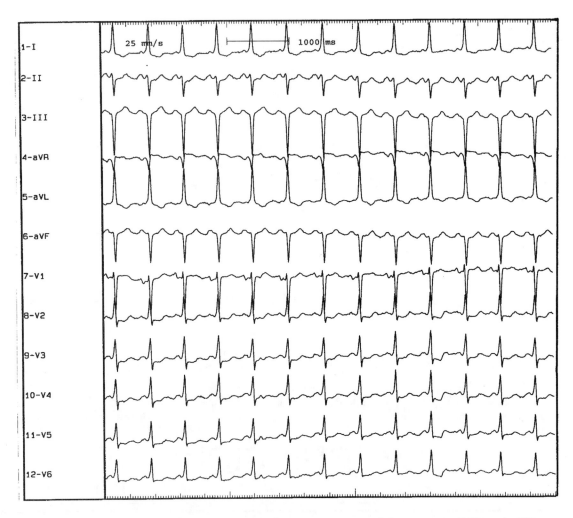

Figure 1. Twelve-lead ECG (25 mm/s) showing negative delta wave in DIII and aVF.

relationship between the presence of the accessory pathway and the occurrence of atrial fibrillation in WPW patients. The low recurrence rate of atrial fibrillation after successful ablation (either surgically or by catheter) tends to confirm this hypothesis. Catheter ablation of an accessory pathway during persistent atrial fibrillation is often difficult. In some cases, external direct current (DC) shock or class Ia/Ic drugs may be needed to restore sinus rhythm and facilitate mapping. In the present case, we used unipolar recordings for mapping the optimal site for ablation. This case also illustrates the utility of pharmacological maneuvers to provoke conduction block through the AV node and therefore to increase ventricular preexcitation. Classically, verapamil is contraindicated in the presence of ventricular preexcitation, because it can shorten the effective refractory period of the accessory pathway

and increase the risk of collapse and ventricular fibrillation. In this case, the risk of verapamil administration was low because the refractory period of the accessory pathway was relatively long (280 ms).

Suggested Reading

Haïssaguerre M, Dartigues JF, Warin JF, et al. Electrogram patterns predictive of successful catheter ablation of accessory pathways. Value of unipolar recording mode. *Circulation* 1991;84:188-202.

Galamhusein S, Ko O, Carruthers G, et al. Acceleration of the ventricular response during atrial fibrillation in the Wolff-Parkinson-White syndrome after verapamil. *Circulation* 1982;65:348-356. Sharma AD, Klein GJ, Guiraudon GM, et al. Atrial fibrillation in patients with Wolff-Parkinson-White syndrome: Incidence after surgical ablation of the accessory pathway. *Circulation* 1985;72:161-169.

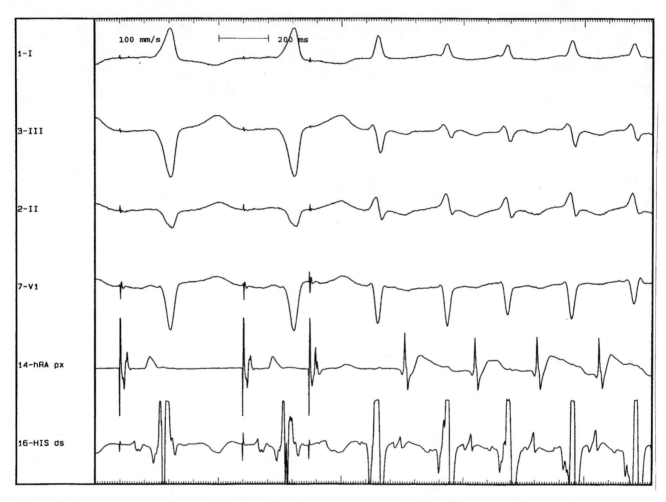

Figure 2. Intracardiac recordings (100 mm/s) showing initiation of atrioventricular reentrant tachycardia (cycle length 250 ms) by programmed atrial stimulation (S1-S1 = 500 ms; S1-S2 = 270 ms). HIS ds = catheter positioned in the His bundle region; hRA px = catheter positioned in the high right atrium.

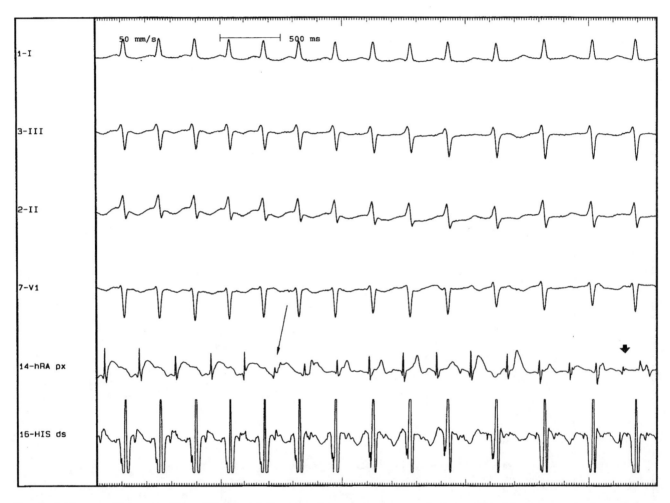

Figure 3. Intracardiac recordings (50 mm/s) showing the spontaneous transformation of atrioventricular reentrant tachycardia into atrial tachycardia (long arrow) and atrial fibrillation (short arrow). During atrial fibrillation the minimal RR interval with preexcitation was 250 ms. Because of the presence of enhanced AV conduction ventricular response during atrial fibrillation was always rapid, with or without ventricular preexcitation. In order to increase the degree of preexcitation (to facilitate mapping) 2.5 mg of intravenous verapamil were administred during atrial fibrillation.

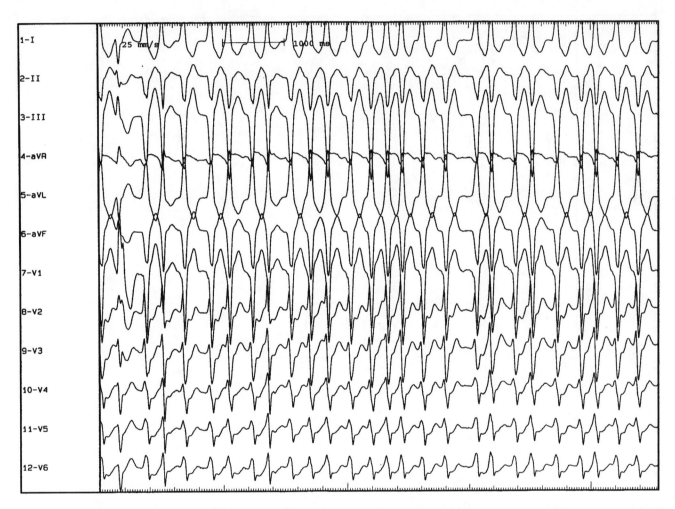

Figure 4. Twelve-lead ECG (25 mm/s) recorded during atrial fibrillation after intravenous administration of 2.5 mg of verapamil. Because of the effects of the drug on the AV node, preexcitation became permanent with a slight acceleration of the ventricular rate (210-240 beats/min; minimal RR interval 230 ms).

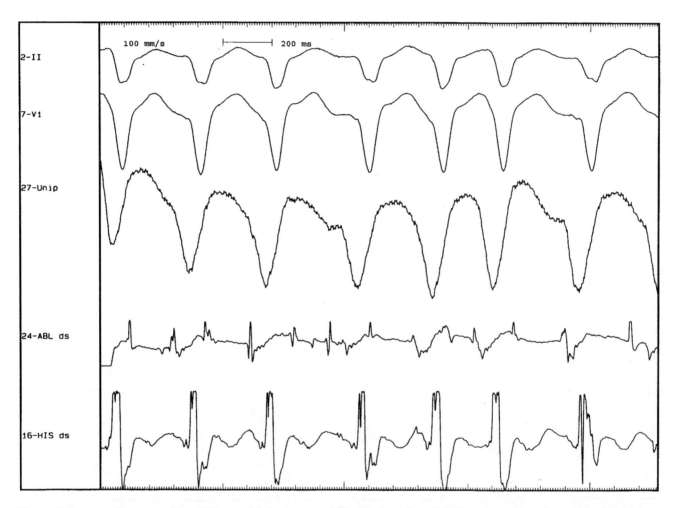

Figure 5. Intracardiac recording (100 mm/s) during atrial fibrillation after the administration of verapamil. Maximal preexcitation was obvious, and mapping was performed using mainly unipolar recordings. At the successful site, unipolar recording (Unip) showed a QS pattern. During atrial fibrillation, the bipolar recording (ABL ds) was of little help in the present case.

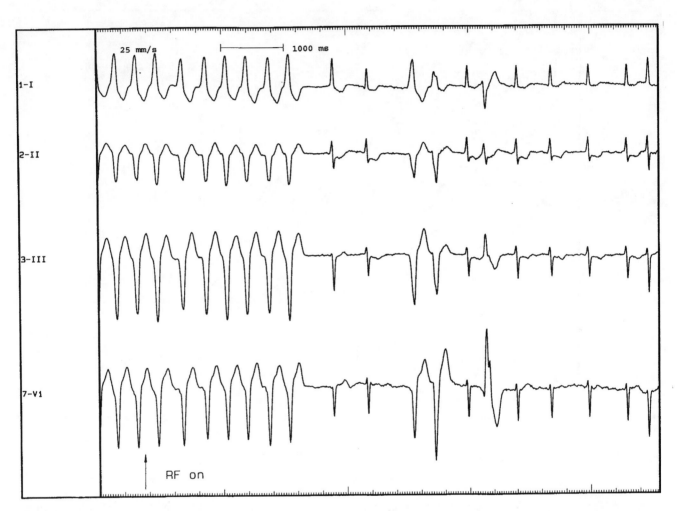

Figure 6. Surface ECG recording (leads DI, DII, DIII, V₁; 25 mm/s) during the first radiofrequency (RF on) current application. Preexcitation disappeared 2 seconds after energy application, which was maintained during 60 seconds.

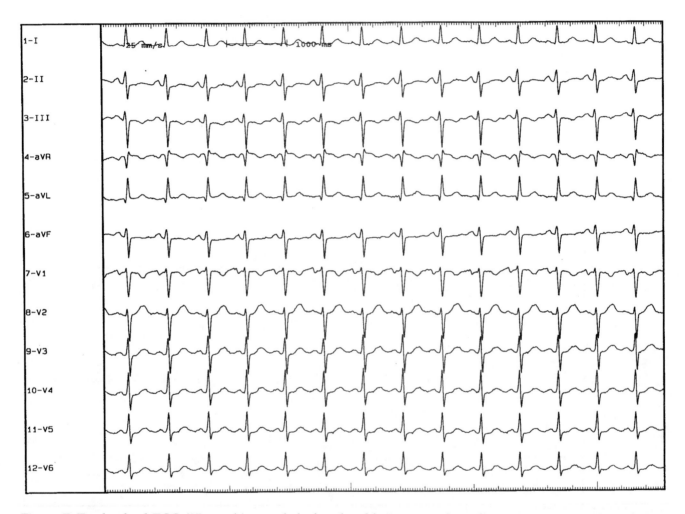

Figure 7. Twelve-lead ECG (25 mm/s) recorded after the ablation procedure. Spontaneous restoration of sinus rhythm occurred 10 minutes after the ablation procedure and no ventricular preexcitation was observed. Follow-up was uneventful with no recurrence of preexcitation, no recurrence of AVRT, and no recurrence of atrial fibrillation.

Chapter 20

Catheter Ablation of a Left Lateral Accessory Pathway through a Patent Foramen Ovale

Medical History

A 20-year-old female patient presented with a history of frequent episodes of palpitations over the last 4 years, associated with chest pain. A 12-lead resting ECG showed a Wolff-Parkinson-White pattern, and she was referred for electrophysiologic testing and radiofrequency catheter ablation.

Comments

Catheter ablation is a highly effective curative treatment for arrhythmias related to the presence of an accessory pathway. Mapping and ablation of left-sided accessory pathways can be accomplished using either a retrograde aortic approach or a transseptal approach. In patients with a patent foramen ovale, the transseptal approach is obviously preferred for technical reasons; special guiding sheaths may be used to adequately position the ablation catheter on the mitral annulus. The transseptal approach allows for greater mobility of the catheter in the left atrium, but overall successes are comparable between the two techniques. In most centers, the decision on which technique is used is based on the experience and preference of the operator. For left-sided accessory pathways, the coro-

From: RETAC: *Radiofrequency Catheter Ablation for the Treatment of Cardiac Arrhythmias: A Practical Atlas with Illustrative Cases.*
© Futura Publishing Company, Inc. Armonk, NY, 2002.

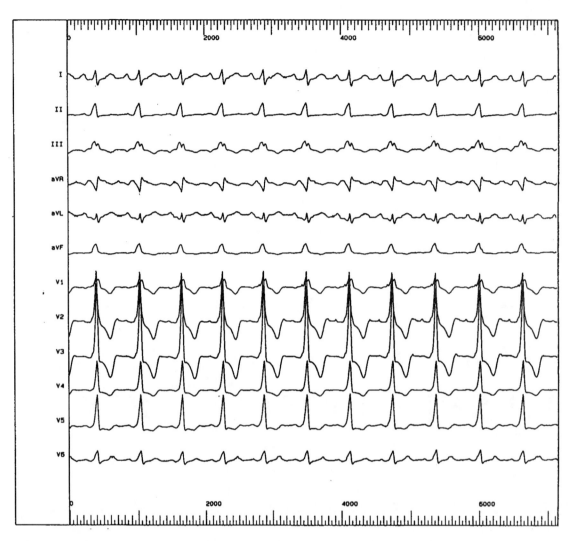

Figure 1. Twelve-lead ECG (25 mm/s) showing normal sinus rhythm with permanent ventricular preexcitation. Delta wave is positive in II, III, aVF, V$_1$ to V$_6$, negative in aVL and isoelectric in DI.

nary sinus should be mapped before ablation and the coronary sinus catheter should be left in place during the ablation procedure to guide precise mapping of the accessory pathway location. Unipolar recordings obtained from the tip of the ablation catheter are highly recommended to precisely locate the accessory pathway.

Suggested Reading

Calkins H, Langberg JJ, Sousa J, et al. Radiofrequency catheter ablation of accessory atrioventricular connections in 250 patients: Abbreviated therapeutic approach to Wolff-Parkinson-White syndrome. *Circulation* 1992;85:133-1346.

Chen X, Borggrefe M, Shenasa M, et al. Characteristics of local electrocardiogram predicting successful transcatheter radiofrequency ablation of left-sided accessory pathways. *J Am Coll Cardiol* 1992;20:656-665.

Deshpande SS, Bremmer S, Sra JS, et al. Ablation of left free-wall accessory pathways using radiofrequency energy at the atrial insertion site. *J Cardiovasc Electrophysiol* 1994;5:219-231.

Lesh MD, Van Hare GF, Scheinman MM, et al. Comparison of retrograde and transseptal methods for ablation of left free wall accessory pathways. *J Am Coll Cardiol* 1993;22:542-549.

Natale A, Wathen M, Yee R, et al. Atrial and ventricular approaches for radiofrequency catheter ablation of left-sided accessory pathways. *Am J Cardiol* 1992;70:114-118.

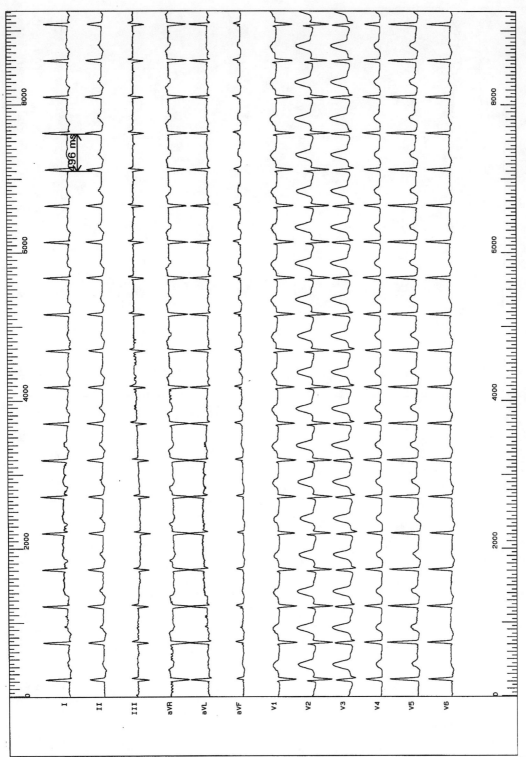

Figure 2. 12-lead ECG (25 mm/s) recorded during an episode of palpitations showing a regular narrow QRS complex tachycardia, at a rate of 122 beats/min (cycle length 496 ms) corresponding to an episode of orthodromic atrioventricular reentrant tachycardia.

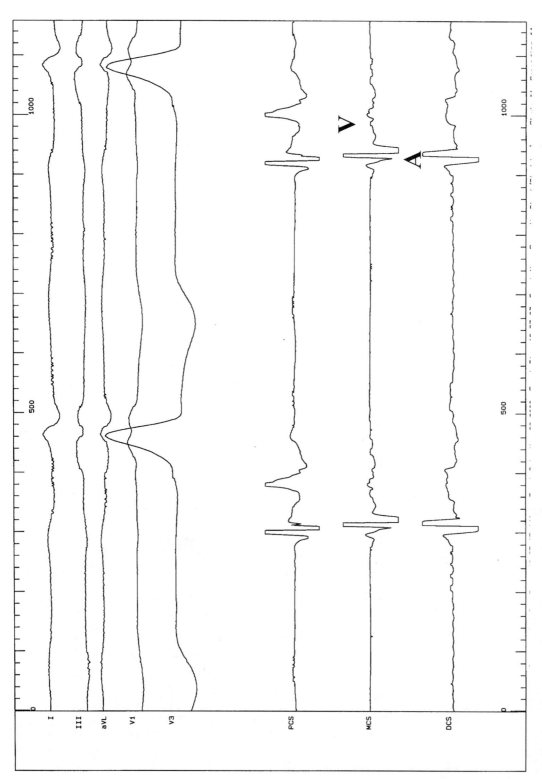

Figure 3. Intracardiac recordings during sinus rhythm. On the figure are shown five surface ECG leads (I, III, aVL, V_1, V_3) together with three bipolar intracardiac recordings (PCS = proximal coronary sinus; MCS = median coronary sinus; DCS = distal coronary sinus). Paper speed 200 mm/s. The shortest AV interval is observed between the median and the distal coronary sinus, suggesting a lateral or postero-lateral location of the accessory pathway.

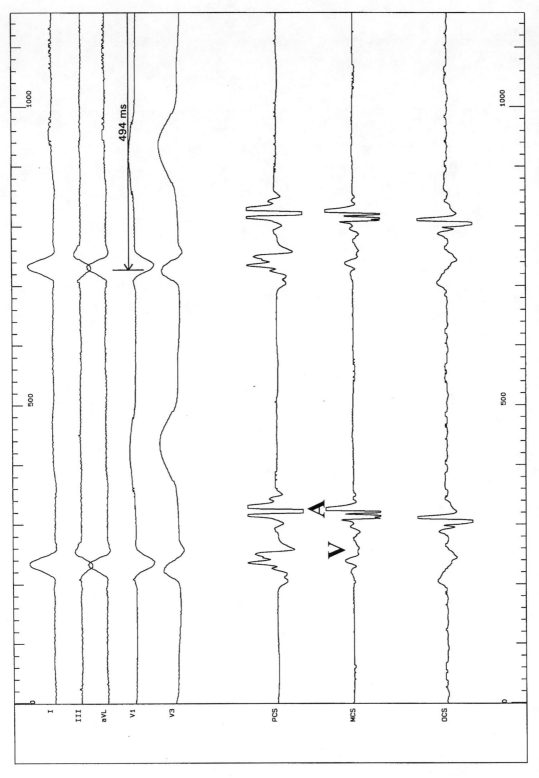

Figure 4. Intracardiac recordings during orthodromic atrioventricular tachycardia. On the figure are shown five surface ECG leads (I, III, aVL, V$_1$, V$_3$) together with three bipolar intracardiac recordings (PCS = proximal coronary sinus; MCS = median coronary sinus; DCS = distal coronary sinus). Paper speed 200 mm/s. The shortest V-A interval is observed in the distal coronary sinus, suggesting a lateral location of the accessory pathway.

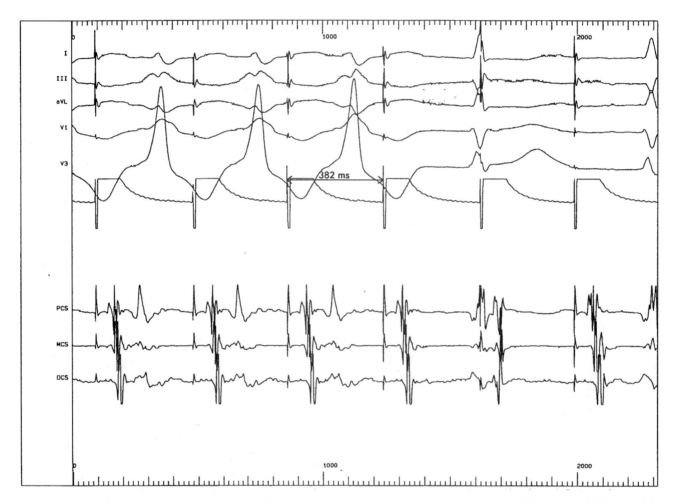

Figure 5. Intracardiac recordings during incremental atrial pacing. On the figure are shown 5 surface ECG leads (I, III, aVL, V_1, V_3) together with three bipolar intracardiac recordings (PCS = proximal coronary sinus; MCS = median coronary sinus; DCS = distal coronary sinus). Paper speed 100 mm/s. There is 1:1 AV conduction over the accessory pathway up to a cycle length of 382 ms (153 beats/min).

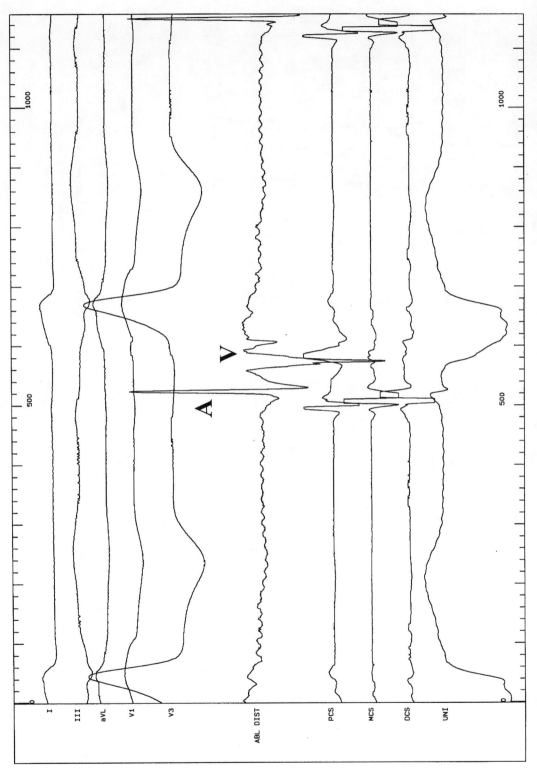

Figure 6. Intracardiac recordings during sinus rhythm at the successful site. On the figure are shown five surface ECG leads (I, III, aVL, V_1, V_3) together with 4 bipolar intracardiac recordings (ABL DIST = bipolar recording from the distal pole of the ablation catheter; PCS = proximal coronary sinus; MCS = median coronary sinus; DCS = distal coronary sinus), and one unipolar recording obtained from the tip of the ablation catheter. Paper speed 200 mm/s. The ablation catheter is introduced into the left atrium through a patent foramen ovale, and is positioned on the atrial side of the mitral annulus. Atrioventricular interval is 30 ms on the ablation catheter.

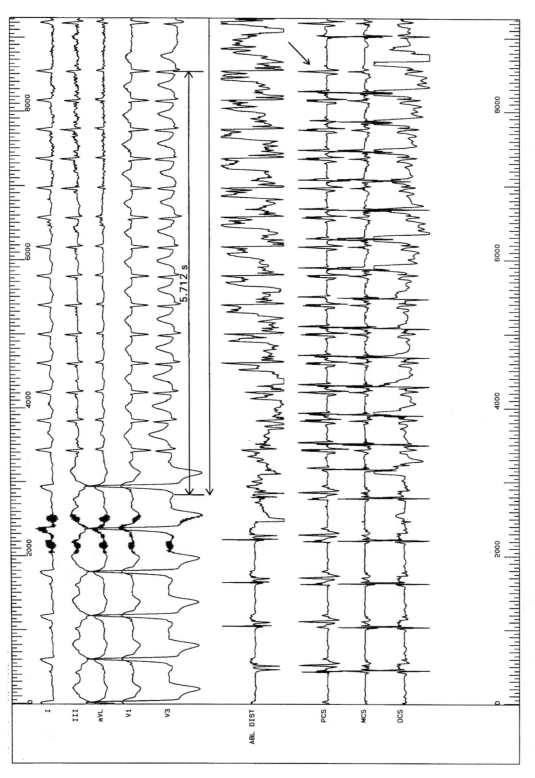

Figure 7. Intracardiac recordings during the first radiofrequency (RF) current application. On the figure are shown five surface ECG leads (I, III, aVL, V₁, V₃) together with four bipolar intracardiac recordings (ABL DIST = bipolar recording from the distal pole of the ablation catheter; PCS = proximal coronary sinus; MCS = median coronary sinus; DCS = distal coronary sinus). Paper speed 25 mm/s. Disappearance of retrograde accessory pathway conduction (arrow) is observed 5.7 seconds after RF current application, which initially induced a short burst of orthodromic atrioventricular reentrant tachycardia.

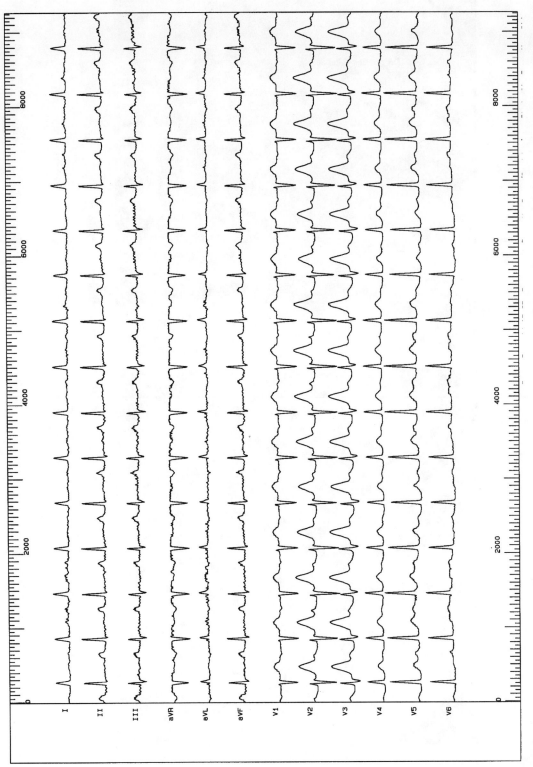

Figure 8. Twelve-lead ECG (25 mm/s) obtained after radiofrequency current application showing normal sinus rhythm without ventricular preexcitation.

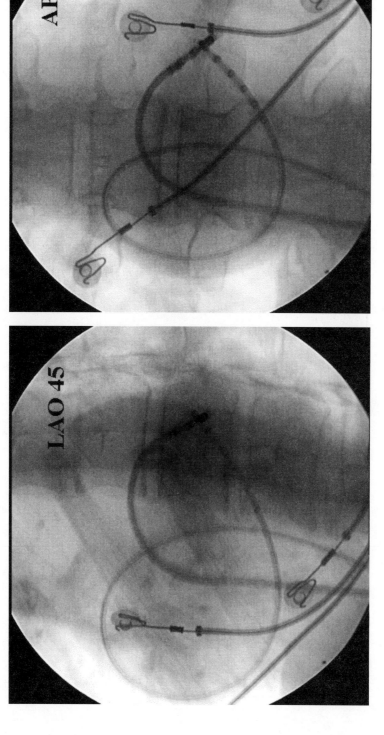

Figure 9. Chest X-rays showing catheter position.

Chapter 21

Catheter Ablation of a Left Posteroseptal Accessory Pathway in a Patient with Aortic Stenosis

Medical History

A 56-year-old male patient presented with a history of paroxysmal supraventricular tachycardia (180 beats/min) for more than 10 years. Ventricular preexcitation was present on the 12-lead resting ECG and the patient experienced several episodes of sustained atrial flutter or fibrillation necessitating amiodarone therapy. Severe aortic stenosis (surface area 0.6 cm^2) and moderate left ventricular dysfunction (left ventricular ejection fraction 45%) were diagnosed during echocardiography.

An electrophysiologic study was proposed.

Comments

Left-sided accessory pathways can be ablated either by a transaortic retrograde approach or, according to personal preferences, by a transseptal approach. In the present case, the transseptal approach was required because of the presence of severe aortic stenosis. Positioning of the ablation catheter in the left posteroseptal region after transseptal puncture is not always technically easy. Moreover, in the present case, the antero-grade and retrograde conduction over the accessory pathway was severely altered by amiodarone, making

From: RETAC: *Radiofrequency Catheter Ablation for the Treatment of Cardiac Arrhythmias: A Practical Atlas with Illustrative Cases.* © Futura Publishing Company, Inc. Armonk, NY, 2002.

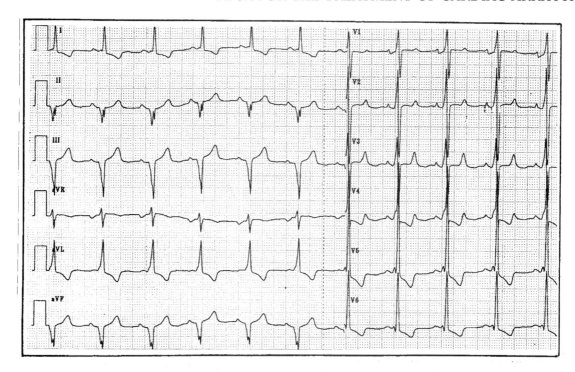

Figure 1. Twelve-lead ECG (25 mm/s) during sinus rhythm showing permanent ventricular preexcitation with a negative delta wave in inferior leads and an initially positive delta wave in V_1.

mapping impossible anterogradely and rather difficult retrogradely. Interruption of all antiarrhythmic drugs is therefore preferred before attempting ablation of an accessory pathway. In the present case, no attempt was made to ablate the flutter circuit; the patient underwent aortic valve replacement without complication, and no arrhythmia recurrence was observed during a follow-up period of 12 months.

Suggested Reading

Chen X, Borggrefe M, Shenasa M, et al. Characteristics of local electrocardiogram predicting successful transcatheter radiofrequency ablation of left-sided accessory pathways. *J Am Coll Cardiol* 1992;20:656-665.

Daoud E, Niebauer M, Bakr O, et al. Placement of electrode catheters into the coronary sinus during electrophysiology procedures. *Am J Cardiol* 1994;74:194-195.

Dhala AA, Deshpande SS, Bremner S, et al. Transcatheter ablation of posteroseptal accessory pathways using a venous approach and radiofrequency energy. *Circulation* 1994;90:1799-1810.

Lesh MD, Van Hare GF, Scheiman MM, et al. Comparison of retrograde and transseptal methods for ablation of left free wall accessory pathways. *J Am Coll Cardiol* 1993;22:542-549.

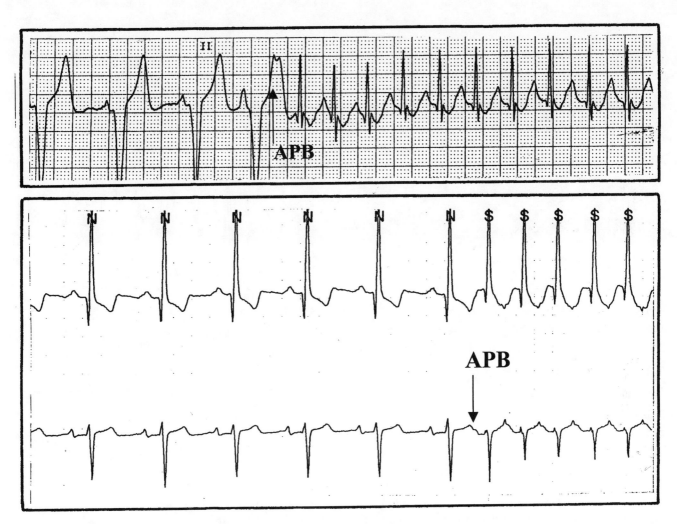

Figure 2. Mode of initiation of the supraventricular tachycardia. **Top**: One-lead ECG monitoring (25 mm/s) showing ventricular preexcitation during sinus rhythm and initiation of atrioventricular reentrant tachycardia (AVRT) by an atrial premature beat (APB) with anterograde block over the accessory pathway. **Bottom**: Two-channel Holter monitoring (25 mm/s) showing normal sinus rhythm without preexcitation and initiation of AVRT by an APB allowing retrograde conduction over the accessory pathway.

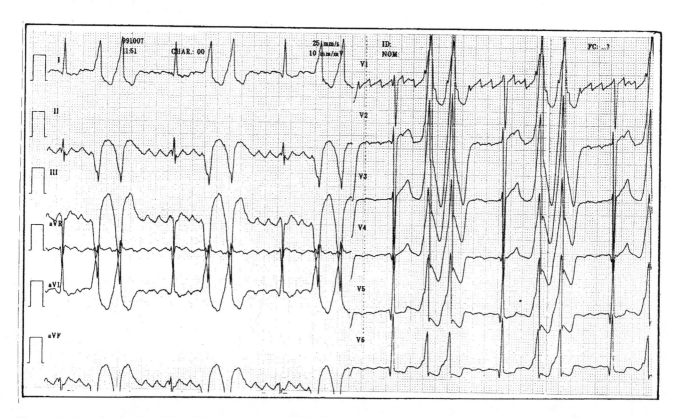

Figure 3. Twelve-lead ECG (25 mm/s) recorded during an episode of severe palpitations showing an atypical atrial flutter with intermittent ventricular preexcitation (pseudo '''ventricular''' trigeminy).

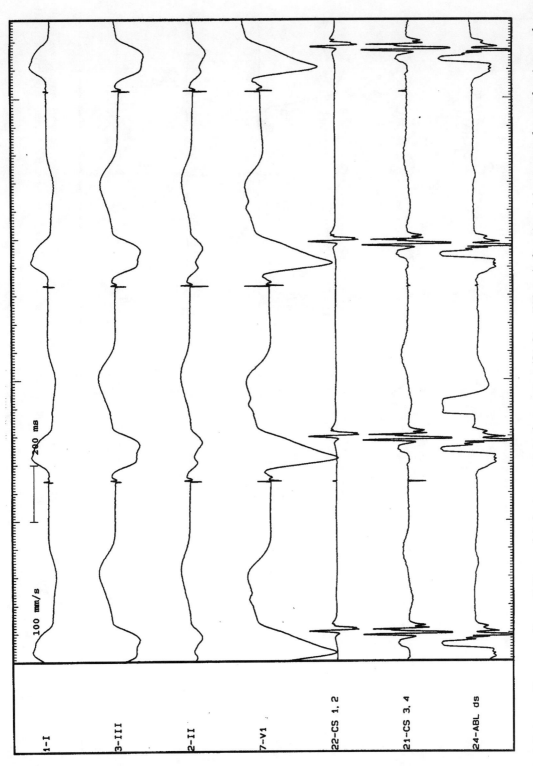

Figure 4. Intracardiac recordings (100 mm/s) during ventricular pacing (S1-S1 = 700 ms) showing 1:1 retrograde conduction and complete V-A fusion in CS 3,4 and on the ablation catheter (ABL ds) positioned in the left posteroseptal region reached by a transseptal approach because of the presence of severe aortic stenosis. During the pre-ablation EP study there was no anterograde conduction over the accessory pathway (probably because of amiodarone therapy) and poor retrograde conduction (retrograde ERP of the accessory pathway = 540 ms). CS 3,4 = proximal coronary sinus; CS 1,2 = distal coronary sinus.

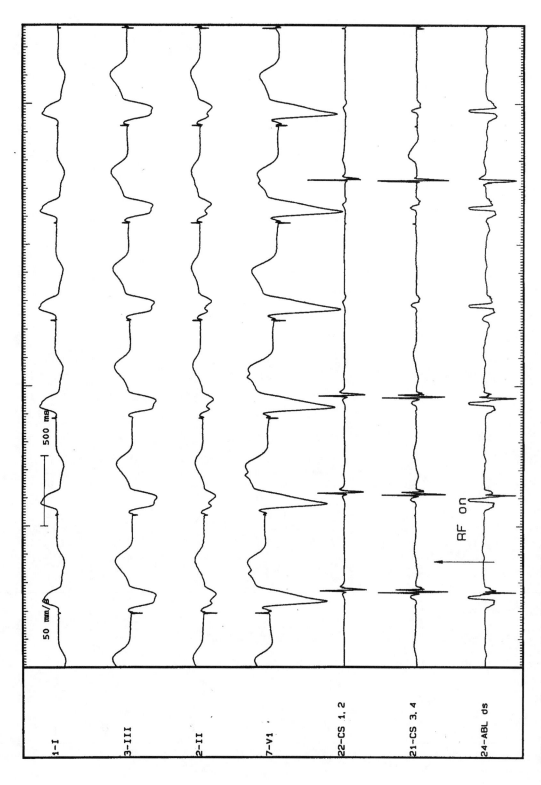

Figure 5. Intracardiac recording (50 mm/s) during the sixth radiofrequency (RF) current application performed during continuous ventricular pacing (S1-S1 : 700 ms). Retrograde conduction over the accessory pathway is interrupted 2 seconds after RF current application, attesting to the success of the procedure.

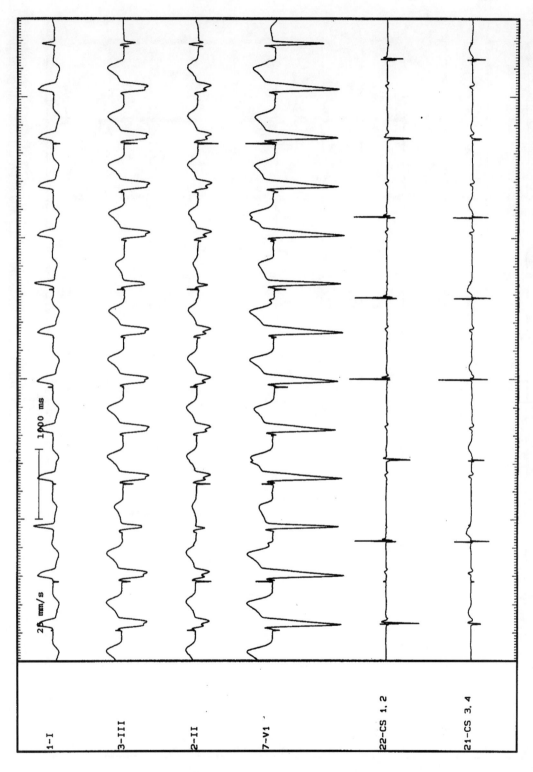

Figure 6. Intracardiac recordings (25 mm/s) after the ablation procedure showing complete V-A dissociation and occasional capture beats.

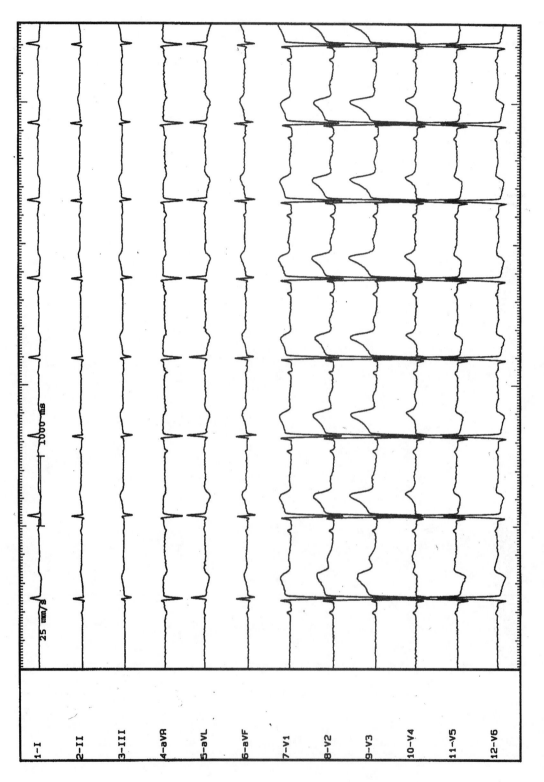

Figure 7. Twelve-lead ECG (25 mm/s) performed after the ablation procedure showing normal sinus rhythm, no ventricular preexcitation, left ventricular hypertrophy, and ST-T changes compatible with left ventricular strain.

Chapter 22

Catheter Ablation of a Left Lateral Accessory Pathway

Medical History

A 45-year-old female patient presented with a history of several episodes of regular tachycardia at a rate of 200 beats/min. Duration of the tachycardia episode was about 1 hour. No antiarrhythmic drug treatment was prescribed because of the patient's refusal. A diagnosis of Wolff-Parkinson-White syndrome was made by another cardiologist, and the patient was referred for electrophysiologic testing and radiofrequency catheter ablation.

Comments

A left lateral location of the accessory pathway is present in up to 45% of patients with the Wolff-Parkinson-White syndrome, and accessory pathways in that location are generally easy to ablate. The site of insertion of an accessory pathway can be grossly determined by analyzing delta-wave polarity on the 12-lead ECG during sinus rhythm. However, precise location can only be assessed by endocardial or epicardial mapping techniques. For left free wall bypass tracts, initial mapping is usually performed using a multipolar electrode catheter positioned in the coronary sinus. To ablate a left free wall accessory pathway, the ablation catheter is positioned on the mitral annulus either using a transaortic retrograde approach (as in the present case) or, less commonly, using a transseptal approach. The mitral annulus is carefully mapped (using the coronary sinus catheter as a guide) by inserting the tip of the ablation catheter beneath the mitral leaflets.

Suggested Reading

Leather RA, Leitch JW, Klein GJ, et al. Radiofrequency catheter ablation of accessory pathways: A learning experience. *Am J Cardiol* 1991;68:1651-1655.

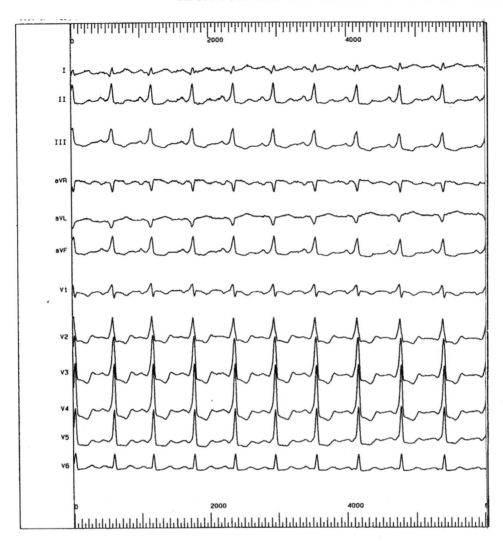

Figure 1. Twelve-lead ECG (25 mm/s) showing normal sinus rhythm with permanent ventricular preexcitation. Delta wave is positive in II, III, aVF, V_1 to V_6, and negative in aVL and DI.

Haïssaguerre M, Dartigues JF, Warin JF, et al. Electrogram patterns predictive of successful catheter ablation of accessory pathways. Value of unipolar recording mode. *Circulation* 1991;84:188-202.

Benito F, Sanchez C. Radiofrequency catheter ablation of accessory pathways in infants. *Heart* 1997;78:160-162.

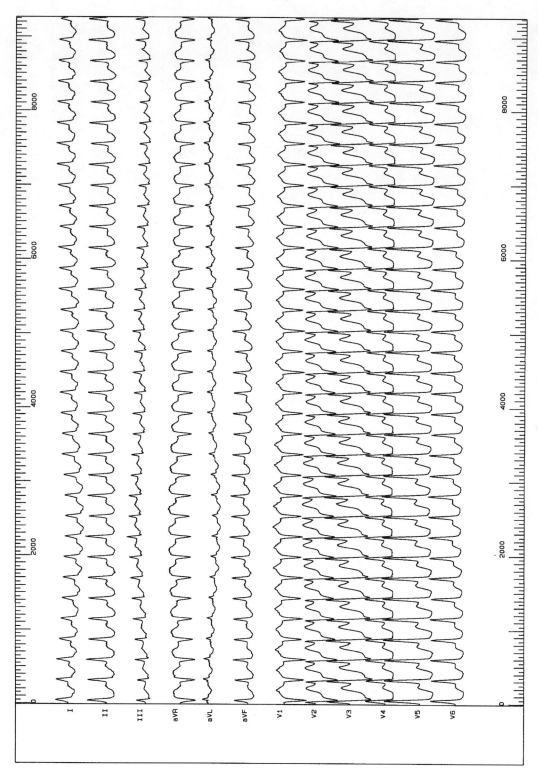

Figure 2. Twelve-lead ECG (25 mm/s) recorded during an episode of clinical tachycardia showing a regular narrow QRS complex tachycardia, at a rate of 210 beats/min (cycle length 288 ms) corresponding to an episode of orthodromic atrioventricular reentrant tachycardia.

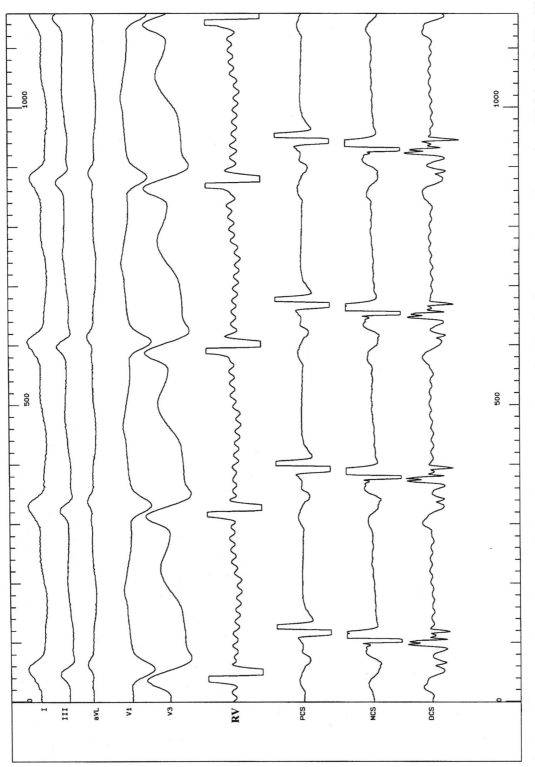

Figure 3. Intracardiac recordings during orthodromic reentrant tachycardia. On the figure are shown five surface ECG leads (I, III, aVL, V$_1$, V$_3$) together with four bipolar intracardiac recordings (RV = right ventricular catheter used for stimulation; PCS = proximal coronary sinus; MCS = median coronary sinus; DCS = distal coronary sinus). Paper speed 200 mm/s. The earliest atrial depolarization occurs in DCS suggesting a left lateral location of the accessory pathway.

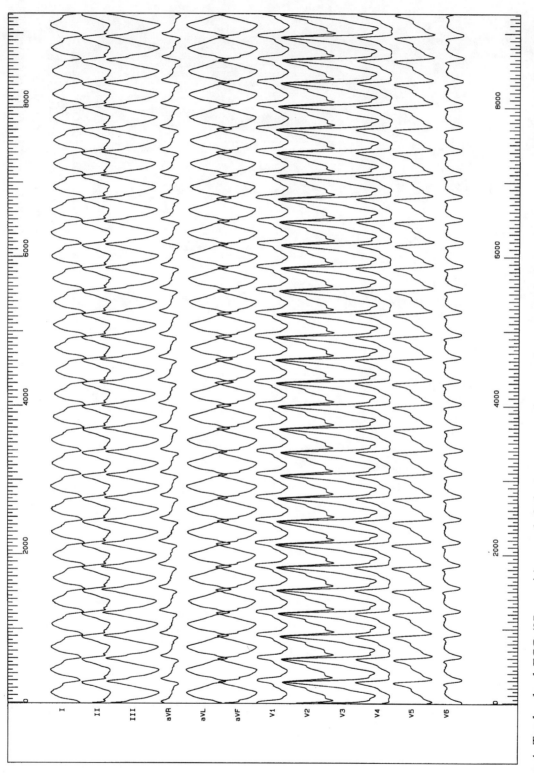

Figure 4. Twelve-lead ECG (25 mm/s) recorded during a second type of reentrant tachycardia showing a regular broad QRS complex tachycardia (maximal preexcitation) at a rate of 200 beats/min (cycle length 302 ms) corresponding to an episode of antidromic atrioventricular reentrant tachycardia.

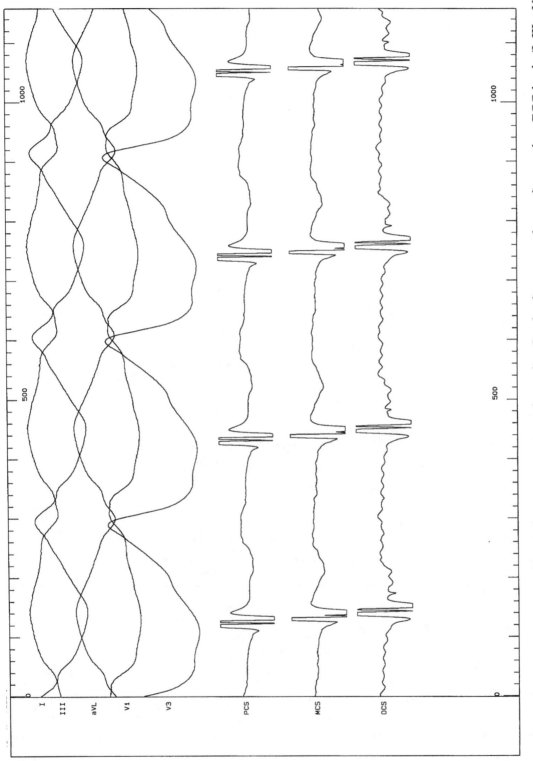

Figure 5. Intracardiac recordings during antidromic reentrant tachycardia. On the figure are shown five surface ECG leads (I, III, aVL, V₁, V₃) together with three bipolar intracardiac recordings (PCS = proximal coronary sinus; MCS = median coronary sinus; DCS = distal coronary sinus). Paper speed 200 mm/s. The earliest atrial depolarization occurs in PCS, suggesting retrograde activation over the normal conduction system and anterograde conduction over the left lateral accessory pathway.

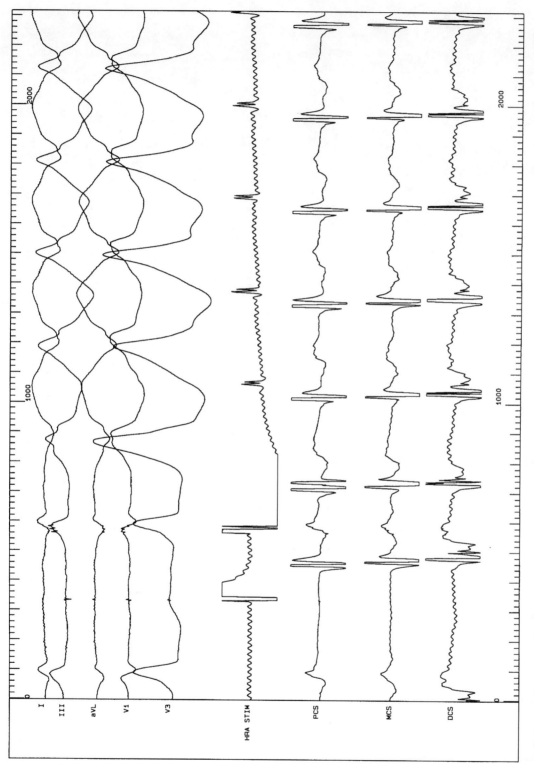

Figure 6. Intracardiac recordings during initiation of antidromic atrioventricular reentrant tachycardia (AVRT). On the figure are shown five surface ECG leads (I, III, aVL, V_1, V_3) together with four bipolar intracardiac recordings (HRA stim = right atrial catheter used for stimulation; PCS = proximal coronary sinus; MCS = median coronary sinus; DCS = distal coronary sinus). Paper speed 100 mm/s. The anterograde effective refractory period of the accessory pathway is < 230 ms, and a short-coupled atrial extrastimulus induces antidromic AVRT.

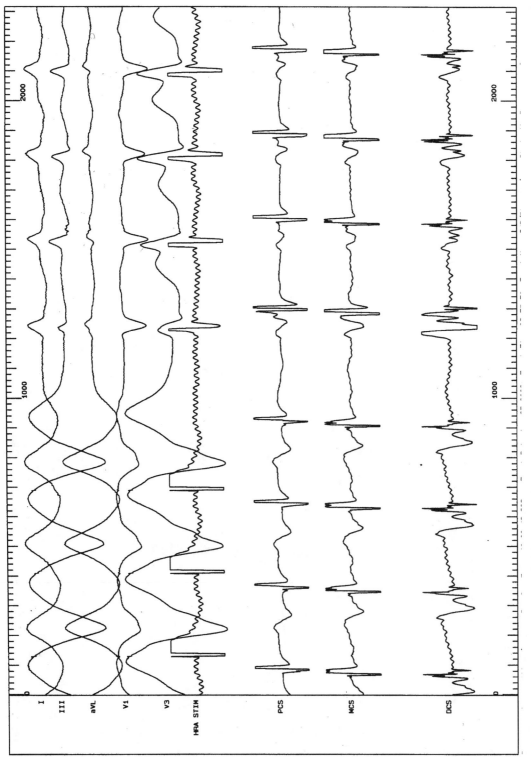

Figure 7. Intracardiac recordings during initiation of orthodromic atrioventricular reentrant tachycardia (AVRT). On the figure are shown five surface ECG leads (I, III, aVL, V₁, V₃) together with four bipolar intracardiac recordings (RV = right ventricular catheter used for stimulation; PCS = proximal coronary sinus; MCS = median coronary sinus; DCS = distal coronary sinus). Paper speed 100 mm/s. Orthodromic atrioventricular reentrant tachycardia is induced during right ventricular pacing (cycle length 280 ms).

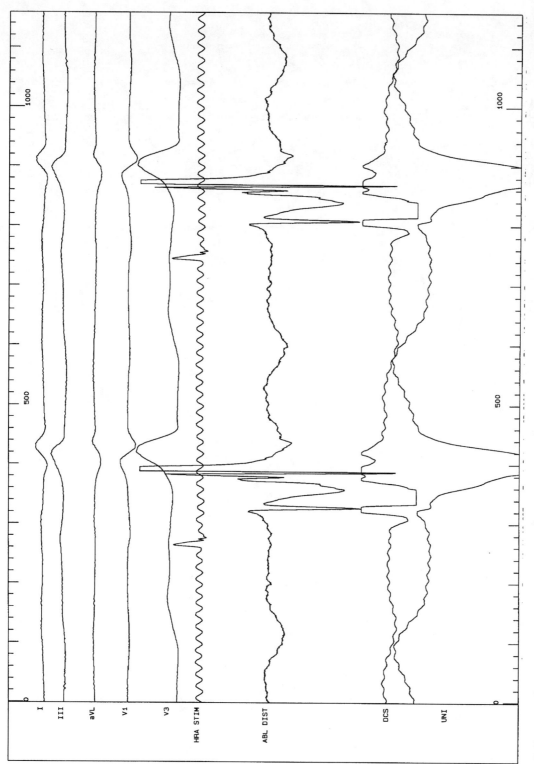

Figure 8. Intracardiac recordings at the successful site during sinus rhythm. On the figure are shown 5 surface ECG leads (I, III, aVL, V_1, V_3) together with four intracardiac recordings (HRA stim : right atrial catheter used for stimulation, ABL DIST : bipolar recording from the distal poles of the ablation catheter positioned on the mitral annulus using a retrograde transaortic approach, DCS : bipolar recording form the distal coronary sinus, UNI : unipolar recording obtained from the distal tip of the ablation catheter). Paper speed 200 mm/s. Of note is the QS aspect of the unipolar recording.

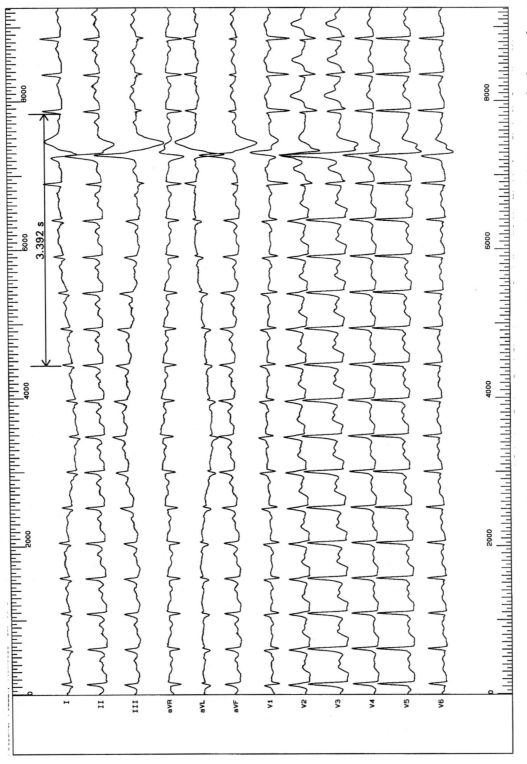

Figure 9. Twelve-lead ECG (25 mm/s) during radiofrequency current application. Ablation is performed during sinus rhythm and ventricular preexcitation disappears 3.4 seconds after initiation of radiofrequency current application with normalization of the 12-lead surface ECG.

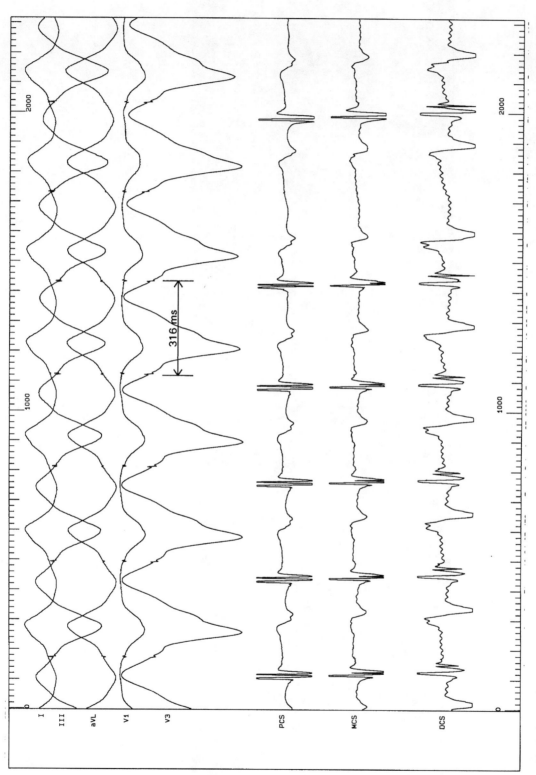

Figure 10. Intracardiac recordings during incremental ventricular pacing after the successful ablation procedure. On the figure are shown five surface ECG leads (I, III, aVL, V$_1$, V$_3$) together with three bipolar intracardiac recordings (PCS = proximal coronary sinus; MCS = median coronary sinus; DCS = distal coronary sinus). Paper speed 100 mm/s. The earliest atrial depolarization occurs now in PCS, suggesting retrograde activation over the normal conduction system, with a progressive increase in ventriculo-atrial interval and retrograde Wenckebach phenomenon (retrograde effective refractory period of the atrioventricular node 316 ms).

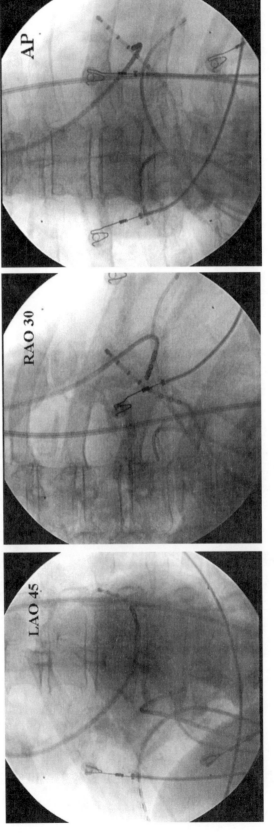

Figure 11. Chest X-rays showing catheter position.

Chapter 23

Left Lateral Concealed Accessory Pathway

Medical History

A 44-year-old male patient presented with a history of paroxysmal regular tachycardia (rate 179 beats/min) since the age of 10 without hemodynamic compromission. The episodes were easily terminated by vagal maneuvers during many years, but tachycardia episodes became more frequent and more prolonged over the last 2 years. The resting 12-lead ECG was normal and no structural heart disease was present. Because of drug intolerance, the patient was referred for radiofrequency catheter ablation.

Comments

By definition, patients with concealed accessory pathways have no ventricular preexcitation on the rest-

ing 12-lead ECG, and the diagnosis can only be suspected (or made) by the electrocardiographic aspect during tachycardia showing distinct P waves after the QRS complexes and an R-P interval shorter than the P-R interval. The precise location of the concealed accessory pathway may be suspected by the polarity of the retrograde P wave during tachycardia, but is usually confirmed during the electrophysiologic study by mapping the sequence of retrograde atrial activation either during orthodromic tachycardia or during ventricular pacing. To ablate a left free wall concealed accessory pathway, the ablation catheter is positioned on the mitral annulus either using a transaortic retrograde approach or using a transseptal approach. Radiofrequency current is applied either during reciprocating tachycardia (as in the present case) or during ventricular pacing. The optimal site for ablation is based on the shortest ventriculo-atrial (V-A) interval,

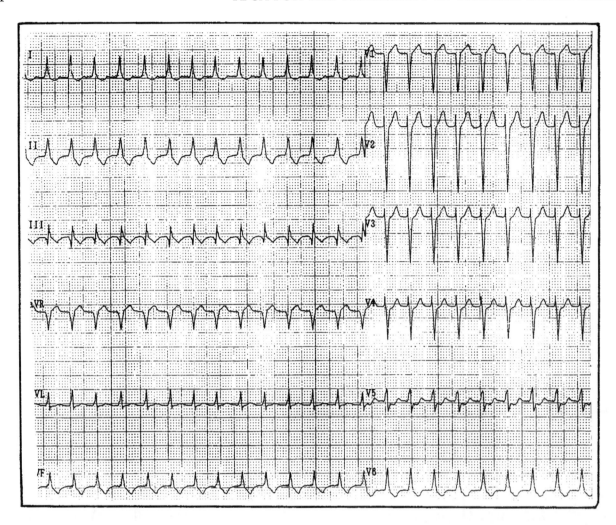

Figure 1. Twelve-lead ECG (25 mm/s) during an episode of palpitations, showing supra-ventricular tachycardia at a rate of 178 beats/min with a negative P wave in inferior leads after the QRS complex (R-P interval < P-R interval).

on the recording of an accessory pathway potential, and/or on the presence of continuous electrical activity between the local ventricular and atrial electrograms.

Suggested Reading

Bardy GH, Poole JE, Coltorti F, et al. Catheter ablation of a concealed accessory pathway. *Am J Cardiol* 1984;54:1366-1367.

Benditt DG, Pritchett ELC, Smith WM, et al. Ventriculoatrials intervals: Diagnostic use in paroxysmal supraventricular tachycardia. *Ann Intern Med* 1979;91:161-170.

Kay GN, Pressley JC, Packer DL, et al. Value of the 12-lead electrocardiogram in discriminating atrioventricular nodal reciprocating tachycardia from circus movement atrioventricular tachycardia utilizing a retrograde accessory pathway. *Am J Cardiol* 1987;59:296-304.

Calkins H, Langberg J, Sousa J, et al. Radiofrequency catheter ablation of accessory atrioventricular connections in 250 patients: Abbreviated therapeutic approach to Wolff-Parkinson-White syndrome. *Circulation* 1992;85:1337-1346.

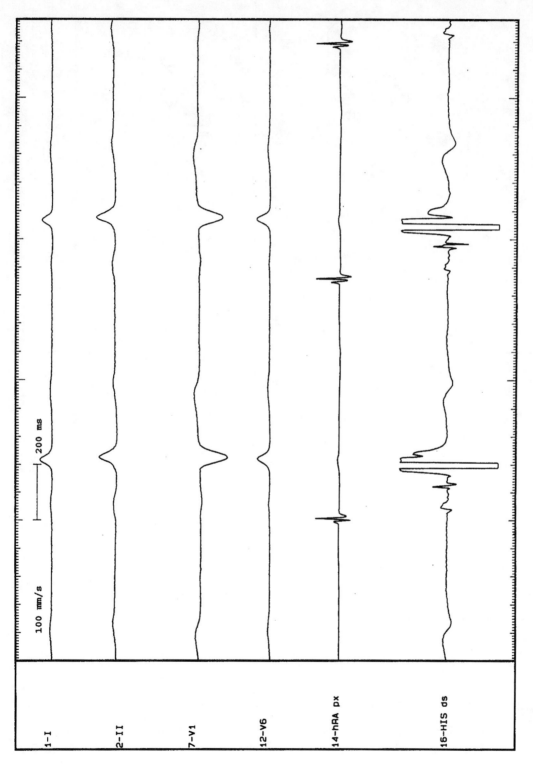

Figure 2. Intracardiac recordings during sinus rhythm (100 mm/s). On the figure are shown four surface ECG leads (I, II, V_1, V_6) together with one bipolar intracardiac recording from the high right atrium (HRA px), and one bipolar intracardiac recording from the His bundle region (HIS ds). A-H interval = 85 ms; H-V interval = 45 ms; no ventricular preexcitation is present.

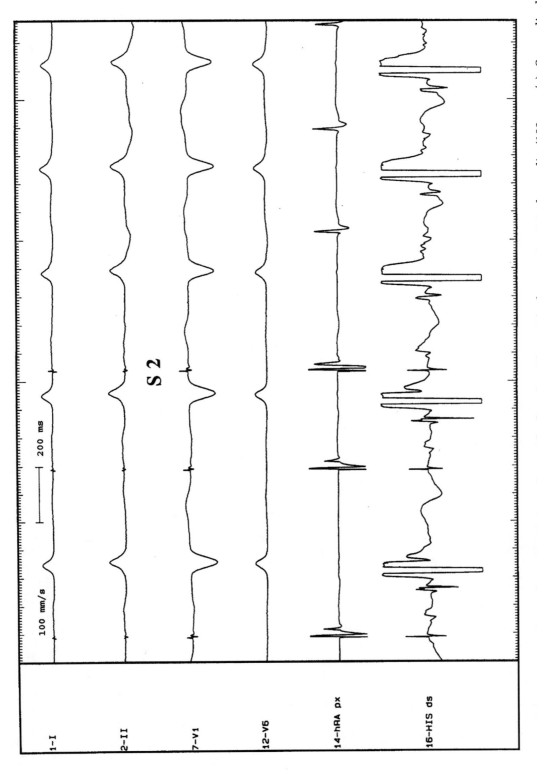

Figure 3. Intracardiac recordings during initiation of an orthodromic atrioventricular reentrant tachycardia (100 mm/s). Same display as Figure 2. An atrial extrastimulus S2 (coupling interval 340 ms) was introduced during atrial pacing (S1-S1 = 600 ms) and induced a reentrant tachycardia with a ventriculo-atrial interval of 190 ms in hRA px and 115 ms in HIS ds.

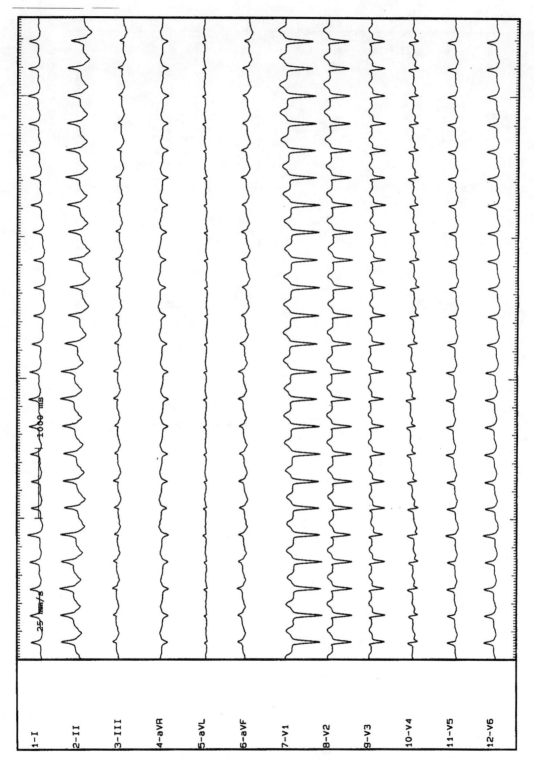

Figure 4. Twelve-lead ECG (25 mm/s) recorded during atrioventricular orthodromic reentrant tachycardia (rate 155 beats/min).

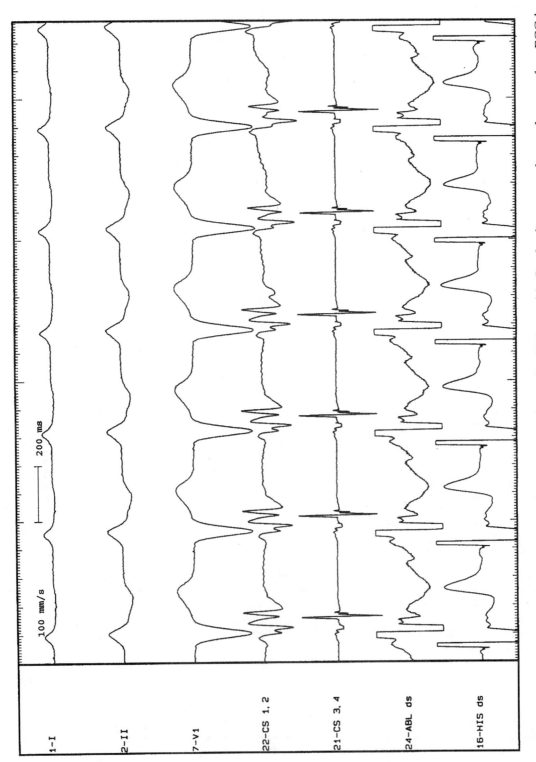

Figure 5. Intracardiac mapping during orthodromic reentrant tachycardia (100 mm/s). On the figure are shown three surface ECG leads (I, II, V₁), two bipolar intracardiac recordings from the coronary sinus (CS 1,2 = distal; CS 3,4 = proximal), one bipolar intracardiac recording obtained from the distal poles of the ablation catheter (ABL ds) introduced in the left ventricle using a transaortic retrograde approach and positioned on the lateral aspect of the mitral annulus, and one bipolar intracardiac recording from the His bundle region (HIS ds). The earliest atrial activation is recorded on the ablation catheter with ventriculo-atrial fusion.

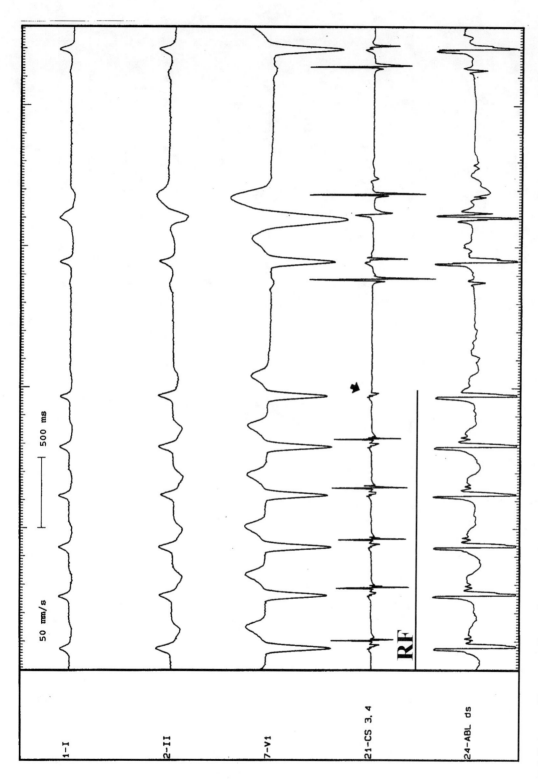

Figure 6. Intracardiac recordings during radiofrequency (RF) current application at the successful site (50 mm/s). On the figure are shown three surface ECG leads (I, II, V₁) one bipolar intracardiac recording from the proximal coronary sinus (CS 3,4), and one bipolar intracardiac recording from the distal poles of the ablation catheter (ABL ds) positioned at the successful site. Five seconds after RF current application, retrograde conduction over the accessory pathway is interrupted (arrow) and tachycardia is terminated. After this RF current application, tachycardia was no longer inducible.

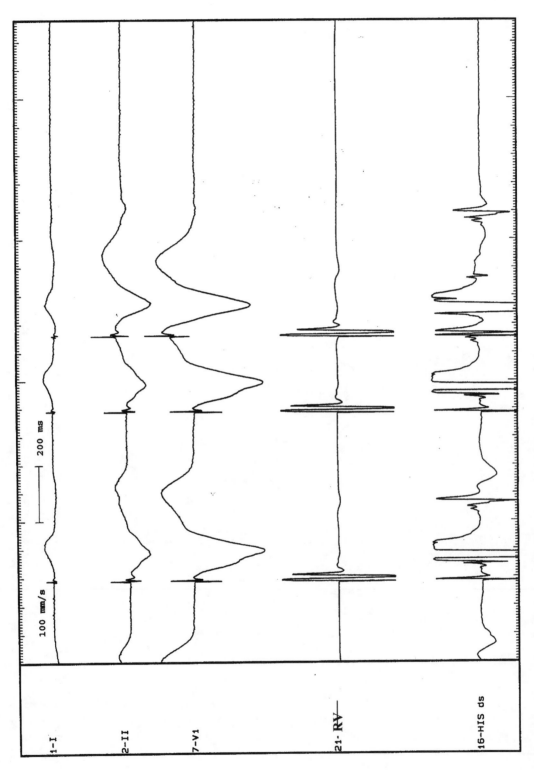

Figure 7. Intracardiac recordings (100 mm/s) during programmed ventricular stimulation (S1-S1 = 600 ms; S1-S2 = 270 ms) after the ablation procedure showing retrograde conduction over the normal conduction system (retrograde His deflection).

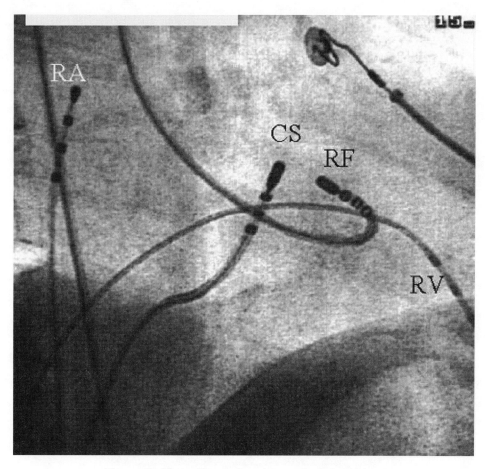

Figure 8. Chest X-ray showing catheter position.

Chapter 24

Catheter Ablation of a Right Posteroseptal Accessory Pathway

Medical History

An 11-year-old female patient with no structural heart disease (normal echocardiography) presented with paroxysmal tachycardia which was hemodynamically poorly tolerated. She experienced two syncopal episodes during very fast (rate > 200 beats/min) but undocumented reentrant tachycardia. The 12-lead resting ECG showed sinus rhythm with permanent ventricular preexcitation. After informed consent, it was decided to map the accessory pathway location, and to perform a radiofrequency catheter ablation if the risk of atrioventricular block was low.

Comments

In the present case, it was impossible to precisely determine the location of the accessory pathway on the basis of the 12-lead resting ECG. The group at Duke University was the first to correlate polarity of the delta wave on the surface ECG with the site of the accessory connection assessed at surgery by epicardial mapping. However, even if the 12-lead resting ECG may be of great help, it has several limitations for the precise location of the accessory pathway: 1) possible existence of multiple accessory pathways; 2) presence of significant fusion of ventricular activation between the accessory pathway and the normal conduction system (a correct interpretation can only be made when preexcitation is maximal as during atrial pacing); and 3) superimposition of the terminal P wave on the initial aspect of the delta wave. Endocardial mapping techniques are always necessary to precisely determine accessory pathway locations and to guide radiofrequency catheter ablation. Unipolar recordings are particularly use-

From: RETAC: *Radiofrequency Catheter Ablation for the Treatment of Cardiac Arrhythmias: A Practical Atlas with Illustrative Cases.*
© Futura Publishing Company, Inc. Armonk, NY, 2002.

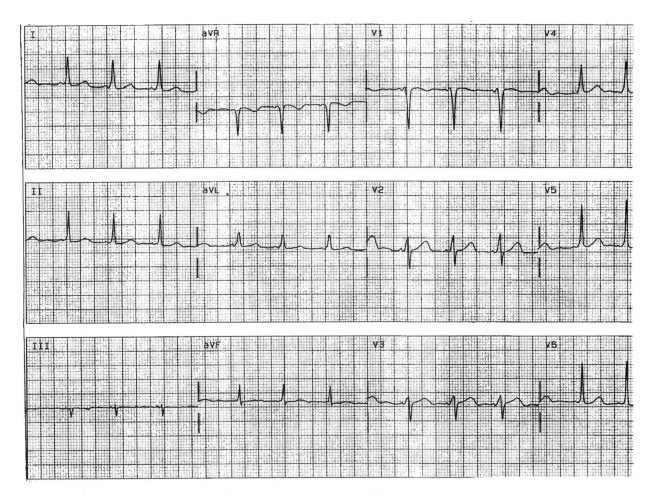

Figure 1. Twelve-lead resting ECG showing permanent ventricular preexcitation (paper speed 25 mm/s). Delta wave is positive in lead I, L, V_2 to V_6; negative in V_1 and isoelectric or slightly positive in II, and aVF.

ful for the precise localization of overt atrioventricular accessory connections. Radiofrequency ablation can be performed either during sinus rhythm, during ventricular pacing or during orthodromic reentrant tachycardia.

Suggested Reading

Tonkin AM, Wagner GS, Gallagher JJ, et al. Initial forces of ventricular depolarization in the Wolff-Parkinson-White syndrome. Analysis based upon localization of the accessory pathway by epicardial mapping. *Circulation* 1975;52:1030-1038.

Gallagher JJ, Pritchett ELC, Sealy WC, et al. The preexcitation syndromes. *Prog cardiovasc Dis* 1978;20:285-299.

Benson DW Jr, Sterba R, Gallagher JJ, et al. Localization of the site of ventricular preexcitation with body surface maps in patients with Wolff-Parkinson-White syndrome. *Circulation* 1982;65:1259-1266.

Haïssaguerre M, Dartigues JF, Warin JF, et al. Electrogram patterns predictive of successful catheter ablation of accessory pathways. Value of unipolar recording mode. *Circulation* 1991;84:188-202.

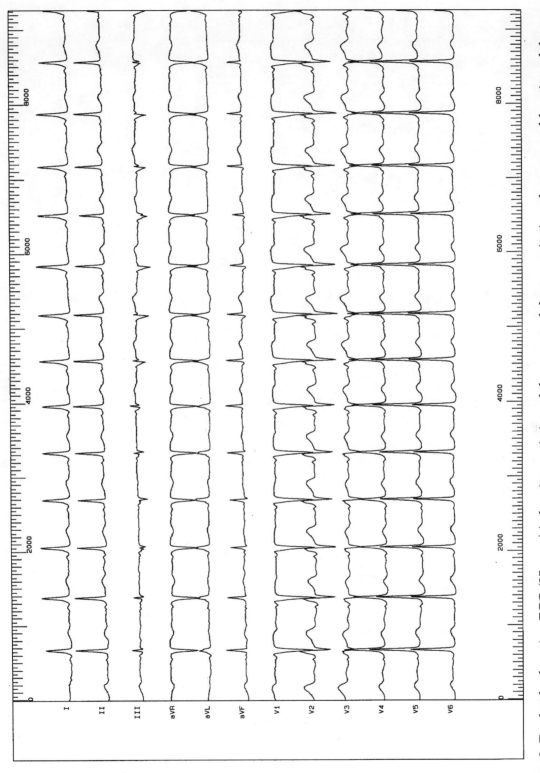

Figure 2. Twelve-lead resting ECG (25 mm/s) showing variation of the aspect of the preexcitation: the supposed location of the accessory pathway was right anteroseptal or midseptal.

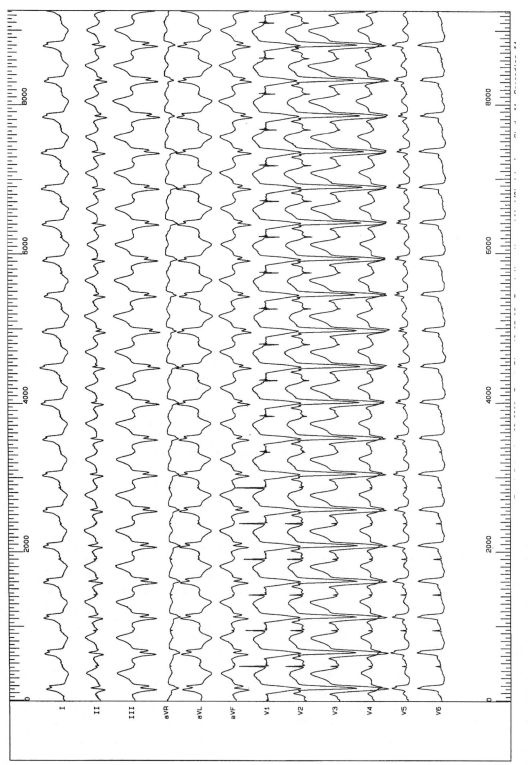

Figure 3. Twelve-lead ECG (paper speed 25 mm/s) during atrial pacing at a rate of 120 beats/min (cycle length 500 ms). Maximal preexcitation is present and the presumed location of the accessory pathway is now right posteroseptal.

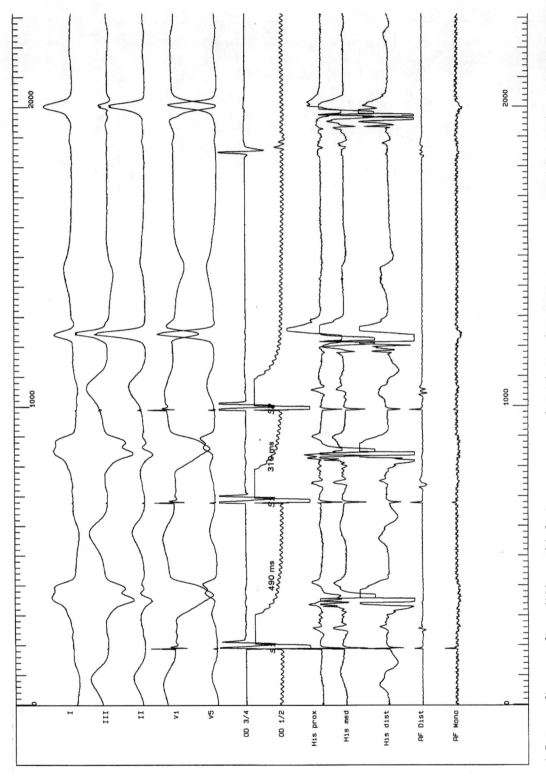

Figure 4. Intracardiac recordings (100 mm/s) during programmed atrial stimulation. Here are represented five surface ECG leads (I, III, II, V₁, V₅), two bipolar recordings from the right atrium (OD 3-4 and OD 1-2), three bipolar recordings from the His bundle region (His prox, His med, and His dist), one bipolar recording from the distal poles of the ablation catheter (RF Dist), and one unipolar recording from the tip of the ablation catheter (RF Mono). Atrial pacing at cycle length of 490 ms and S1-S2 310 ms. The figure shows the value of the anterograde refractory period of the accessory pathway (310 ms). With shorter coupling intervals, orthodromic atrioventricular reentrant tachycardia was easily induced.

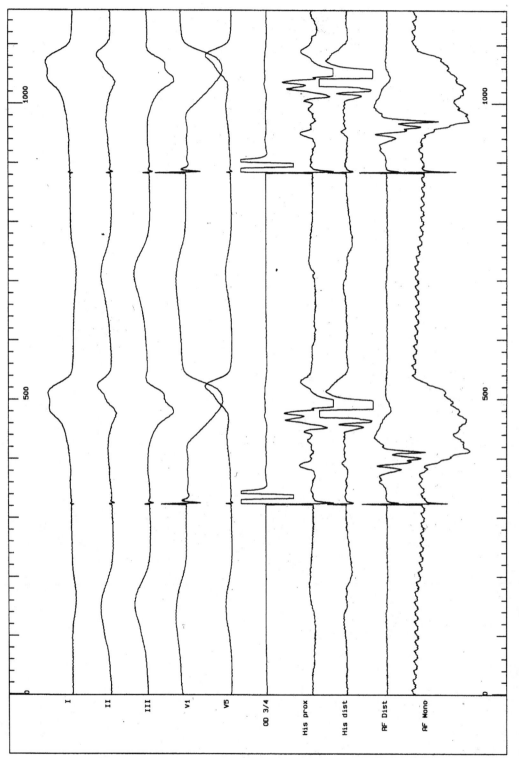

Figure 5. Intracardiac recordings (200 mm/s) during programmed atrial pacing in the posterolateral region of the tricuspid annulus. Here are represented five surface ECG leads (I, II, III, V_1, V_5), one bipolar recording from the right atrium (OD 3-4), two bipolar recordings from the His bundle region (His prox and His dist), one bipolar recording from the distal poles of the ablation catheter (RF Dist), and one unipolar recording from the tip of the ablation catheter (RF Mono). The ablation catheter is positioned on the atrial side of the tricuspid annulus, atrioventricular fusion is present on the bipolar recording (RF Dist) and there is a QS pattern on the unipolar recording.

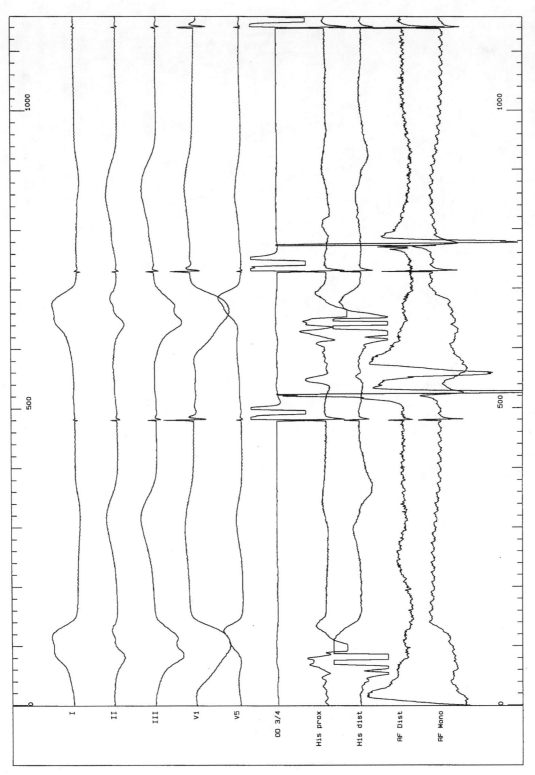

Figure 6. Intracardiac recordings (200 mm/s) during programmed atrial stimulation. Same display as Figure 5. During atrial pacing (S1-S1 = 500 ms and S1-S2 = 300 ms) the atrial and ventricular electrograms are clearly separated and identified.

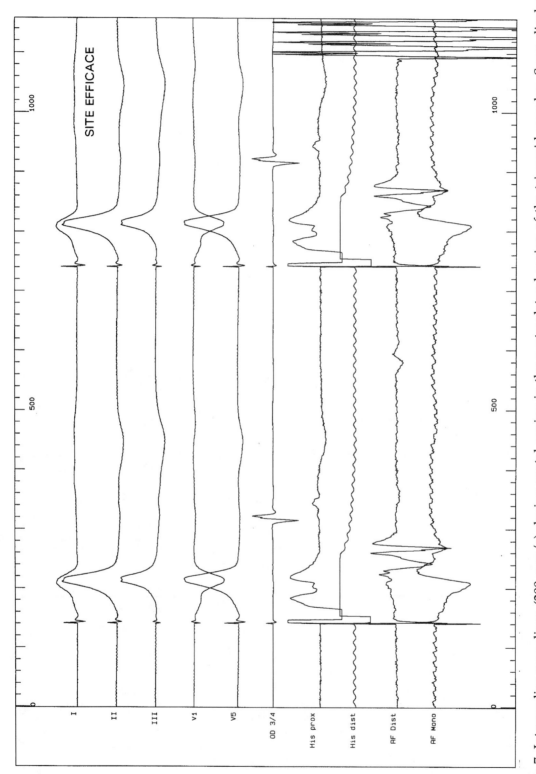

Figure 7. Intracardiac recordings (200 mm/s) during septal pacing in the posterolateral region of the tricuspid annulus. Same display as Figure 5. During ventricular pacing (S1-S1 600 ms), ventriculo-atrial fusion was observed, and this site was considered optimal for radiofrequency ablation.

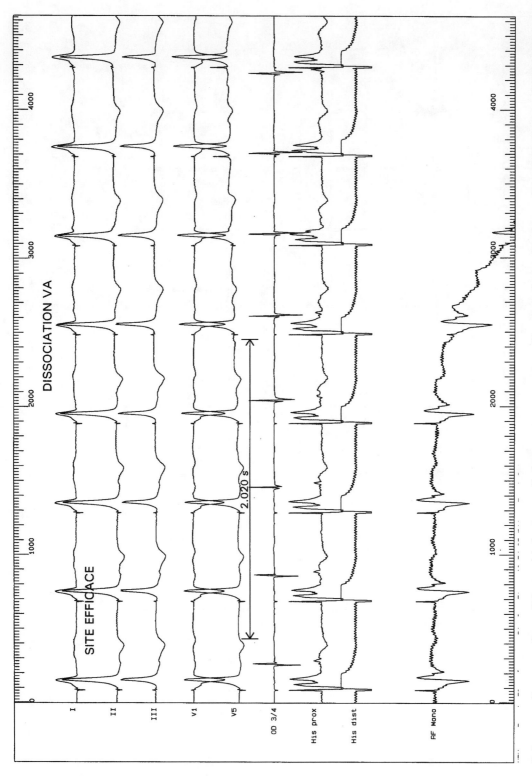

Figure 8. Intracardiac recordings (50 mm/s) during radiofrequency current application. Same display as figure 5. Ventriculo-atrial dissociation occurred 2 seconds after the onset of radiofrequency current application.

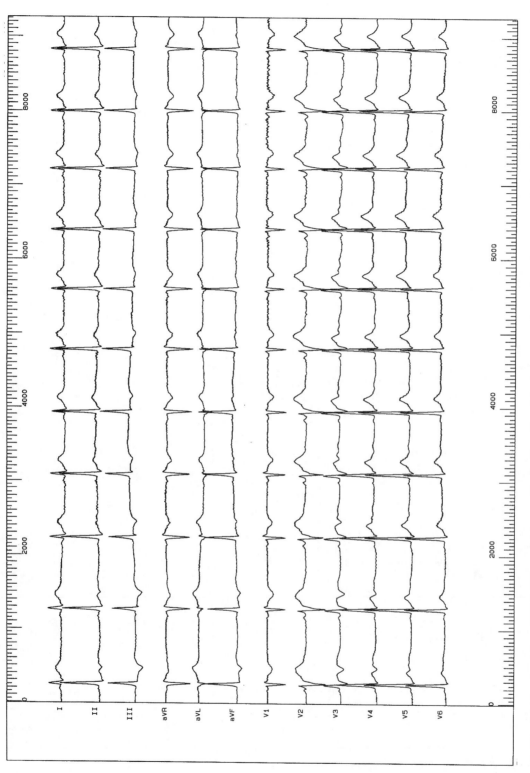

Figure 9. Twelve-lead surface ECG (25 mm/s) recorded after the ablation procedure showing normal sinus rhythm and disappearance of ventricular preexcitation.

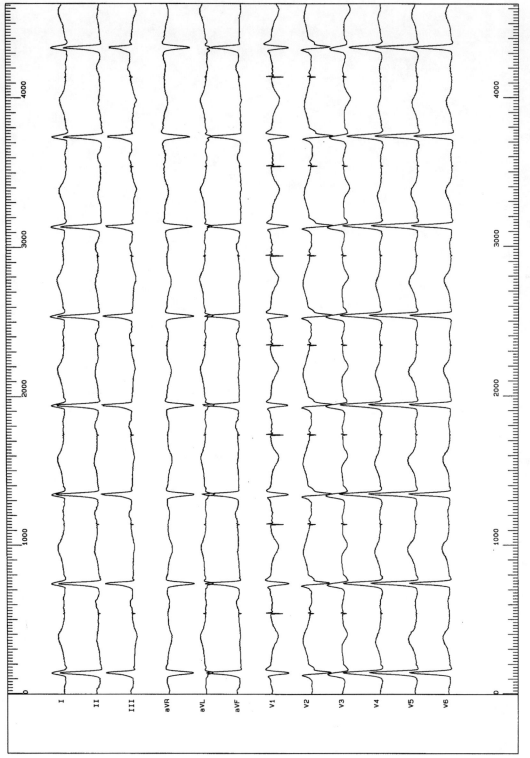

Figure 10. Twelve-lead surface ECG (50 mm/s) recorded after the ablation procedure during atrial pacing confirming the absence of ventricular preexcitation.

Chapter 25

Permanent Junctional Reciprocating Tachycardia

Medical History

An 18-year-old female patient was referred for palpitations and shortness of breath occurring during exercise for many years. An ECG was obtained during palpitations showing a narrow complex tachycardia at a rate of 150 beats/min, with a long R-P interval. The differential diagnosis for such a tachycardia is:

1. atrial tachycardia
2. atypical form of atrioventricular node reentrant tachycardia (AVNRT, "fast-slow" type)
3. atrioventricular reentrant tachycardia using an accessory pathway with slow and decremental retrograde conduction ("permanent junctional reciprocating tachycardia" or PJRT).

Comments

As stated above, the differential diagnosis of a narrow QRS complex tachycardia with a long R-P interval includes: 1) atrial tachycardia; 2) the permanent form of junctional reciprocating tachycardia described by Coumel (PJRT); or 3) the atypical ("fast-slow") form of AVNRT. By definition, the PJRT is permanent or incessant as in the present case, it occurs usually in children and young adults, and in this particular form of macroreentry the retrograde conduction is slow and exhibits decremental conduction properties. Patients with PJRT do not have a manifest delta wave during sinus rhythm, either because no anterograde conduction exists over the accessory pathway, or because the anterograde conduction is so much prolonged that it

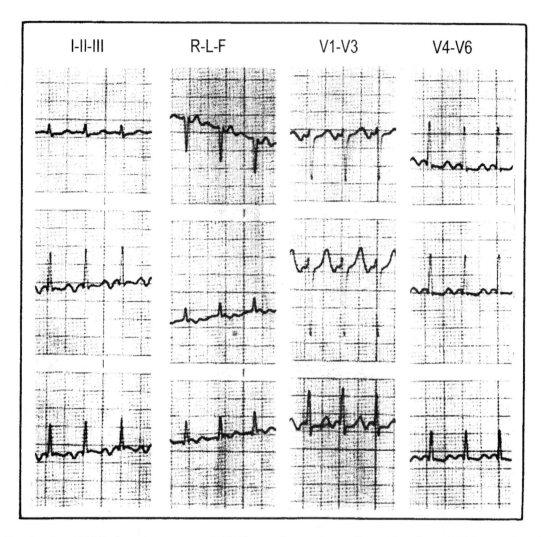

Figure 1. Twelve-lead ECG showing a narrow QRS complex tachycardia with a long R-P interval and negative P waves in inferior leads (paper speed 25 mm/s).

can never be demonstrated because of AV nodal conduction. Most of these slowly conducting retrograde accessory pathways are located in the posterior septum. This form of incessant/permanent tachycardia is most often resistant to antiarrhythmic drugs and may lead to tachycardia-induced cardiomyopathy. Radiofrequency catheter ablation is the treatment of choice, and the ablation should be guided by identifying the earliest retrograde atrial activation during tachycardia, as in the present case.

Suggested Reading

Coumel P, Cabrolo C, Fabiato A, et al. Tachycardie permanente par rythme réciproque.1. Preuves du diagnostic par stimulation auriculaire et ventriculaire. *Arch Mal C{{oe}}ur* 1967;60:1830-1838.

Chein WW, Cohen TJ, Lee MA, et al. Electrophysiological findings and long-term follow-up of patients with the permanent form of junctional reciprocating tachycardia treated by catheter ablation. *Circulation* 1992;85:1329-1336.

Critelli G, Gallagher JJ, Monda V, et al. Anatomic and electrophysiologic substrate of the permanent form of reciprocating tachycardia. *J Am Coll Cardiol* 1984;4:601-610.

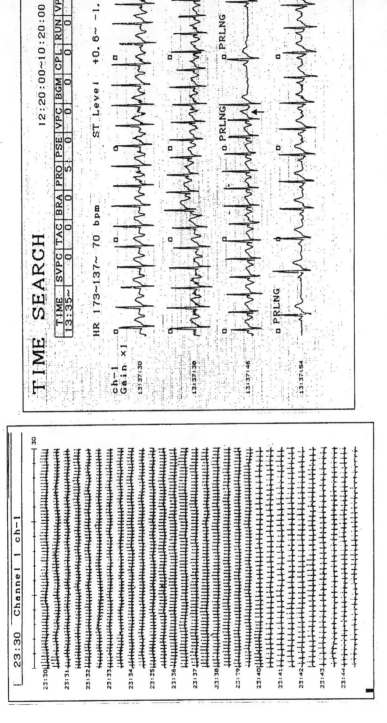

Figure 2. **Left**: 15-minute recording from the Holter obtained while the patient was taking β-blockers and verapamil. Supraventricular tachycardia is almost incessant and normal sinus rhythm is observed only during sleep or at rest. **Right**: spontaneous interruption of the tachycardia by an atrial premature beat (arrow). Interruption of the long R-P tachycardia by an atrial premature beat does not help to define the mechanism of the tachycardia. When the long R-P tachycardia is systematically interrupted by a ventricular premature beat, atrial tachycardia can almost be ruled out.

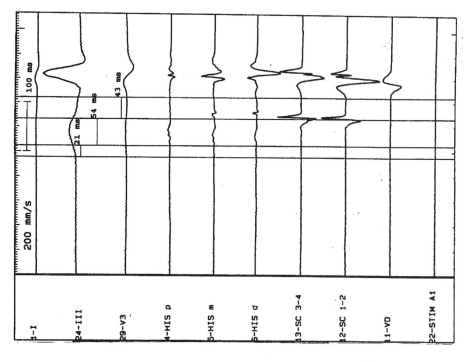

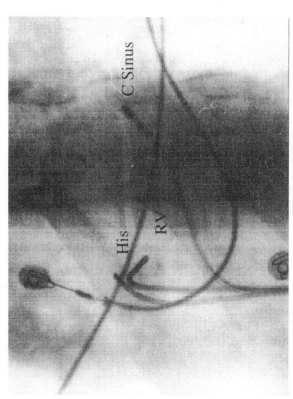

Figure 3. Intracardiac recordings at baseline (200 mm/s). Here are represented three surface ECG leads (I, III, V$_3$), three bipolar recordings from the His bundle region (proximal = His p; median = His m; distal = His d), two bipolar recordings from the coronary sinus (distal = SC 1-2; proximal = SC 3-4), and one bipolar recording from the right ventricular apex (VD). During sinus rhythm, AH interval is 54 ms, HV interval is 43 ms and atrial activation occurs in the His bundle region before occurring in the coronary sinus region. Catheter position is shown at left.

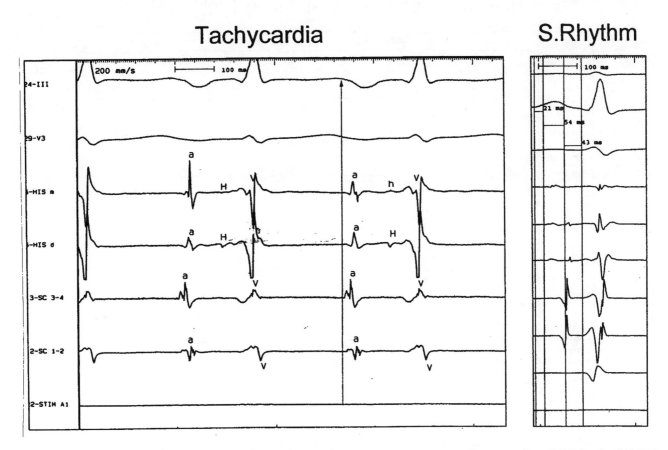

Figure 4. Intracardiac recordings at baseline (200 mm/s). Here are represented two surface ECG leads (III, V$_3$), two bipolar recordings from the His bundle region (median = His m; distal = His d), and two bipolar recordings from the coronary sinus (distal = SC 1-2; proximal = SC 3-4). During tachycardia, the proximal coronary sinus is activated first (vertical arrow), and conduction intervals are normal.

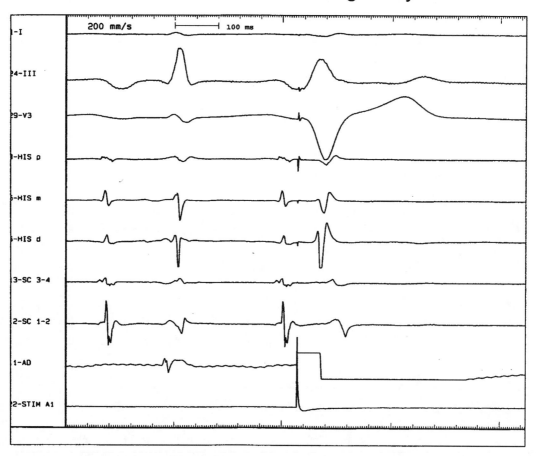

Figure 5. Intracardiac recordings during programmed ventricular stimulation (200 mm/s). Same display as Figure 3, except that the bipolar recording from the right ventricle is labeled AD. Tachycardia is interrupted by a ventricular premature beat not capturing the atrium, thus ruling out atrial tachycardia.

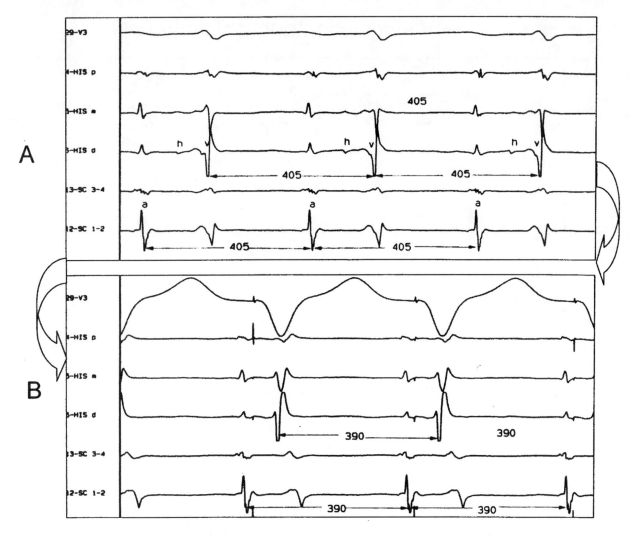

Figure 6. Intracardiac recordings during ventricular pacing (200 mm/s). Here are represented one surface ECG lead (V₃), three bipolar recordings from the His bundle region (proximal = His p; median = His m; distal = His d), and two bipolar recordings from the coronary sinus (distal = SC 1-2; proximal = SC 3-4). Tachycardia can be entrained by pacing the right ventricular septum (panel **B**) at a cycle length 15 ms shorter (390 ms) than the tachycardia (405 ms; panel **A**).

RV stimulation during Tachycardia

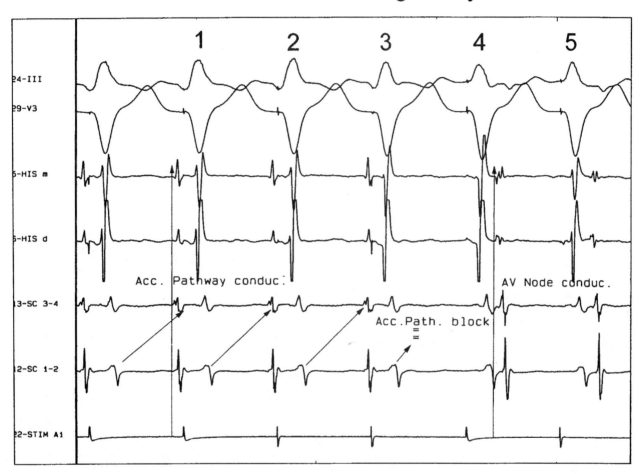

Figure 7. Intracardiac recordings during right ventricular stimulation (100 mm/s). Same display as Figure 4. Beat 1 and 2 show a prolonged ventriculo-atrial (V-A) interval and an earliest atrial activation in CS 3-4 (Acc. Pathway conduc). V-A conduction is blocked on beat 3 (Acc. Path. block). On beat 4 and 5, retrograde conduction is again present but with a much shorter V-A interval and with an earliest atrial activation in His m (retrograde conduction through the atrioventricular node). The presence of a dual retrograde conduction pattern does not allow to differentiate an atypical atrioventricular node reentry from a slow conducting retrograde accessory pathway.

RV stimulation during Tachycardia

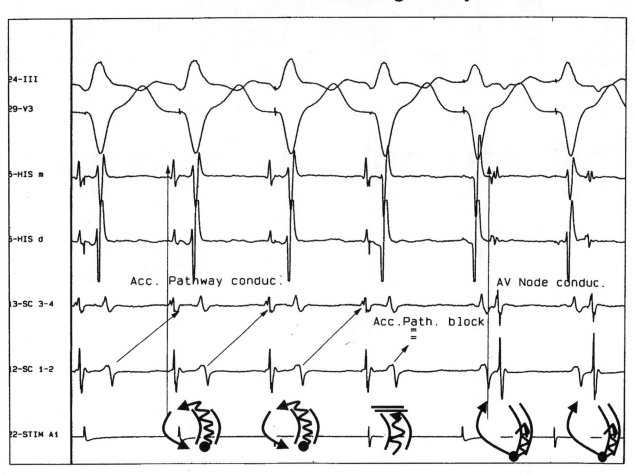

Figure 8. Intracardiac recordings during right ventricular stimulation (100 mm/s). Same display as Figure 7 with a schematic representation of the retrograde conduction. See Figure 7 legend for explanation.

VPB with refractory His during tachycardia

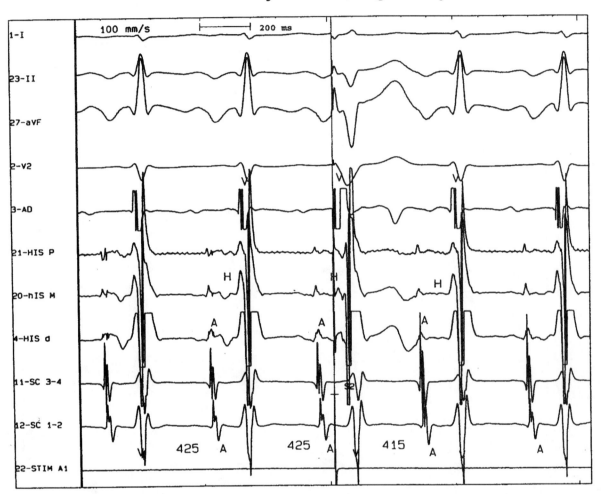

Figure 9. Intracardiac recordings during programmed ventricular stimulation (100 mm/s). Here are represented four surface ECG leads (I, III, aVF, V₂), one bipolar recording from the right ventricular apex (AD), three bipolar recordings from the His bundle region (proximal = His p; median = His m; distal = His d), and two bipolar recordings from the coronary sinus (distal = SC 1-2; proximal = SC 3-4). A late ventricular extrastimulus S2 is applied during tachycardia (cycle length 425 ms) at a time when the His bundle is refractory (S2 is simultaneous to H) and preexcitation of the atrium is observed (A-A interval = 415 ms compared to the A-A interval of 425 ms during tachycardia) confirming that the retrograde conduction occurs over an accessory pathway, and ruling out an atypical form of atrioventricular node reentrant tachycardia.

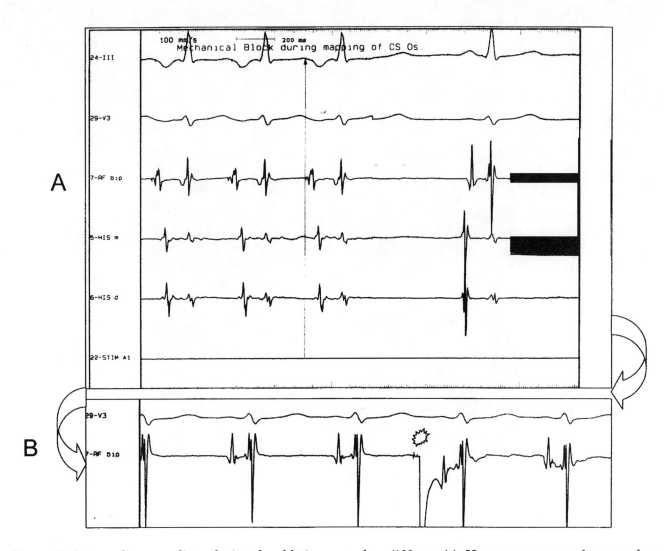

Figure 10. Intracardiac recordings during the ablation procedure (100 mm/s). Here are represented two surface ECG leads (III, V₃), one bipolar recording obtained from the distal poles of the ablation catheter (RF bip), and two bipolar recordings from the His bundle region (median = His m; distal = His d). Mapping was performed during tachycardia and the earliest atrial activation was observed at the os of the coronary sinus (panel **A** and fluoroscopic image in the LAO projection). During mapping, mechanical block was observed (**A**), and radiofrequency current was applied at that site during sinus rhythm (panel **B**).

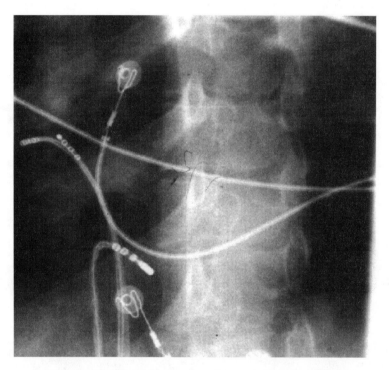

Figure 11. Chest X-ray showing catheter position.

Chapter 26

Permanent Junctional Reciprocating Tachycardia

Medical History

A 20-year-old male patient presented with a history of palpitations lasting for many years. Episodes of palpitations were mainly related to stress and emotions, but could occur even at rest or during the night. A regular tachycardia (rate 120 beats/min) has been observed on several occasions. During Holter monitoring, an incessant supraventricular tachycardia with a long R-P interval was diagnosed. Clinical examination was normal, as well as the 12-lead resting ECG and the echocardiogram. Palpitations persisted despite treatment with atenolol, and the patient was referred for an electrophysiologic study.

Comments

The permanent form of junctional reciprocating tachycardia (PJRT) was initially described by Coumel and coworkers. It may occur in any age group and the ventricular rate is usually between 100 and 200 beats/min. The retrograde accessory pathway with decremental conduction properties is most often located in the right posteroseptal region. However, as in the present case, the accessory pathway may be located more laterally or even on the left side. The incessant nature of the tachycardia is related to the slow conduction and to the decremental conduction properties of both sides of the reentrant circuit. The decremental conduction properties are probably related to a very serpiginous accessory pathway, although it has been hypothesized that this particularity represents displaced atrioventricular node tissue. Because this type of arrhythmia is either permanent or incessant, radiofrequency catheter ablation of the accessory pathway is mandatory in order to avoid a tachycardiomyopathy.

From: RETAC: *Radiofrequency Catheter Ablation for the Treatment of Cardiac Arrhythmias: A Practical Atlas with Illustrative Cases.*
© Futura Publishing Company, Inc. Armonk, NY, 2002.

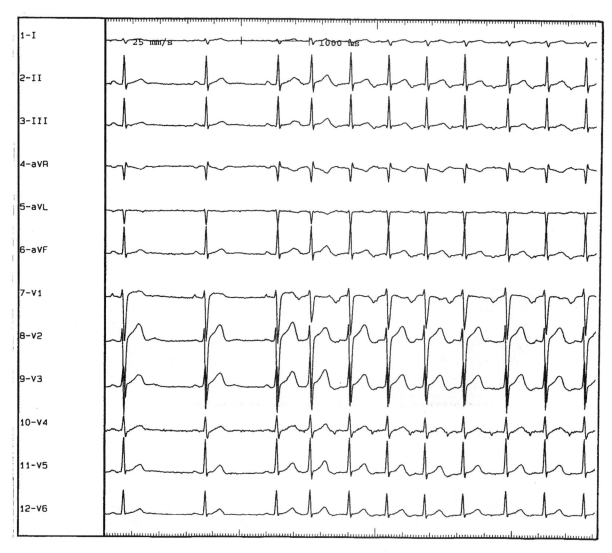

Figure 1. Twelve-lead ECG (25 mm/s) during an episode of palpitations, showing supra-ventricular tachycardia at a rate of 118 beats/min with a long R-P interval and a negative P wave in inferior leads.

Suggested Reading

Gallagher JJ, Sealy WC. The permanent form of junctional reciprocating tachycardia: Further evaluation of the underlying mechanism. *Eur Heart J* 1978;8:413-420.

Klein GJ, Kostuk WJ, Ko P, et al. Permanent junctional reciprocating tachycardia in an asymptomatic adult. Further evidence for an accessory ventriculoatrial nodal structure. *Am Heart J* 1981;102:282-284.

Critelli G, Gallagher JJ, Thiene G, et al. Electrophysiologic and histopathologic correlation in a case of permanent form of reciprocating tachycardia. *Eur Heart J* 1985;6:130-136.

Li HG, Klein GJ, Thakur RK, et al. Radiofrequency ablation of decremental accessory pathways mimicking nodoventricular conduction. *Am J Cardiol* 1994;74:829-833.

Murdock CJ, Leitch JW, Teo WS, et al. Characteristics of accessory pathways exhibiting decremental conduction. *Am J Cardiol* 1991;67:506-510.

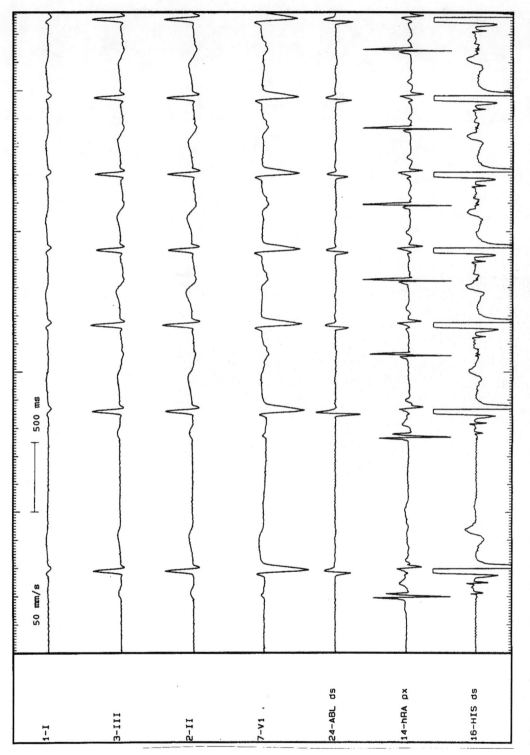

Figure 2. Intracardiac recordings during the spontaneous occurrence of the arrhythmia (50 mm/s). On the figure are shown four surface ECG leads (I, III, II, V_1) together with one bipolar intracardiac recording from the ablation catheter positioned here in the right ventricle (ABL ds), one intracardiac bipolar recording from the high right atrium (hRA px), and one bipolar intracardiac recording from the His bundle region (HIS ds). The tachycardia was incessant. Note the long R-P interval during tachycardia and the negative P waves in III, II and V_1.

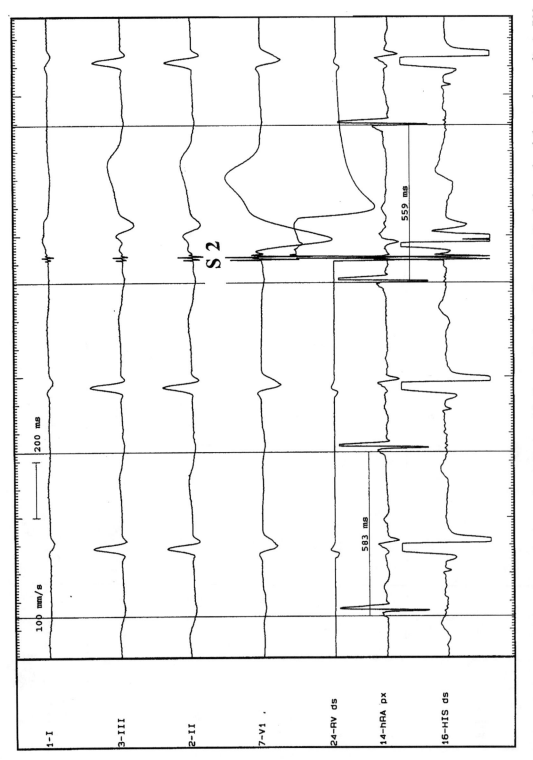

Figure 3. Intracardiac recordings during tachycardia (100 mm/s). Same display as Figure 2. Cycle length of the tachycardia is 583 ms. A ventricular extrastimulus (S2, coupling interval 510 ms) was introduced at a time when the His bundle was refractory and lead to atrial preexcitation (A-A 559 ms). This observation argues for the presence of an accessory atrioventricular connection.

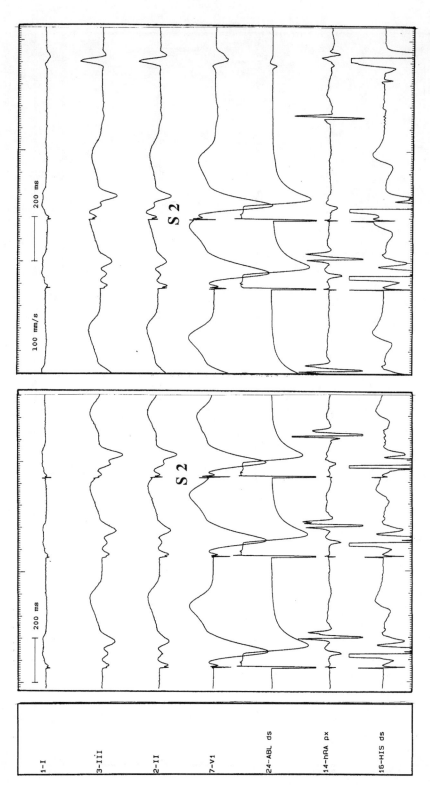

Figure 4. Intracardiac recordings during ventricular programmed stimulation (100 mm/s). Same display as Figure 2. A ventricular extrastimulus (S2) was introduced during ventricular pacing at a rate of 100 beats/min (S1-S1 = 600 ms). At a coupling interval of 320 ms, retrograde conduction occurred over the atrioventricular node (**left**: V-A interval = 310 ms); at a coupling interval of 300 ms, retrograde conduction occurred over a slow retrograde pathway (**right**: V-A = 400 ms) with an echo beat. The slow retrograde pathway showed decremental conduction properties, with a V-A interval progressively increasing from 400 to 460 ms.

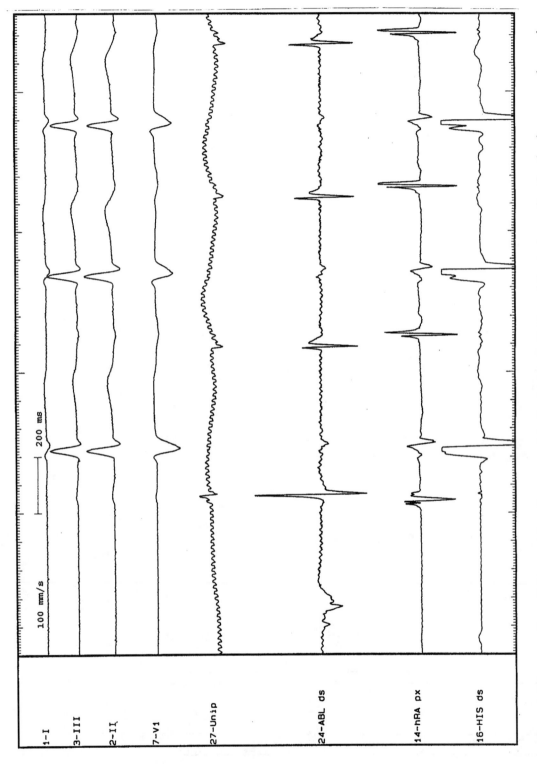

Figure 5. Intracardiac recordings (100 mm/s) at the successful site during initiation of the tachycardia. On the figure are shown four surface ECG leads (I, III, II, V₁), one unipolar recording from the tip of the ablation catheter (Unip) positioned on the atrial side of the right atrioventricular groove in the inferolateral region, one bipolar recording from the distal poles of the ablation catheter (ABL ds), one bipolar recording from the high right atrium (hRA px), and one bipolar recording from the region of the His bundle (HIS ds). During tachycardia, the bipolar recording from the ablation catheter preceded the onset of the P wave by 50 ms, and a QS potential was observed on the unipolar recording.

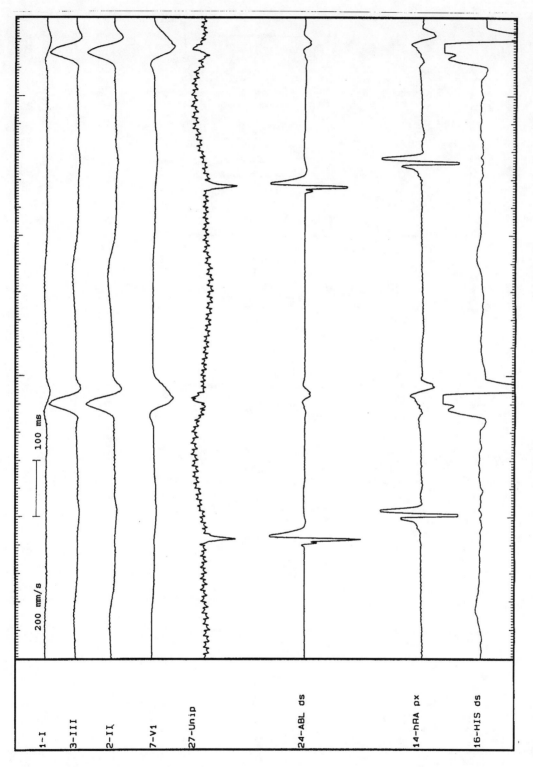

Figure 6. Intracardiac recordings (200 mm/s) at the successful site during tachycardia. Same display as Figure 5. Note the QS pattern of the atrial electrogram on the unipolar recording. The ablation procedure was performed at this site, on the atrial insertion of the atrioventricular connection.

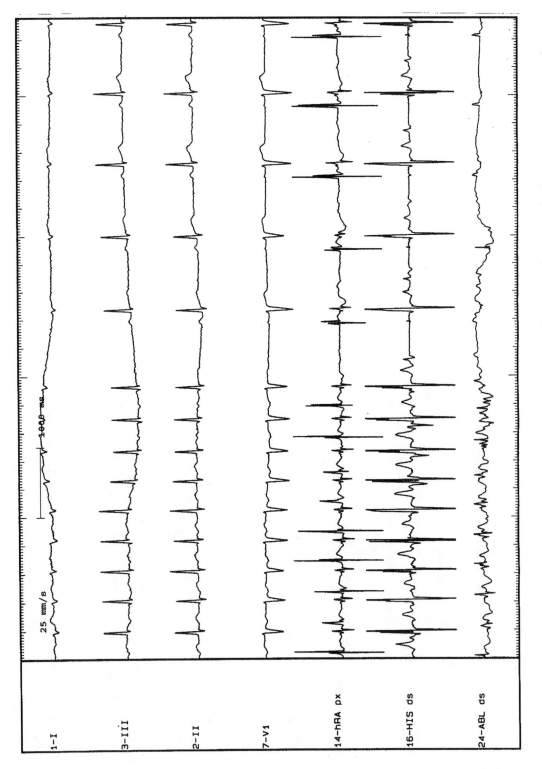

Figure 7. Intracardiac recordings (25 mm/s) showing interruption of the tachycardia during radiofrequency current application at the successful site with restoration of sinus rhythm. After this first radiofrequency current application, the tachycardia was no longer inducible even during isoproterenol infusion.

Chapter 27

Mahaim-Type Ventricular Preexcitation

Medical History

A 15-year-old boy presented with a history of palpitations and rapid heart beats since the age of 10. Physical examination was normal and echocardiography could not reveal any cardiac abnormality.

Comments

Mahaim-fibers represent a rare kind of accessory pathways connecting the right-sided atrioventricular (AV) ring with the distal portions of the right bundle ('atriofascicular connections''). Consequently, reciprocating tachycardias involving Mahaim-fibers always have a left bundle branch block morphology and a left axis deviation in the frontal plane.

In contrast to typical accessory AV connections (Kent bundles), Mahaim-type connections conduct anterogradely only, and show decremental conduction properties somewhat similar to the AV node. Successful ablation can be achieved by targeting the atrial insertion, usually at the postero-lateral aspect of the tricuspid annulus, or by mapping the earliest endocardial ventricular potential relative to the preexcited QRS complex. The most successful approach appears to be to look for an accessory pathway potential at the atrial insertion site and to ablate there.

Suggested Reading

Haïssaguerre M, Warin JF, Le Metayer P, et al. Catheter ablation of Mahaim fibers with preservation of atrioventricular nodal conduction. *Circulation* 1990;82:418-427.

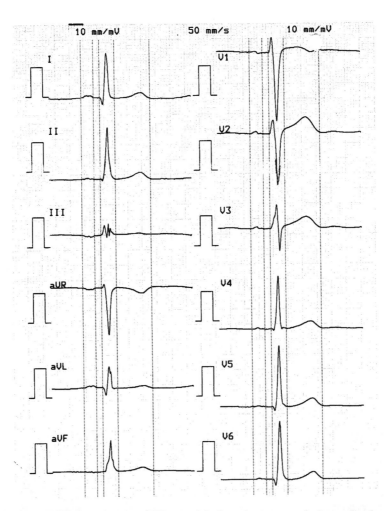

Figure 1. Twelve-lead resting ECG (paper speed 50 mm/s) showing normal sinus rhythm, a normal P-R interval (130 ms), a QRS-axis in the frontal plane of 40°, and a QRS-width of 100 ms without evidence of preexcitation.

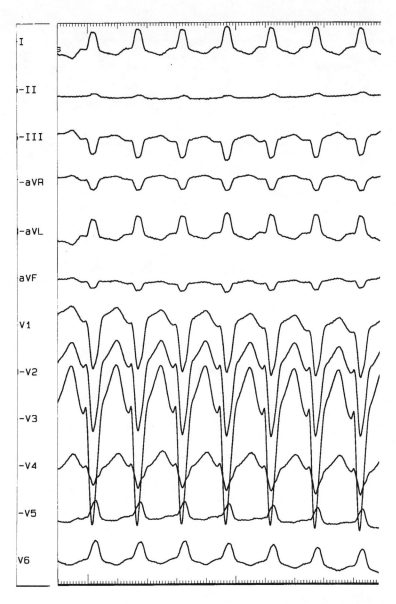

Figure 2. Twelve-lead ECG (50 mm/s) during an acute attack of palpitations. A wide QRS complex tachycardia (cycle length 290 ms) is present with left bundle branch block morphology, a superior axis and late R wave transition (V4-V5); P waves are not discernible; the differential diagnosis includes: 1) supraventricular tachycardia with LBBB aberrancy (e.g., atrioventricular node reentrant tachycardia); 2) ventricular tachycardia; and 3) antidromic atrioventricular reentrant tachycardia incorporating a right-sided accessory pathway not visible during resting conditions (see Figure 1).

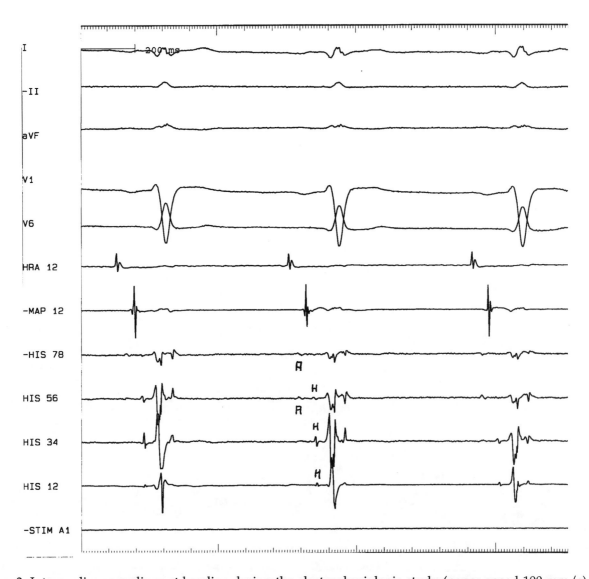

Figure 3. Intracardiac recordings at baseline during the electrophysiologic study (paper speed 100 mm/s). Here are represented five surface ECG leads (I, II, aVF, V_1, V_6), one bipolar recording from the high right atrium (HRA 12), one bipolar recording from the distal poles of the ablation catheter (MAP 12) positioned in the coronary sinus, and four bipolar recordings from the His bundle region (HIS 12, 34, 56,78). Intracardiac time-intervals are normal (P-A interval 23 ms, A-H interval 72 ms, and H-V interval 35 ms) and there is no evidence of ventricular preexcitation. Note the normal proximal-to-distal activation of the His bundle.

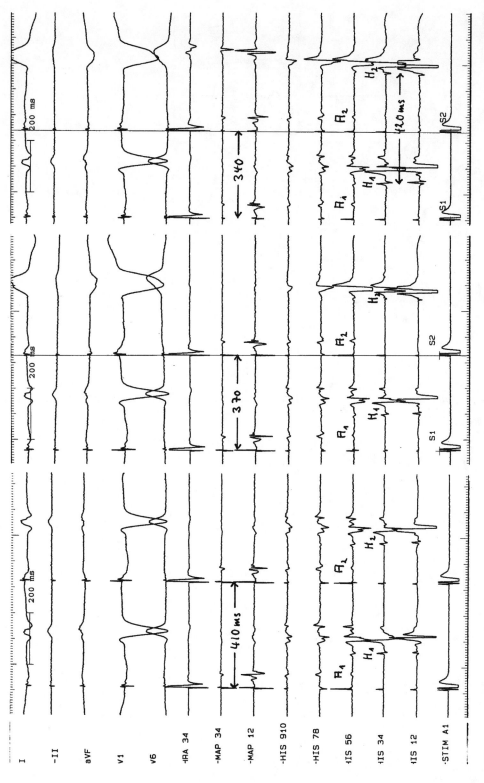

Figure 4. Intracardiac recordings (paper 100 mm/s) during programmed atrial stimulation with progressive shortening of the coupling interval. (**A**) The *first extrastimulus* (S2) has a coupling interval of 410 ms, but without aberrancy or alteration of the intracardiac activation sequence. (**B**) The *second S2* has a coupling interval of 370 ms, and is conducted to the ventricles with a left bundle branch block (LBBB) pattern; there is prolongation of the A-H interval, but clear shortening of the H-V interval with the proximal and distal His being activated simultaneously. (**C**) The *third S2* has a coupling interval of 340 ms and a LBBB tachycardia induced; again, there is prolongation of the A-H interval and further shortening of the H-V interval; the activation sequence of the His-bundle is now reversed with the distal H being activated first. The atria are activated retrogradely via the atrioventricular node. This figure clearly demonstrates the presence of a preexcited (antidromic) atrioventricular reentrant tachycardia. Note that the H1-H2 interval is 420 ms, proving that the anterograde pathway has decremental properties.

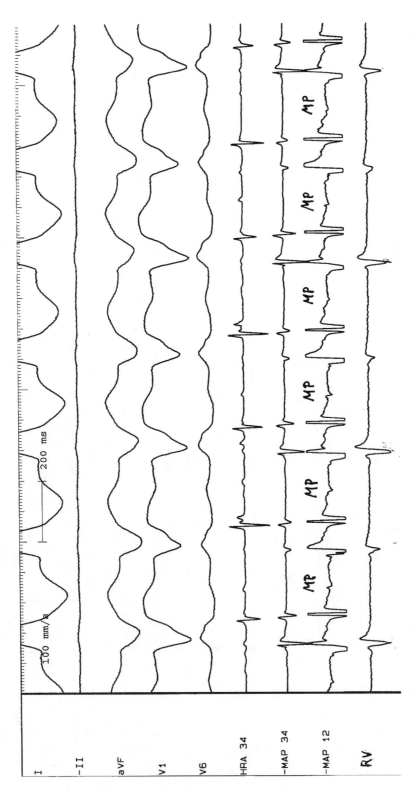

Figure 5. Intracardiac recordings during tachycardia (paper speed 100 mm/s). Mapping the right-sided atrioventricular ring (tricuspid annulus) during antidromic tachycardia revealed the presence of a "Mahaim-potential"(MP). RV = right ventricle.

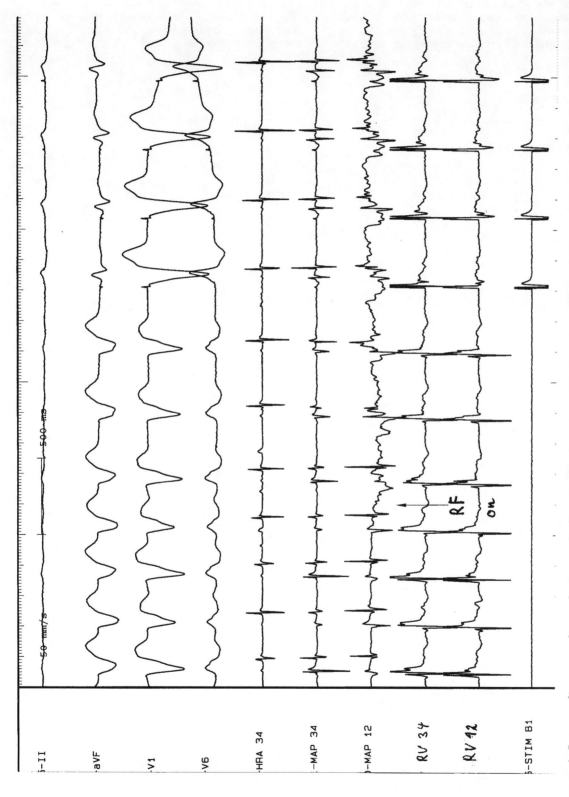

Figure 6. Intracardiac recordings during radiofrequency current application (paper speed 50 mm/s). Radiofrequency delivery (RF on) terminates the reentrant tachycardia immediately; ventricular pacing is initiated; the retrograde conduction is the same as during the tachycardia. After 60 seconds of RF current application, conduction via the accessory pathway was totally eliminated.

Heald SC, Davies DW, Ward DE, et al. Radiofrequency catheter ablation of Mahaim tachycardia by targeting Mahaim potentials at the tricuspid annulus. *Br Heart J* 1995;73:250-257.

Klein GJ, Guiraudon GM, Kerr CR, et al. "Nodoventricular" accessory pathway: Evidence for a distinct accessory atrioventricular pathway with atrioventricular node-like properties. *J Am Coll Cardiol* 1988;11:1035-1040.

Klein LS, Hackett FK, Zipes DP, et al. Radiofrequency catheter ablation of Mahaim fibers at the tricuspid annulus. *Circulation* 1992;87:738-747.

Chapter 28

Atriofascicular Mahaim Fibers and Ebstein's Anomaly

Medical History

A 46-year-old woman presented with a first episode of paroxysmal atrial fibrillation resistant to procainamide and necessitating external direct current (DC) shock for cardioversion. The QRS morphology during atrial fibrillation suggested the presence of ventricular preexcitation, but the 12-lead resting ECG during sinus rhythm was normal. The work-up performed revealed Ebstein's anomaly of the tricuspid valve and the presence of a patent foramen ovale. Atrial fibrillation with a rapid ventricular response recurred, and radiofrequency catheter ablation of the presumed accessory pathway was proposed.

Comments

This case illustrates the presence of an accessory connection corresponding to an atriofascicular pathway (Mahaim fibers) located on the posterior right ventricular wall in a patient with Ebstein's anomaly. The site of this accessory pathway had been deduced from the 12-lead ECG which shows, during prexcitation, a left bundle branch block morphology and a superior axis indicating a right posterior position, which is quite uncommon for Mahaim fibers. A more precise definition of the anatomic site of the accessory pathway was obtained from the Halo catheter, and by mapping with the ablation catheter. A distinct and sometimes huge Mahaim potential could be recorded at a specific site. This Mahaim potential could be traced for several centimeters from the atrioventricular (AV) groove and the atrio-Mahaim (A-M) interval could be prolonged by pacing during long-short sequences. Another particularity of this case is the long ventriculo-atrial (V-A) interval during antidromic tachycardia with the earliest occurrence of atrial activation in the proximal coronary sinus, suggesting the presence of a

From: RETAC: *Radiofrequency Catheter Ablation for the Treatment of Cardiac Arrhythmias: A Practical Atlas with Illustrative Cases.*
© Futura Publishing Company, Inc. Armonk, NY, 2002.

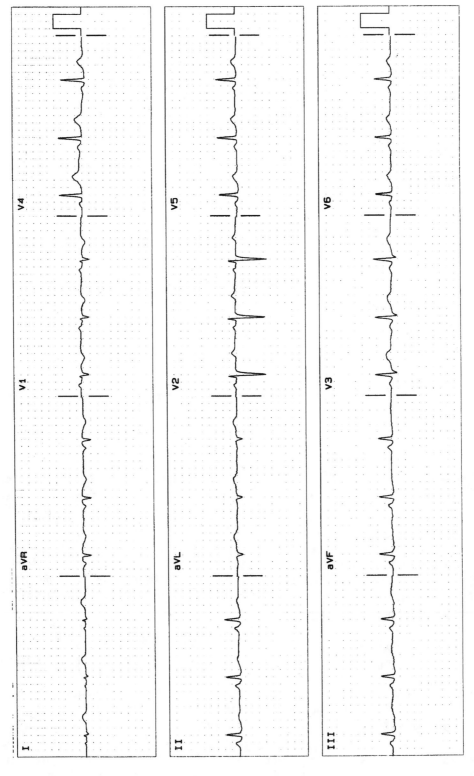

Figure 1. Twelve-lead resting ECG showing normal sinus rhythm without any ventricular preexcitation (paper speed 25 mm/s).

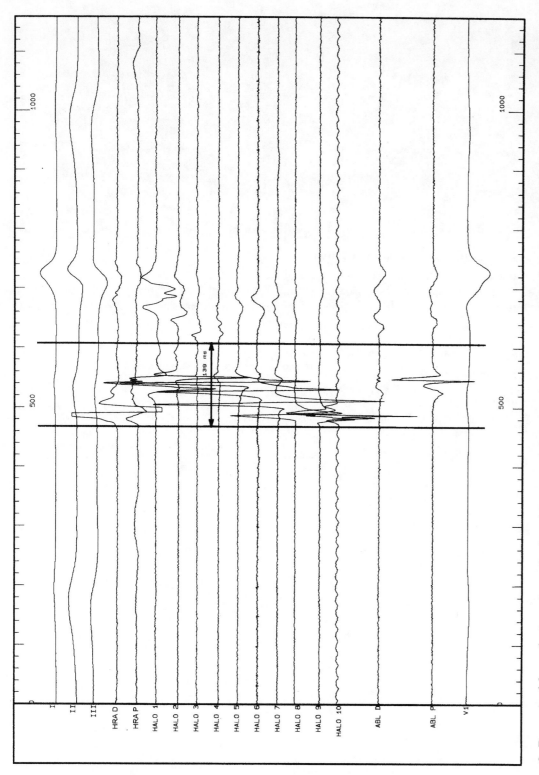

Figure 2. Preexcited beat during sinus rhythm (paper speed 200 mm/s). Here are represented four surface ECG leads (I, II, III, V_1), two bipolar recordings from the high right atrium (HRA D for distal and HRA P for proximal), ten bipolar recordings obtained from a 20-poles halo catheter (HALO 1 to 10) positioned in the right atrium with the distal dipole 1 near the os of the coronary sinus and proximal dipole 10 on the roof of the right atrium, and two bipolar recordings obtained from the ablation catheter (ABL D for distal and ABL P for proximal). The ablation catheter is positioned at the posterior atrioventricular (AV) annulus of the right heart. A spontaneous sinus beat shows partial ventricular preexcitation identified by the presence of a Q wave in II and III. The earliest ventricular activation appears at "HALO 3" positioned at the right posterior AV annulus.

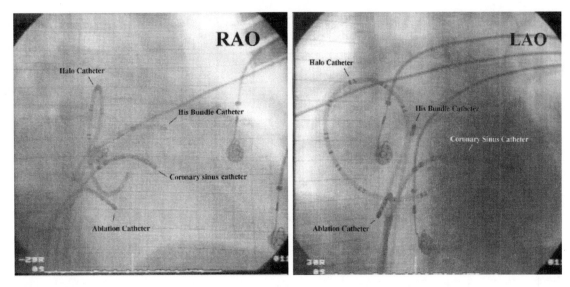

Figure 3. X-Ray image of the catheters position (left = RAO 30°; right = LAO 30°). The halo catheter (HALO) is positioned in the right atrium. A multipolar catheter is positioned in the His bundle region (HBE) and another multipolar catheter in the proximal part of the coronary sinus (CS). The ablation catheter (ABL) is at the site where Mahaim potentials were recorded, at the right posterior part of the atrioventricular groove, 1-2 cm away from the septum.

slow retrograde conduction over the AV node (slow pathway). Radiofrequency catheter ablation on the precise site of the Mahaim potential interrupted the preexcitation. A second application completely abolished the preexcitation after a first recurrence. The ablation procedure was then completed by interrupting the slow pathway, because a "fast-slow" or "slow-slow" type of AV node reentrant tachycardia with a Mahaim pathway bystander could not totally be excluded.

Suggested Reading

Okishige K, et al. New electrophysiologic features and catheter ablation of atrioventricular and atriofascicular accessory pathways: Evidence of decremental conduction and the anatomic structure of the Mahaim pathway. *J Cardiovasc Electrophysiol* 1998;9:22-33.

Berntsen RF, et al. Radiofrequency catheter ablation of two right Mahaim-like accessory pathways in a patient with Ebstein's anomaly. *J Interv Card Electrophysiol* 1998;2:293-299.

Reich JD, et al. The pediatric radiofrequency ablation registry's experience with Ebstein's anomaly. Pediatric Electrophysiology Society. *J Cardiovasc Electrophysiol* 1998;9:1370-1377.

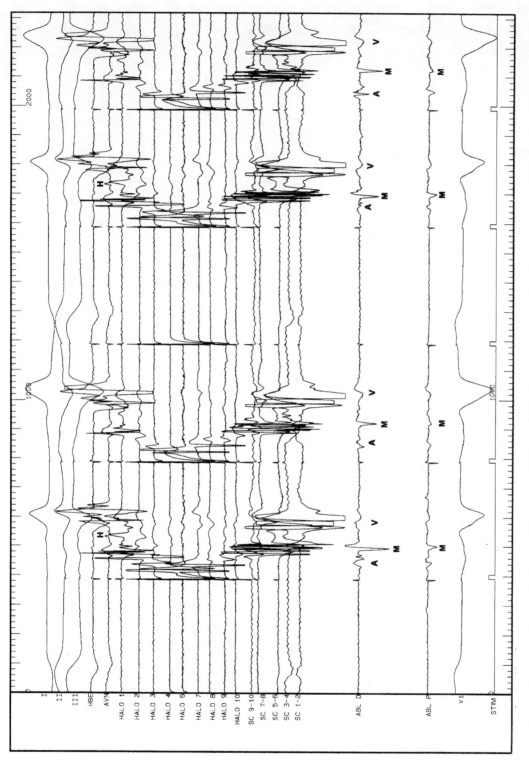

Figure 4. Intracardiac recordings during atrial pacing (100 mm/s). Here are represented four surface ECG leads (I, II, III, V_1), two bipolar recordings from the His bundle region (HBE and AVN), ten bipolar recordings from the halo catheter, five bipolar recordings from the coronary sinus (CS 1-2 to SC 9-10), and two bipolar recordings from the ablation catheter (distal = ABL D; proximal = ABL P). Halo 5 has been skipped (used for pacing). Pacing from the lower lateral right atrium modifies the QRS morphology, with a clear prematurity of the endocardial ventricular potential in HALO 2. This precedes the His potential in HBE, indicating ventricular preexcitation in the right posteroseptal region (shifting of the H potential into the QRS complex with increased preexcitation on the surface ECG). On the ablation catheter (ABL D) the amplitude of V is lower, but a distinct Mahaim potential (M) is recorded and there is a progressive increase in A-M interval.

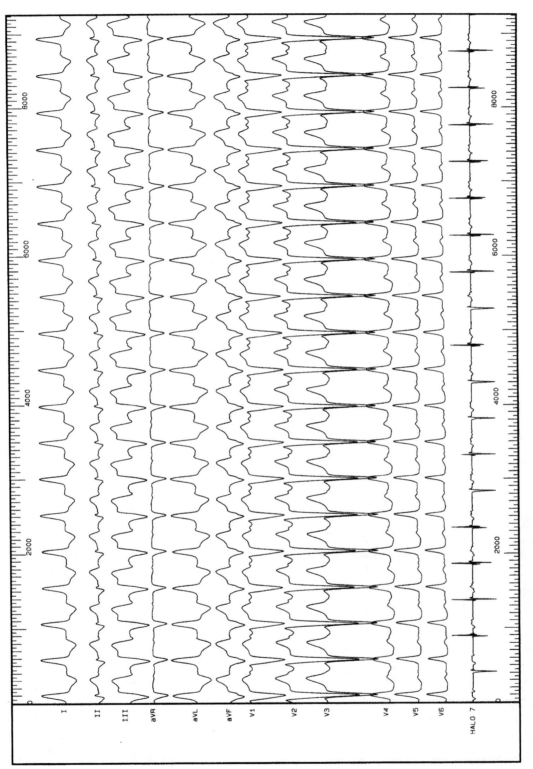

Figure 5. Twelve-lead ECG (25 mm/s) recorded during an episode of reciprocating tachycardia at a rate of 125 beats/min. HALO 7 is a reference atrial electrogram. The QRS is preexcited with a left bundle branch mrophology, a transition between V_3 and V_4, and a left upward axis. Note the Q wave in II and III is markedly different from the basal QRS complex during sinus rhythm shown in Figure 1. Negative P waves are present in II, III and aVF and the R-P interval is longer than the P-R interval (R-P = 325 ms). This long R-P is unusual and suggests a slowed retrograde conduction over the AV node. Another explanation could be a "fast-slow" or a "slow-slow" type of AV node reentrant tachycardia with anterograde conduction over a bystander Mahaim pathway.

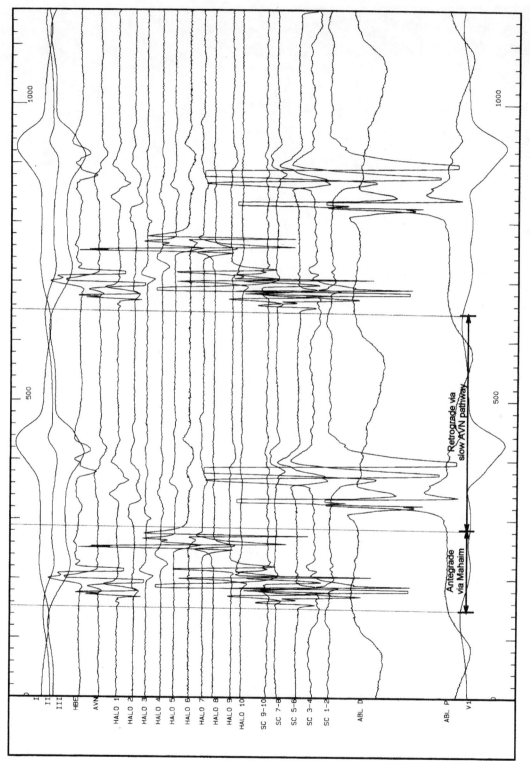

Figure 6. Intracardiac recordings during reciprocating antidromic tachycardia (200 mm/s). Same display as Figure 4, but the His bundle catheter has shifted somewhat posteriorly with a more pronounced A deflection. Note again the early occurrence of the ventricular electrogram on HALO 2. The ablation catheter is slightly away from the accessory pathway and V occurs slightly later. Retrograde atrial activation is observed earliest in SC 5-6 (proximal to median coronary sinus), earlier than at the atrioventricular (AV) node level, with a marked ventriculo-atrial delay indicating the presence of a slow AV node pathway conducting retrogradely.

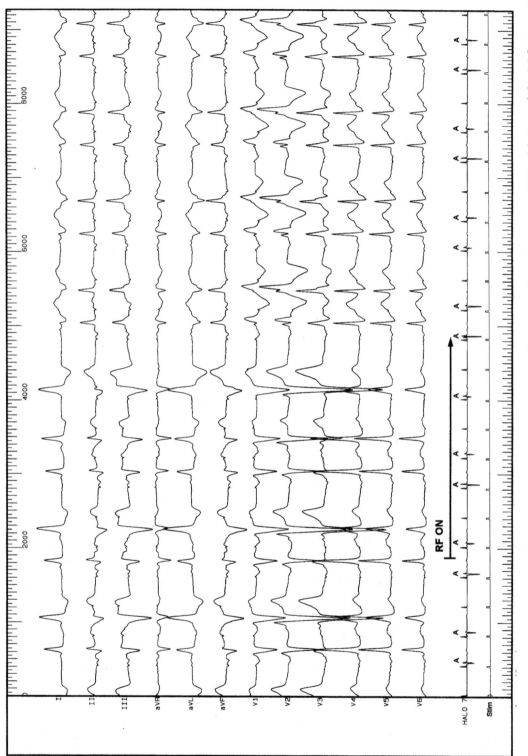

Figure 7. Twelve-lead ECG during ablation of the atriofascicular pathway (25 mm/s). Radiofrequency (RF) ablation of the Mahaim pathway on the atrial insertion site is performed during atrial pacing in order to enhance preexcitation. Due to intermittent capture of the right atrium, the sequences are irregular with a maximal preexcitation after the long-short cycles. Less than 3 seconds after RF current application (RF ON) preexcitation disappears and normal conduction is restored with a right bundle branch block pattern (due to mechanical block by the HBE catheter) and a right axis. HALO 7 is the reference atrial endocardial lead.

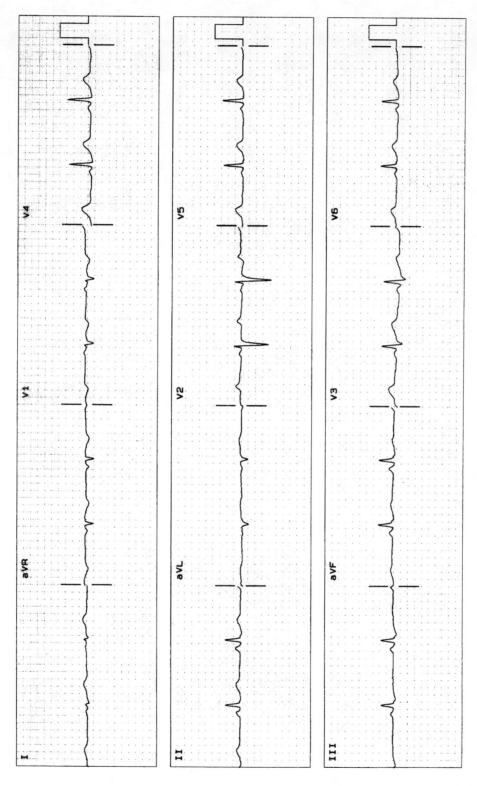

Figure 8. Twelve-lead ECG (25 mm/s) obtained after ablation of the Mahaim pathway and of the slow atrioventricular nodal pathway. There is no difference between this tracing and the 12-lead ECG of Figure 1 recorded before the ablation procedure.

Chapter 29

Catheter Ablation of Mahaim Fibers

Medical History

A 47-year-old male patient without any detectable structural heart disease presented with a history of palpitations since childhood. All ECGs recorded during palpitation showed a wide QRS complex tachycardia with a left bundle branch block pattern. The arrhythmia was always sustained and external direct current (DC) shock was necessary on three occasions to restore sinus rhythm. Pharmacologic treatment (including amiodarone and propafenone) was unsuccessful, and the two last episodes of tachycardia were reported to be faster than usual and badly tolerated.

Comments

The electrophysiologic features of nodoventricular accessory pathways are as follows: 1) minimal (like in the present case) or absent preexcitation during sinus rhythm; 2) rate dependent anterograde conduction time; 3) left bundle branch block morphology; 4) right ventricular apical electrogram usually early during maximal preexcitation; 5) no retrograde conduction over the accessory connection; and 6) frequent association with multiple pathways or atrioventricular (AV) node reentrant tachycardia. When Mahaim fibers are found in association with AV node reentry, they are not always necessary to the reentrant circuit and may act as an innocent bystander. Recent observations from surgical or radiofrequency catheter ablation suggest that so-called "nodoventricular" fibers are, in fact, decremental right-sided accessory pathways.

Suggested Reading

Josephson ME. Nodoventricular and fasciculoventricular bypass tracts. In: Josephson ME, ed. Clinical Cardiac Electro-

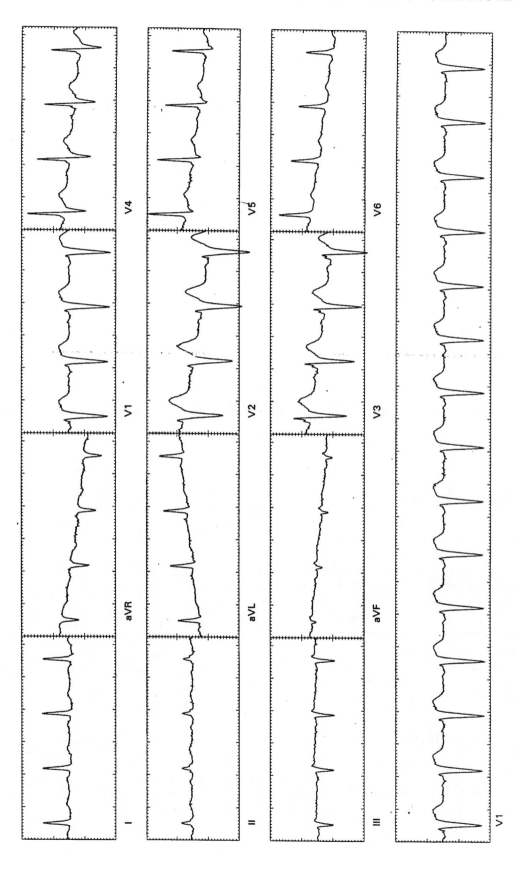

Figure 1. Twelve-lead resting ECG (paper speed 25 mm/s) showing normal sinus rhythm, a normal P-R interval (170 ms), and a QRS width of 100 ms with slight slurring of the initial portion of the QRS.

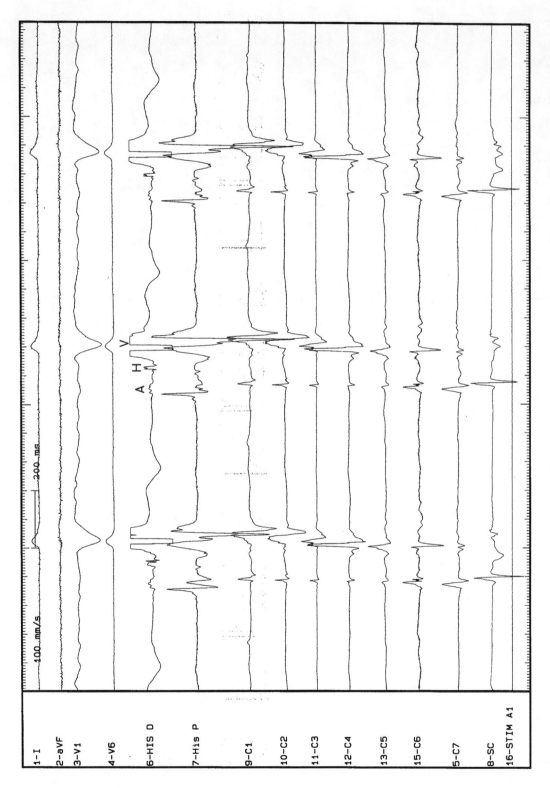

Figure 2. Intracardiac recordings at baseline during the electrophysiologic study (paper speed 100 mm/s). Here are represented four surface ECG leads (I, aVF, V_1, V_6), two bipolar recordings from the His bundle region (HIS D for distal and HIS P for proximal), seven bipolar recordings from the epicardial side of the tricuspid annulus obtained by means of a Cardima catheter (Cardima/Medtronic, Fremont, CA, USA) (positioned in the right coronary artery (C1 to C7), and one bipolar recording from the coronary sinus (SC). AH interval is 80 ms and HV interval 30 ms.

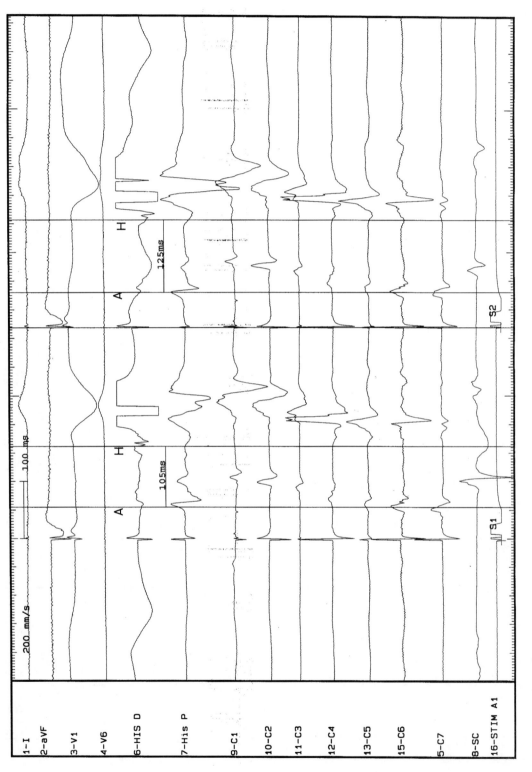

Figure 3. Intracardiac recordings during programmed atrial stimulation (paper speed 200 mm/s). Same display as Figure 2. During programmed atrial stimulation (coupling interval between S1 and S2: 375 ms), A-H interval increased from 105 to 125 ms, H-V interval decreased from 30 to 10 ms, and the QRS complex on the surface ECG became wider with a left bundle branch block morphology.

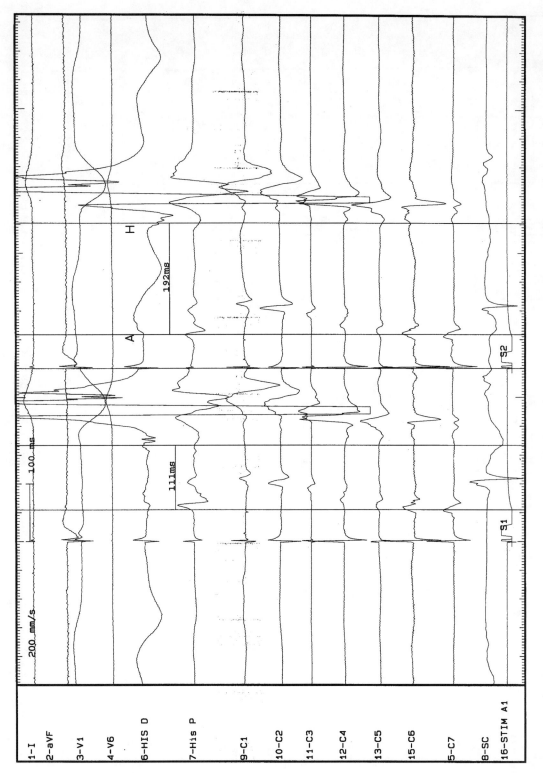

Figure 4. Intracardiac recordings during programmed atrial stimulation (paper speed 200 mm/s). Same display as Figure 2. At a coupling interval of 300 ms, atrioventricular node duality was demonstrated, with an A-H interval increasing suddenly from 111 to 192 ms.

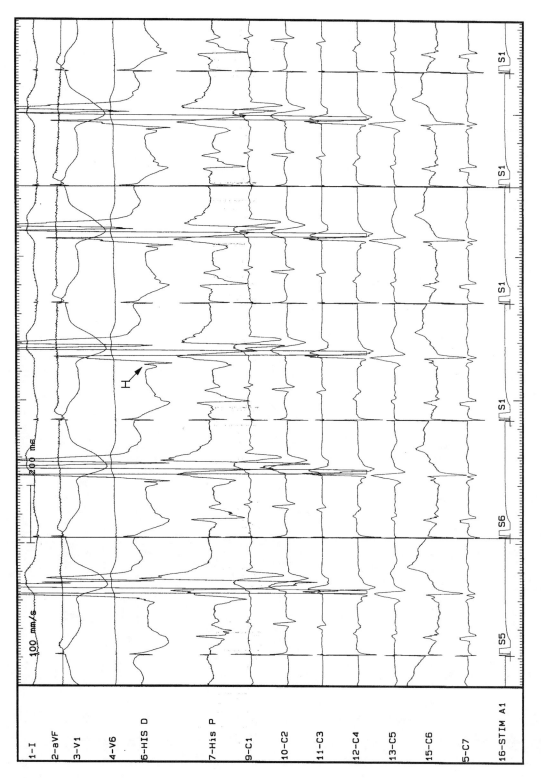

Figure 5. Intracardiac recordings during atrial stimulation (cycle length 410 ms; paper speed 100 mm/s). Same display as Figure 2. Ventricular preexcitation is present, with a negative (-10 ms) H-V interval, a His bundle potential identified at the very beginning of the QRS complex, and a left bundle branch block morphology on the surface ECG.

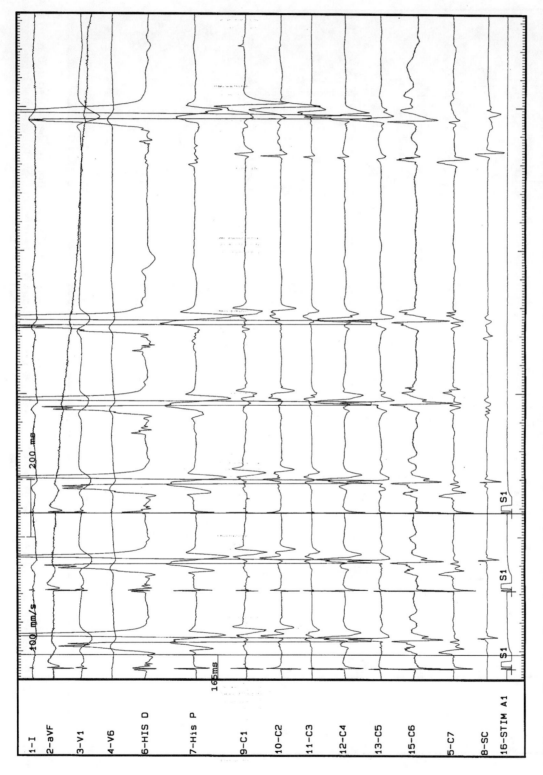

Figure 6. Intracardiac recordings during atrial stimulation (paper speed 100 mm/s). Same display as Figure 2. When atrial pacing at a cycle length of 270 ms is abruptly interrupted, two atrioventricular node echoes appeared (slow-fast type).

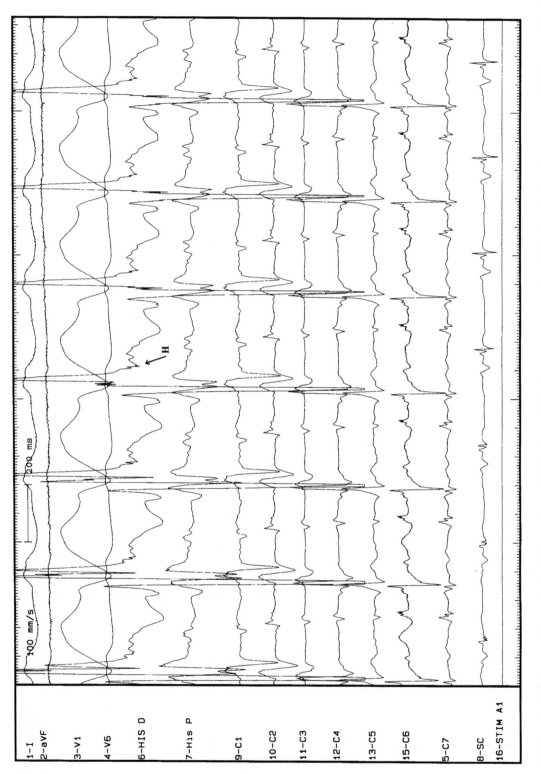

Figure 7. Intracardiac recordings during the tachycardia induced during programmed atrial stimulation (paper speed 100 mm/s). Same display as Figure 2. The tachycardia had a cycle length of 330 ms and a left bundle branch block morphology. Intracardiac recordings showed that the earliest atrial activation occurred in the His bundle region with a retrograde His deflection.

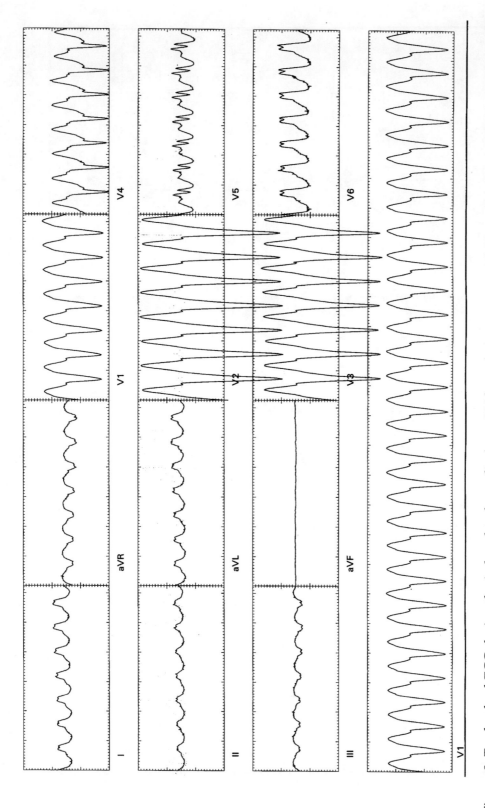

Figure 8. Twelve-lead ECG during the induced tachycardia (rate: 186 beats/min; paper speed 25 mm/s) showing left bundle branch block morphology. In fact, the aspect of the 12-lead ECG is identical to the one observed during rapid atrial stimulation (see Figure 5).

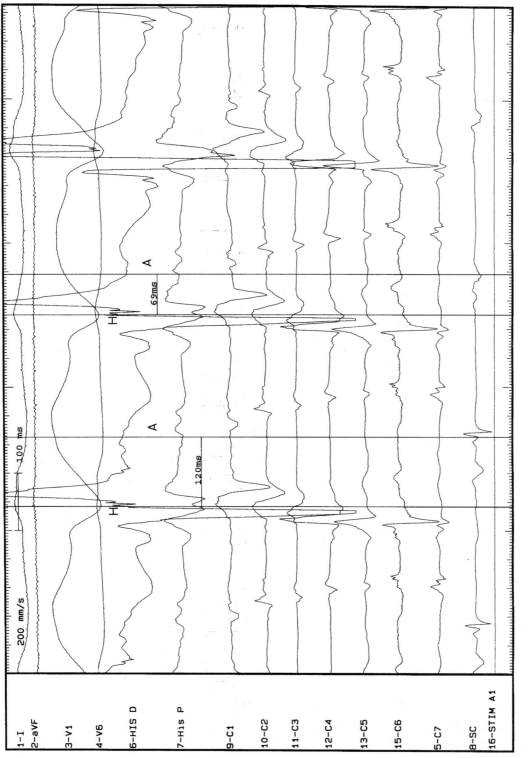

Figure 9. Intracardiac recordings during the tachycardia (paper 200 mm/s). Same display as Figure 2. A spontaneous change in H-A interval was observed (from 120 to 69 ms) without any change in atrial retrograde activation pattern but with a shortening in tachycardia cycle length (from 670 ms to 570 ms). This figure illustrates an abrupt switch from the slow to the fast retrograde pathway, excluding slow-fast atrioventricular node reentrant tachycardia as the mechanism of the induced tachycardia.

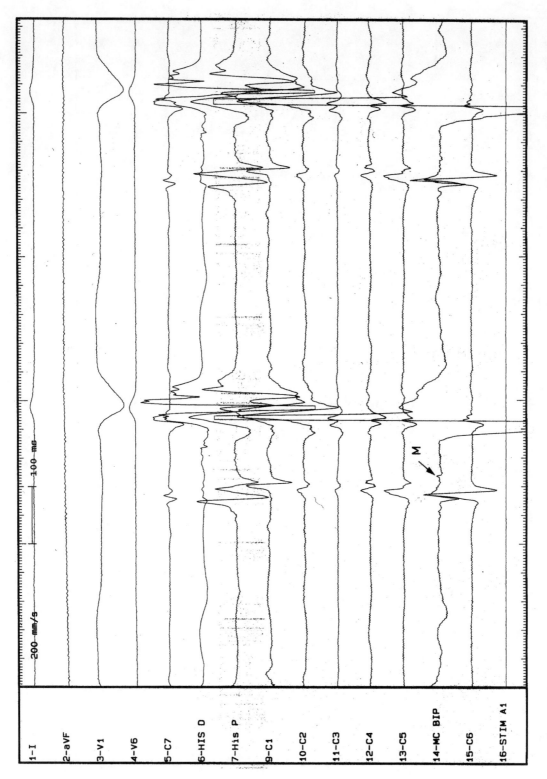

Figure 10. Intracardiac recordings during mapping of the tricuspid annulus during sinus rhythm. Same representation as Figure 2, except that a bipolar recording obtained from the tip of the ablation catheter (MC BIP) is now displayed. In the lateral region of the tricuspid annulus a specific potential was recorded (M potential).

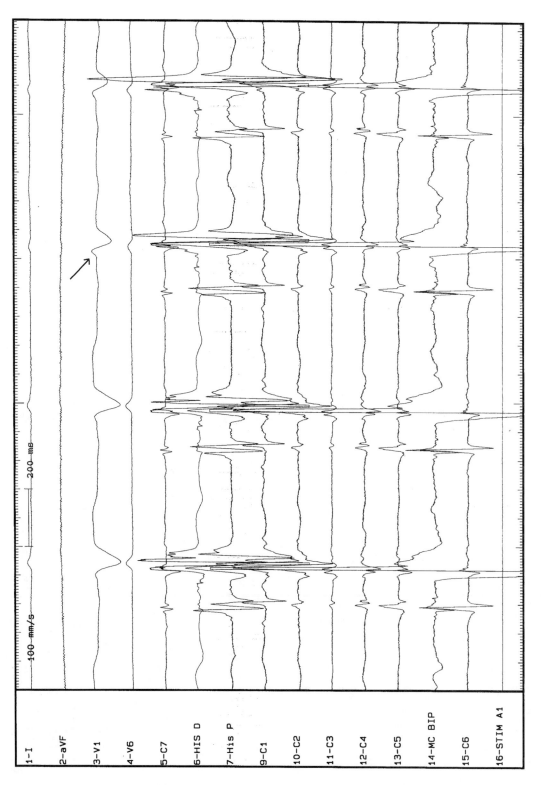

Figure 11. Intracardiac recordings during mapping of the tricuspid annulus during sinus rhythm. Same representation as Figure 2. When mapping the region where the M potential was recorded, mechanical block occurred (normalization of the QRS complex on the surface ECG, normalization of H-V interval) (arrow). Ablation was performed at this site.

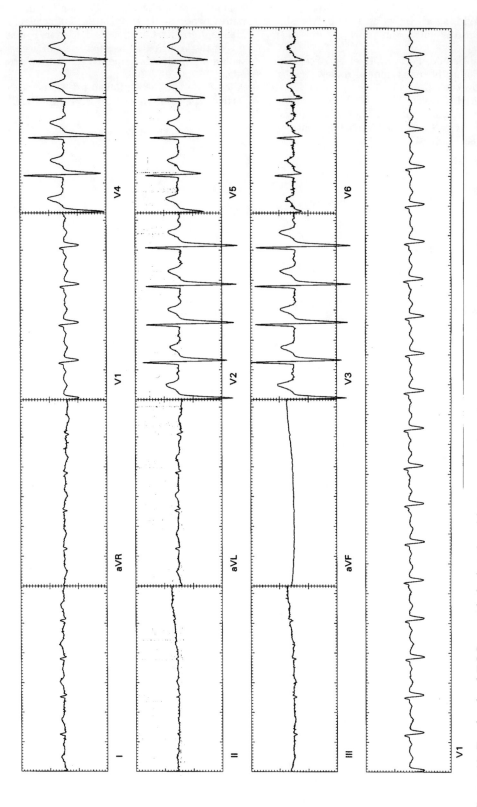

Figure 12. Twelve-lead ECG recorded after the ablation procedure (paper speed 25 mm/s). Radiofrequency current was applied on the site shown in Figure 11. The 12-lead ECG is now totally normal without any ventricular preexcitation.

physiology: Techniques and Interpretation, 2nd edition. Malvern, Pennsylvania: Lea & Febiger 1993: pp 396-416.

Gallagher JJ, Smith WM, Kasell JH, et al. Role of Mahaim fibers in cardiac arrhythmias in man. *Circulation* 1981;64:176-184.

Ellenbogen KA, Ramirez NM, Packer DL, et al. Accessory nodoventricular (Mahaim) fibers: A clinical review. *Pacing Clin Electrophysiol* 1986;9:868-875.

Tchou P, Lehmann MH, Jazayeri M, et al. Atriofascicular connections or a nodoventricular Mahaim fiber? Electrophysiologic elucidation of the pathway and associated reentrant circuit. *Circulation* 1988;77:837-841.

Mounsey JP, Griffith MJ, McComb JM, et al. Radiofrequency ablation of Mahaim fiber following localization of Mahaim pathway potentials. *J Cardiovasc Electrophysiol* 1994;5:432-434.

Haissaguerre M, Cauchemez B, Marcus F, et al. Characteristics of the ventricular insertion sites of accessory pathways with anterograde decremental conduction properties. *Circulation* 1995;91:1077-1085.

Aliot E, de Chillou C, Revault d'Allones G, et al. Mahaim tachycardias. *Eur Heart J* 1998;19(suppl E):E25-31.

Chapter 30

Slow-Fast Atrioventricular Node Reentrant Tachycardia

Medical History

A 54-year-old female patient presented with frequent episodes of sustained paroxysmal supraventricular tachycardia. The duration of the episodes varied from several minutes to several hours, and the arrhythmia was characterized by palpitation and dizziness. Personal history was unremarkable and physical examination was normal, as was the 12-lead electrocardiogram. Treatment with β-blockers and calcium antagonists failed to prevent paroxysmal supraventricular tachycardia. Because the tachycardia episodes were poorly tolerated radiofrequency catheter ablation was considered.

Comments

Slow-fast atrioventricular node reentrant tachycardia (AVNRT) is the most common form of regular paroxysmal supraventricular tachycardia. This arrhythmia is more common in women and may become clinically evident at any age. Most patients with AVNRT have no structural heart disease and the rate of the tachycardia may vary from 130 to more than 250 beats/min. The most common form of AVNRT is called "slow-fast" because a slow pathway is used for anterograde conduction and a fast pathway for retrograde conduction. Therefore, during tachycardia the atrium is activated almost simultaneously to the ventricle and P waves are obscured by the QRS complex. In fact, in many cases, the P wave is visible in the terminal portion of the QRS complex (pseudo s wave in inferior leads; r' aspect in V_1).

Ablation or modification of the slow pathway is the method of choice to cure patients with AVNRT. The approach may be purely anatomical or electrophysiologically guided (using specific potentials of the slow pathway as those described by Jackman or by

From: RETAC: *Radiofrequency Catheter Ablation for the Treatment of Cardiac Arrhythmias: A Practical Atlas with Illustrative Cases.*
© Futura Publishing Company, Inc. Armonk, NY, 2002.

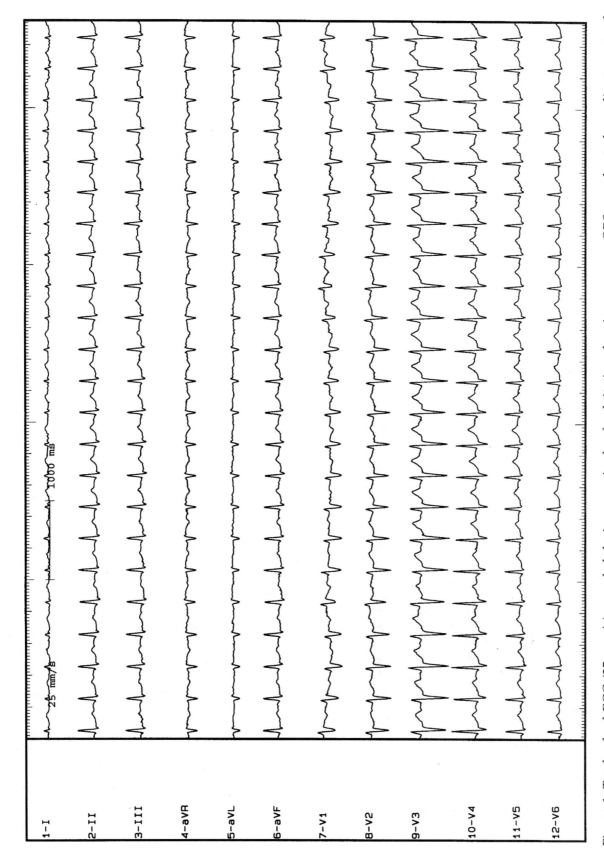

Figure 1. Twelve-lead ECG (25 mm/s) recorded during an episode of palpitation showing a narrow QRS complex tachycardia at a rate of 170 beats/min. P waves are not clearly identified, but there is an rSr′ aspect in V_1 and pseudo s wave in inferior leads, suggesting the presense of a P wave in the terminal portion of the QRS complex.

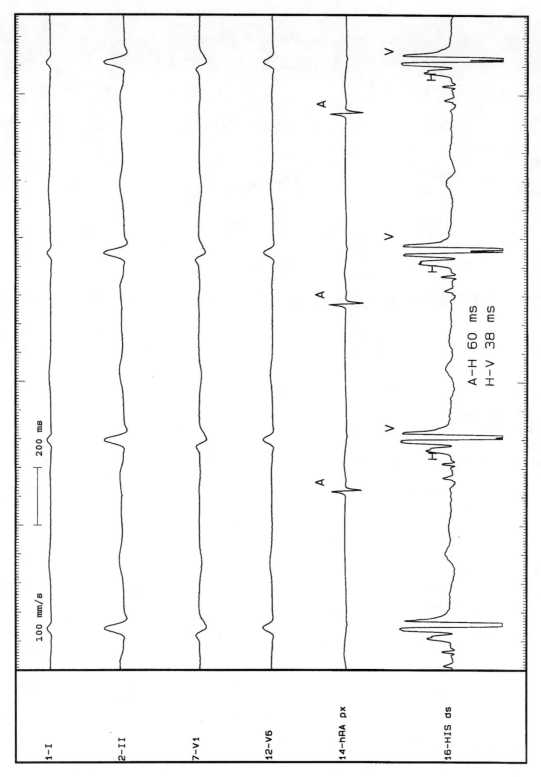

Figure 2. Intracardiac recordings (100 mm/s) at baseline. Here are displayed four surface ECG leads (I, II, V₁, V6), one bipolar recording obtained from the high right atrium (hRA px), and one bipolar recording obtained from the His bundle region (HIS ds). During sinus rhythm no ventricular preexcitation is present, A-H interval is 60 ms and H-V interval 38 ms.

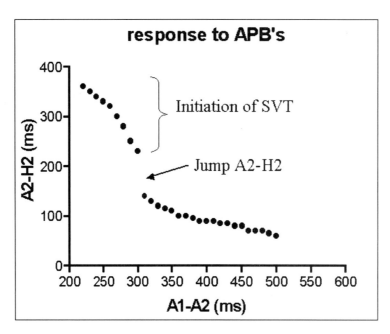

Figure 3. Response of A2-H2 interval to atrial premature beats (A1-A2), with demonstration of dual atrioventricular node pathways. At long A1-A2 intervals, conduction occurs over the fast pathway (A2-H2 interval 60 to 120 ms). At an A1-A2 interval of 310 ms, there is a marked increase in A2-H2 interval (jump in A2-H2 interval) as fast pathway refractoriness is reached. Conduction then proceeds over the slow pathway with immediate initiation of supraventricular tachycardia.

Haïssaguerre). Junctional ectopy occurs during radiofrequency (RF) current application in 90% to 100% of effective sites. Radiofrequency application should be immediately interrupted if ventriculo-atrial (V-A) block is observed during junctional ectopy in order to avoid complete AV block. This type of complication is uncommon but not exceptional (incidence of 0.5% to 1.0 % in reported series). Complete ablation of the slow pathway is not essential for clinical cure, and a simple modification of the slow pathway conduction properties is usually sufficient to prevent AVNRT recurrences in the long term. Endpoint for the ablation procedure should be noninducibility of AVNRT at baseline and after isoproterenol infusion, and persistance of dual AV node physiology (with or without a single AV nodal echo) should not be an indication for continued ablation attempts. Recurrence rate of AVNRT after ablation or modification of the slow pathway varies between 4% and 8%, depending on length of follow-up.

Suggested Reading

Haïssaguerre M, Warin JF, Lemetayer P. Closed-chest ablation of retrograde conduction in patients with atrioventricular nodal reentrant tachycardia. *N Engl J Med* 1989;320:426-433.

Lee MA, Morady F, Kadish A, et al. Catheter modification of the atrioventricular junction with radiofrequency energy for control of atrioventricular nodal reentry tachycardia. *Circulation* 1991;83:827-835.

Haïssaguerre M, Gaita F, Fischer B, et al. Elimination of atrioventricular nodal reentrant tachycardia using discrete slow potentials to guide application of radiofrequency energy. *Circulation* 1992;85:2162-2175.

Jackman WM, Beckman KJ, McClelland JH, et al. Treatment of supraventricular tachycardia due to atrioventricular node reentry by radiofrequency catheter ablation of the slow pathway conduction. *N Engl J Med* 1992;327:313-318.

Wathen M, Natale A, Wolfe K, et al. An anatomically guided approach to atrioventricular node slow pathway ablation. *Am J Cardiol* 1992;70:886-889.

Kalbfleisch SJ, Strickberger SA, Williamson B, et al. Randomized comparison of anatomic and electrogram mapping approaches to ablation of the slow pathway of atrioventricular node reentrant tachycardia. *J Am Coll Cardiol* 1994;23:716-723.

Man KC, Kalbfleisch SJ, Hummel JD, et al. The safety and cost of outpatient radiofrequency ablation of the slow pathway in patients with atrioventricular nodal reentrant tachycardia. *Am J Cardiol* 1993;72:1323-1324.

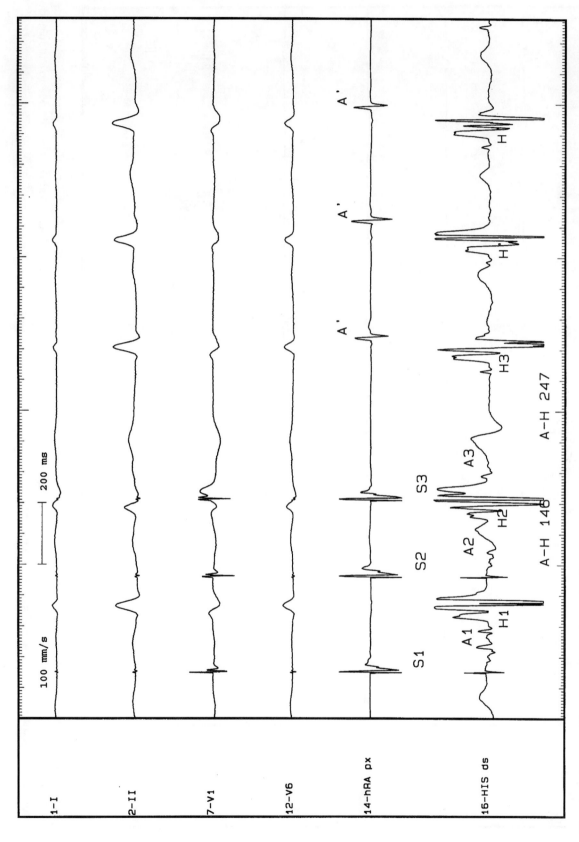

Figure 4. Intracardiac recordings (100 mm/s) during initiation of supraventricular tachycardia (SVT). Same display as Figure 2. The basic cycle length (S1-S1) is 600 ms (not shown). A first atrial premature beat (S2, coupling interval 320 ms) is conducted over the fast pathway (A2-H2 interval 146 ms), whereas the second atrial premature beat (S3, coupling interval 260 ms) is conducted over the slow pathway (A2-H2 interval 247 ms) immediately initiating an episode of SVT. During the tachycardia, retrograde conduction (A') occurs over the fast pathway ("slow-fast" atrioventricular node reentrant tachycardia).

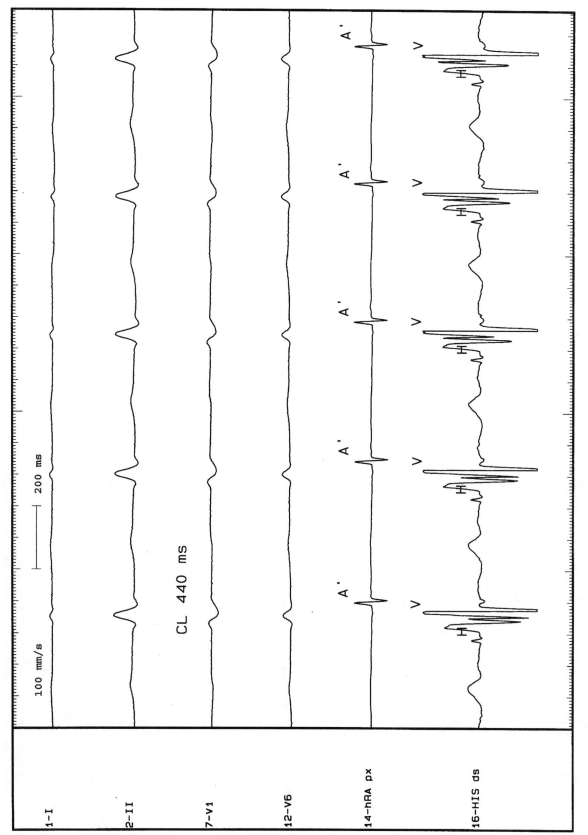

Figure 5. Intracardiac recordings (100 mm/s) during supraventricular tachycardia (cycle length 440 ms). During the tachycardia, retrograde conduction (A') occurs over the fast pathway and anterograde conduction over the slow slow pathway ("slow-fast" atrioventricular node reentrant tachycardia). H-V interval is normal (40 ms).

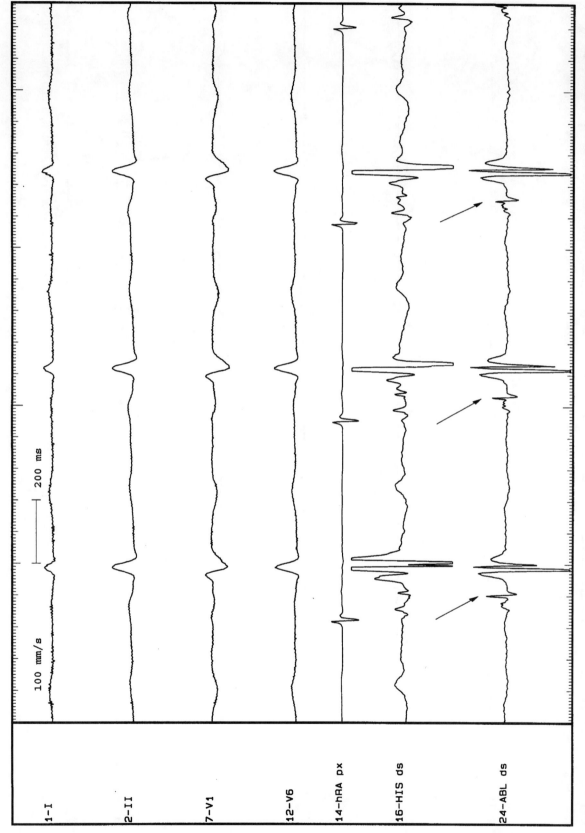

Figure 6. Intracardiac recordings (100 mm/s) at the successful site during sinus rhythm. Same display as Figure 2, with the ablation catheter (ABL ds) located in the inferior part of Koch's triangle just anteriorly to the os of the coronary sinus. A sharp potential (arrow) is recorded in that site, resembling the potential described by Jackman in the early 1990s. This type of potential recorded at a distance from the His bundle is thought to represent specific activity from the slow pathway region.

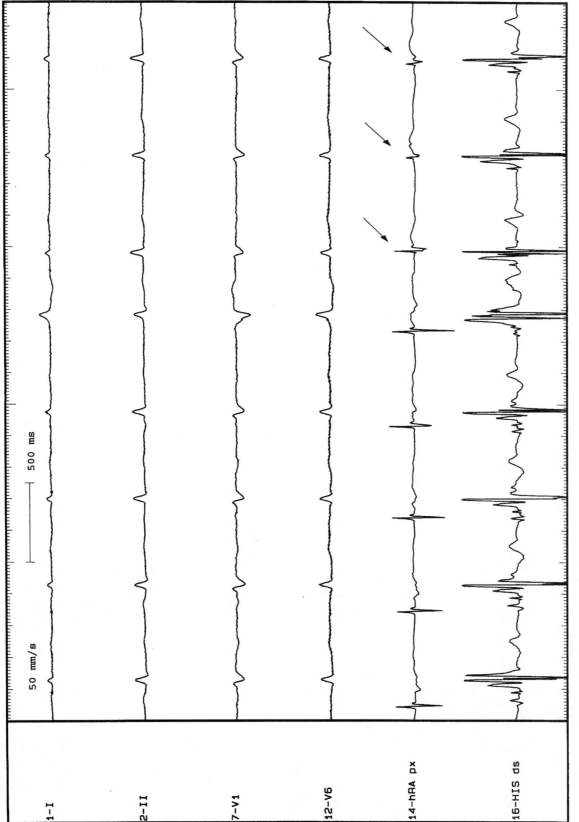

Figure 7. Intracardiac recordings (50 mm/s) during radiofrequency (RF) application at the successful site. The RF current is applied during sinus rhythm and junctional beats are observed (arrows).

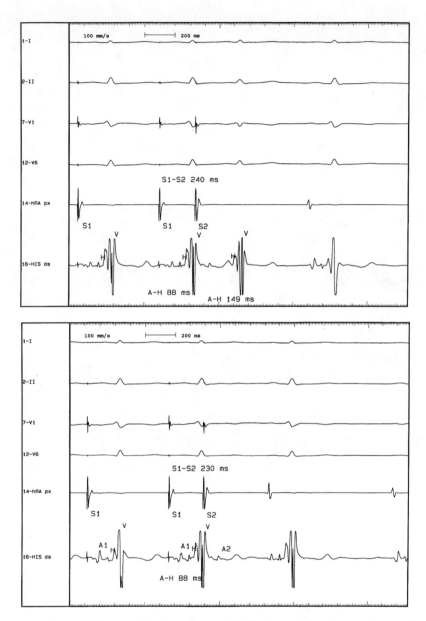

Figure 8. Intracardiac recordings (100 mm/s) after successful ablation of the slow pathway. Same display as Figure 2. Post ablation control during isoproterenol infusion. **Left**: After a premature atrial beat S2 with a coupling interval of 240 ms, conduction proceeds over the fast pathway with an A2-H2 interval of 149 ms. **Right**: After a premature atrial beat S2 with a coupling interval of 230 ms, conduction is blocked after A2 (complete ablation of the slow pathway).

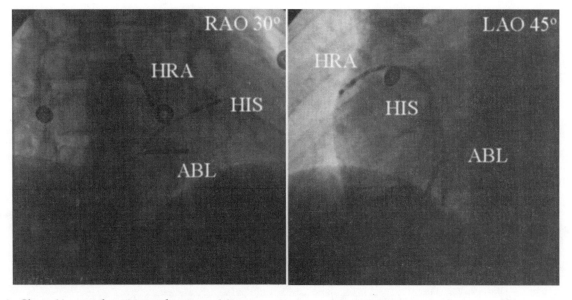

Figure 9. Chest X-rays showing catheter position.

Chapter 31

Three Forms of Atrioventricular Nodal Reentrant Tachycardia in the Same Patient

Medical History

A 50-year-old woman had frequent episodes of tachycardia for more than 10 years, sometimes lasting several hours. Physical examination, echocardiography and exercise stress testing were all within normal limits.

Comments

Typical ("slow-fast") atrioventricular node reentrant tachycardia (AVNRT) is currently the most common indication for radiofrequency catheter ablation.

Slow pathway ablation can be performed with a high success rate and a very low recurrence and/or complication rate. If there is a doubt about precise diagnosis, pacing maneuvers can be helpful to rule out atrioventricular reentrant tachycardia or atrial tachycardia. Atypical ("fast-slow") and "slow-slow" AVNRTs are less common, and it is quite rare to see all three forms of AVNRT in the same patient.

In the case of atypical AVNRT, mapping of the slow pathway for the earliest retrograde atrial activation during "fast-slow" tachycardia or during ventricular pacing may be an alternative to an anatomically guided approach.

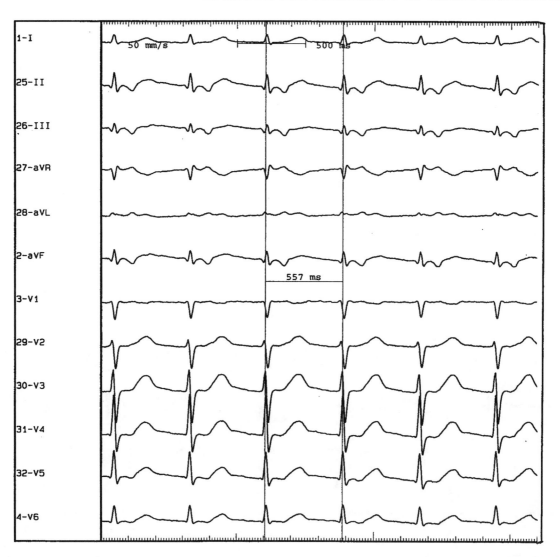

Figure 1. Twelve-lead ECG recorded during an episode of palpitations. Paper speed 50 mm/s. A regular tachycardia with narrow QRS complexes is present at a rate of only 112 beats/min (cycle length 557 ms). Note the presence of negative P-waves just after the QRS complex in lead I, III, and aVF. The differential diagnoses are: atrioventricular reentrant tachycardia (AVRT), slow-slow atrioventricular node reentrant tachycardia (AVNRT) or typical slow-fast AVNRT with slow retrograde/fast pathway conduction.

Suggested Reading

Haissaguerre M, Gaita F, Fischer B, et al. Elimination of atrioventricular nodal reentrant tachycardia using discrete slow pathway potentials to guide application of radiofrequency energy. *Circulation* 1992;85:2162-2175.

Jackman WM, Beckman KJ, McClelland JH, et al. Treatment of supraventricular tachycardia due to atrioventricular node reentry by radiofrequency catheter ablation of slow-pathway conduction. *N Engl J Med* 1992;327:313-318.

Jazayeri MR, Hempe SL, Sra JS, et al. Selective transcatheter ablation of the fast and slow pathways using radiofrequency energy in patients with atrioventricular nodal reentry tachycardia. *Circulation* 1992;85:1318-1328.

Jackman WM, Nakagawa H, Heidbüchel H, et al. Three forms of atrioventricular nodal (junctional) reentrant tachycardia: Differential diagnosis, electrophysiological characteristics, and implications for anatomy of the reentrant circuit. In Zipes D, Jalife J (eds): Cardiac Electrophysiology: From Cell to Bedside, Philadelphia, WB Saunders 1995, p.620-637.

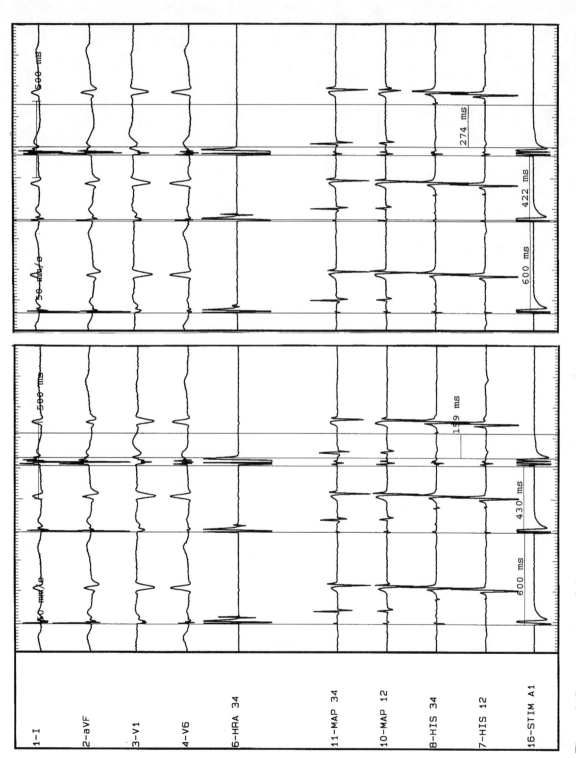

Figure 2. Demonstration of the jump phenomenon. Paper speed 50 mm/s. Here are represented four surface ECG leads (I, aVF, V$_1$, V$_6$); one bipolar recording from the high right atrium (HRA 34); two bipolar recordings from the His bundle region (HIS 12, HIS 34) and two bipolar recordings from the coronary sinus (MAP 12 and MAP 34). Note the increment of atrioventricular nodal conduction time with sudden increase ("jump") of A-H interval (from 159 ms to 274 ms) during programmed atrial stimulation (A1-A1 600 ms; A1-A2 430 ms on the left panel and A1-A2 422 ms on the right panel), when anterograde conduction changes from the fast to the slow pathway.

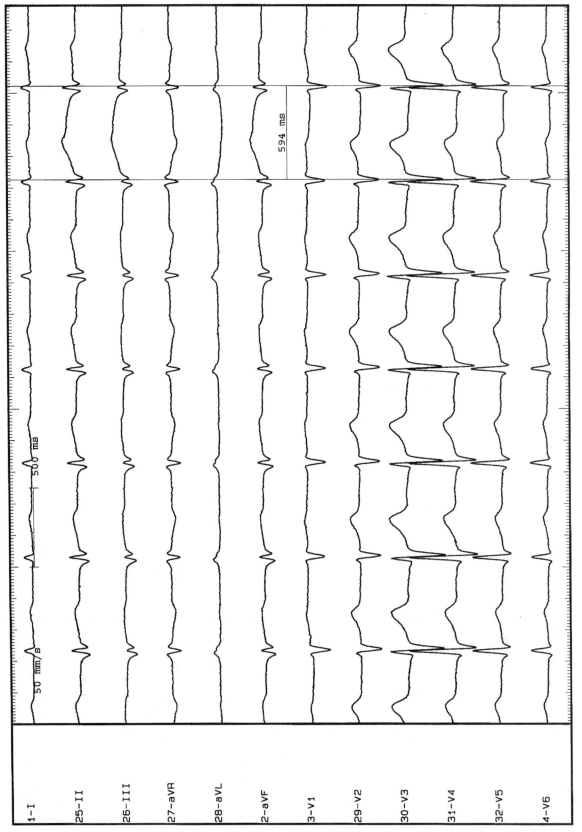

Figure 3. Twelve-lead ECG (Paper speed 50 mm/s) showing typical "slow-fast" AVNRT induced during the electrophysiological study, at a rate of 102 beats/min (cycle length 594 ms). Note the presence of negative P-waves immediately before the QRS complex.

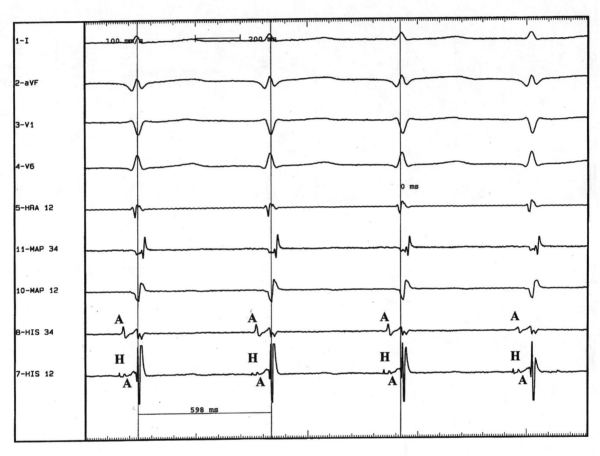

Figure 4. Intracardiac recordings during "slow-fast" AVNRT. Paper speed 100 mm/s. Here are represented four ECG leads (I, aVF, V_1, V_6), one bipolar recording from the high right atrium (HRA 12), two bipolar recordings from the His bundle region (HIS 12 and HIS 34), two bipolar recordings from the coronary sinus (MAP 12 and MAP 34). The earliest atrial activation is reecorded in HIS 3-4, indicating retrograde conduction over the fast pathway during typical ("slow-fast") AVNRT. Atrial depolarization in HRA is simultaneous to the QRS complex.

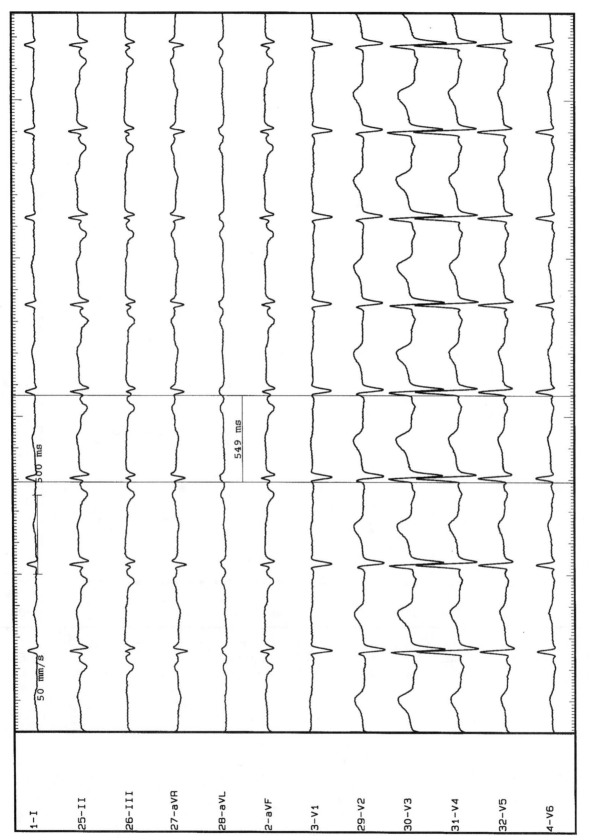

Figure 5. Twelve-lead ECG (paper speed 50 mm/s) during atypical atrioventricular node reentrant tachycardia ("fast-slow" AVNRT) at a rate of 110 beats/min (cycle length 549 ms). Note the presence of negative P waves in lead II, III, AVF 400 ms after the preceding QRS complex (long R-P interval). The differential diagnosis of supraventricular tachycardia with a long R-P interval includes atypical ("fast-slow") AVNRT, permanent junctional reciprocating tachycardia (PJRT) or atrial tachycardia.

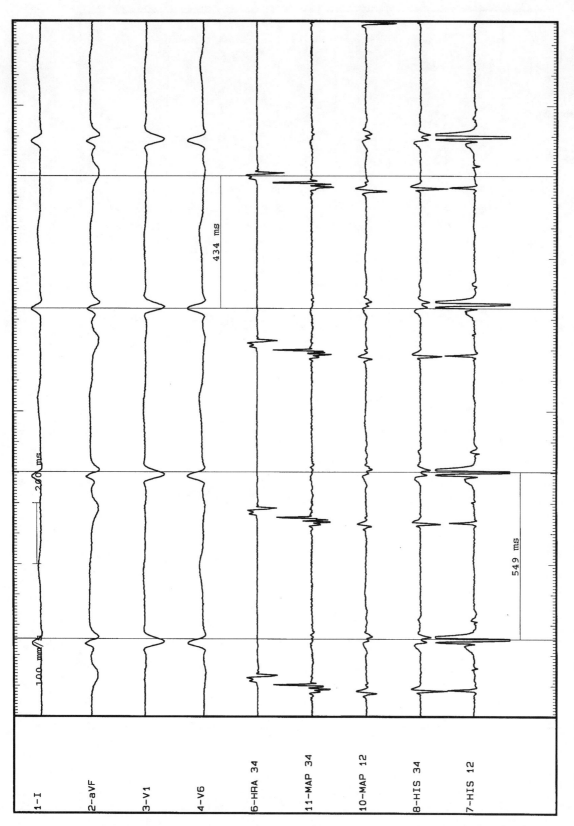

Figure 6. Intracardiac recordings during atypical "fast-slow" AVNRT. Paper speed 100 mm/s. Here are represented four ECG leads (I, aVF, V_1, V_6), one bipolar recording from the high right atrium (HRA 34), two bipolar recordings from the His bundle region (HIS 12 and HIS 34), and two bipolar recordings from the posterior region of the coronary sinus os (MAP 12 and MAP 34). The earliest atrial activation is in MAP 12, indicating retrograde conduction over the slow pathway during atypical ("fast-slow") AVNRT. Note the long interval (434 ms) measured from QRS onset to atrial depolarization in HRA due to retrograde conduction over the slow pathway.

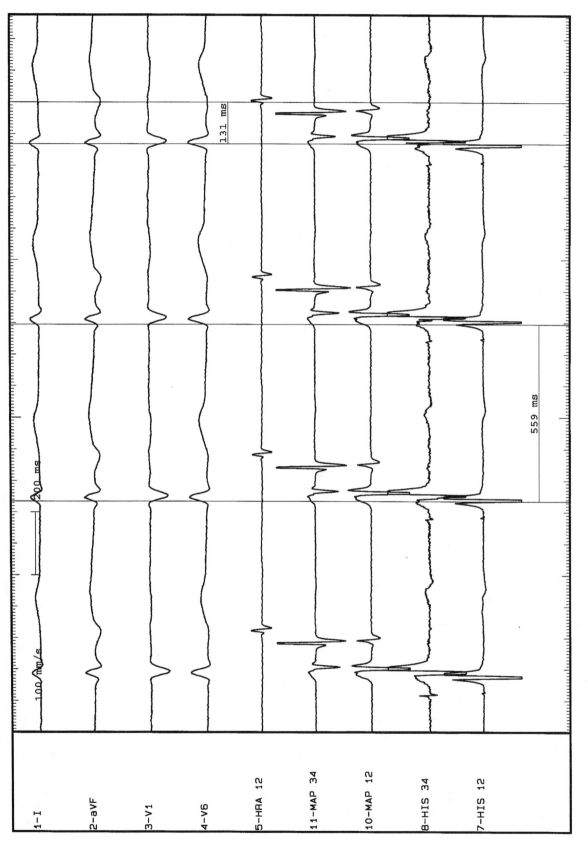

Figure 7. Intracardiac recordings during "slow-slow" AVNRT. Paper speed 100 mm/s. Same representation as Figure 6. The surface ECG is identical as the one recorded during palpitations (see Figure 1). Note that the atrial depolarization in the high right atrium (HRA) is now occurring 131 ms after the QRS complex in this "slow-slow" form of AVNRT, using two different slow pathways.

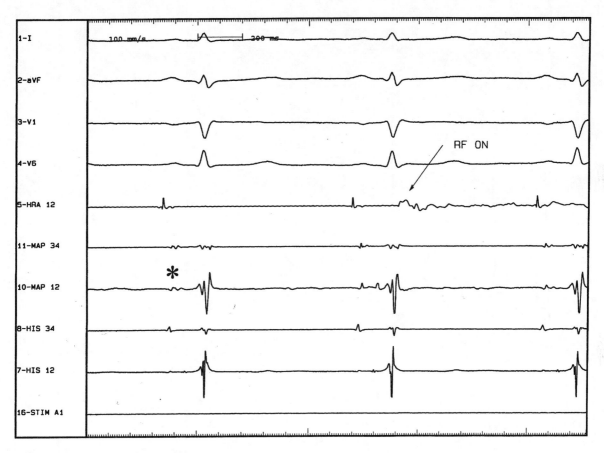

Figure 8. Intracardiac recordings (paper speed 100 mm/s) showing the position of the ablation catheter (MAP 12) just before successful application of radiofrequency energy (RF ON). Note the small fragmented atrial potential (*) (first described by Haïssaguerre as a slow pathway potential) and the much bigger ventricular potential at the successful site. This demonstrates the ventricular position near coronary sinus os. More posteriorly located ablation sites, with atrial potentials in MAP 12 recorded 30 ms after atrial potentials in HIS 34 were not successful.

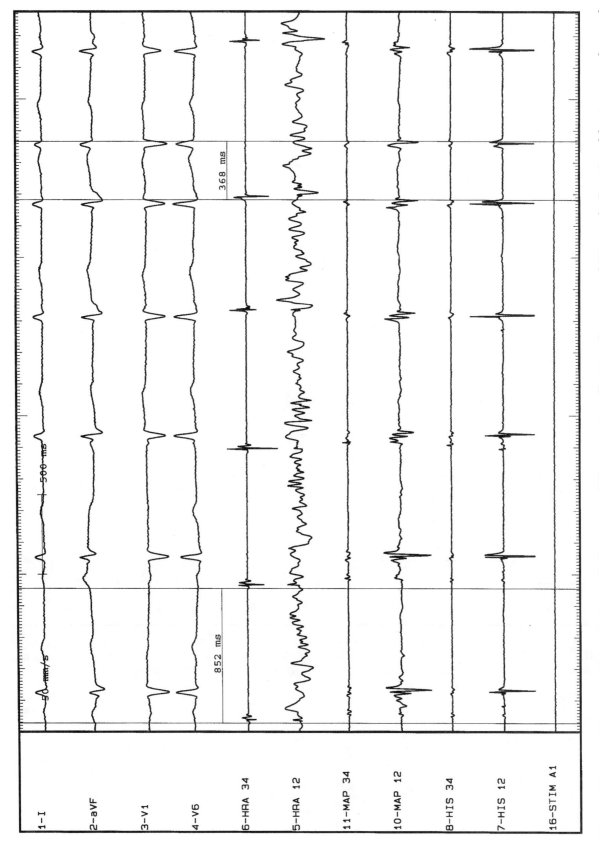

Figure 9. Intracardiac recordings during radiofrequency (RF) current application. Paper speed 50 mm/s. Junctional beats were observed during successful RF application on the slow pathway. Note simultaneous atrial activation in HRA 34 on junctional beats indicating preserved retrograde conduction over the fast pathway. One premature (368 ms) junctional beat (the fourth one) has no retrograde conduction, due to fast pathway refractoriness.

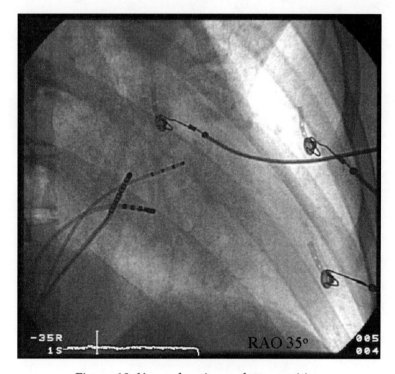

Figure 10. X-ray showing catheter position.

Chapter 32

Atrioventricular Node Reentrant Tachycardia in a Patient with Dextrocardia

Medical History

A 34-year-old male patient with situs inversus including dextrocardia presented with recurrent episodes of tachycardia at a rate of 210 beats/min. The tachycardia was successfully terminated by adenosine and the 12-lead resting ECG disclosed atypical right bundle branch block pattern with left axis deviation and very small R waves from V_3 to V_6. Pseudo-normalization of the precordial aspect was obtained by recording right precordial leads (V_1R-V_6R). At the age of 27, the patient had undergone closure of a ventricular septal defect with resection of a muscular ring in the mid right ventricular cavity. Physical examination was compatible with situs inversus. Echocardiography confirmed dextrocardia with slight right ventricular dilatation but no residual left-to-right shunt.

Comments

Radiofrequency (RF) ablation in patients with dextrocardia has been only rarely reported. Hatala et al. reported successful RF ablation of an incessant atrial tachycardia originating within the inferolateral pulmonary vein. In that case, transesophageal echocardiography was used in addition to fluoroscopy for catheter guidance during the transseptal puncture and ablation site was identified by activation mapping and by the

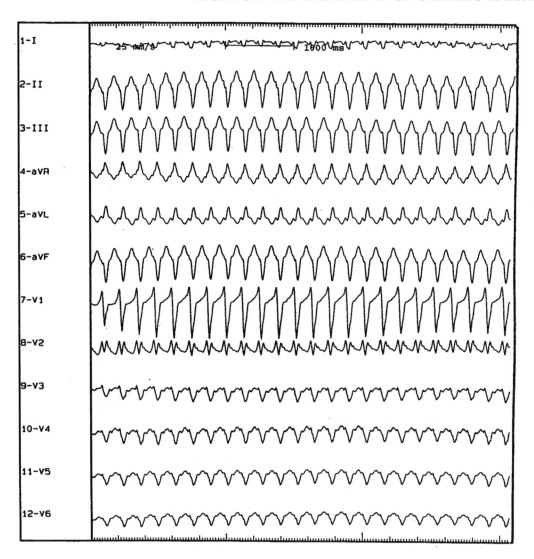

Figure 1. Twelve-lead ECG recorded during tachycardia: rate is 210 beats/min, QRS width is 120 ms, and there is left axis deviation with an atypical right bundle branch block pattern with rsr′ in V_2 and nearly absence of R waves from V_3 to V_6. The morphologic appearance of the QRS complex is identical to the one observed during sinus rhythm (see Figure 2A).

identification of a fragmented potential in the pulmonary vein. Wu et al. reported successful ablation of a reentrant right atrial tachycardia in a patient with dextrocardia and corrected secundum type atrial septal defect. These authors proposed adjustement of biplane fluoroscopy to the RAO 60° and LAO 30° positions to facilitate endocardial mapping. Finally, Abe et al. described a case with successful ablation of a left posteroseptal accessory pathway in a patient with dextrocardia using standard fluoroscopic positions (RAO 30°, LAO 45°).

By simply rotating the fluoroscopic image 180°, positioning of the RF ablation catheter is easy and allows the operator to use familiar anatomical landmarks. Because of the abnormal anatomy, detailed preablation echocardiography is necessary. The ablation procedure has to be conducted in a very prudent way using a progressive increase of power, progressive ascent of the RF ablation catheter in the low septal region, and immediate cessation of RF application in case of rapid junctional rhythm or presence of ventriculo-atrial block during junctional rhythm as usual.

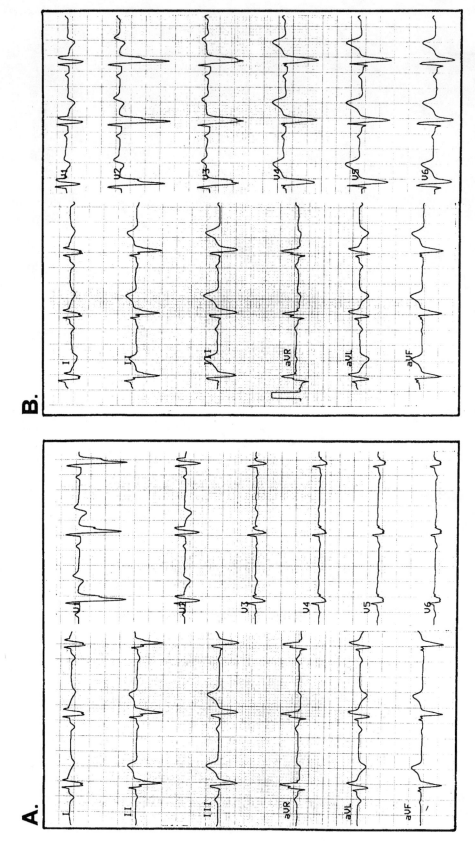

Figure 2. Twelve-lead resting ECG during sinus rhythm. (**A**) Normal electrode position. (**B**) With right precodial leads, but without reversal of limb leads. Paper speed 25 mm/s.

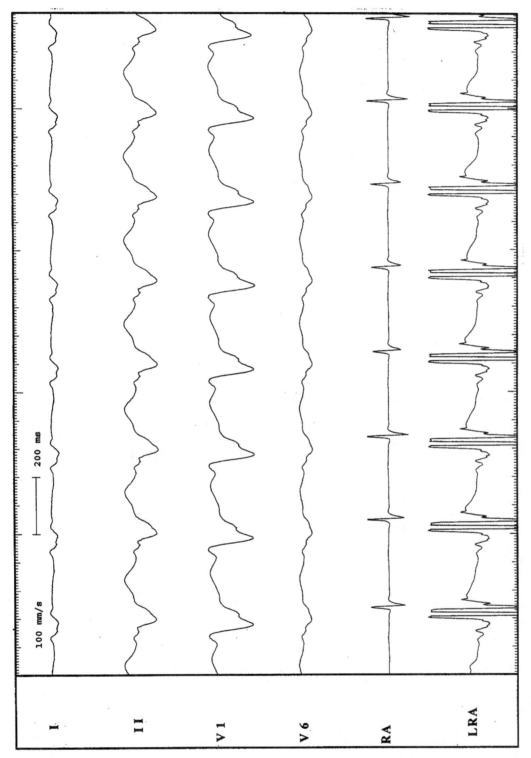

Figure 3. The tachycardia was easily inducible by programmed atrial stimulation. The figure shows intracardiac recordings during tachycardia: here are represented four surface ECG leads (DI, DII, V₁, V₆), one bipolar intracardiac electrogram from the mid right atrium (RA), and one bipolar intracardiac electrogram from the low right atrium, close to the His bundle region (LRA). Atrial activation occurs simultaneously to ventricular activation. A diagnosis of atrioventricular nodal reentrant tachycardia (AVNRT) was confirmed by the presence of dual AV node physiology and tachycardia induction with a jump in A-H interval. A retrograde septal accessory pathway was ruled out by right ventricular stimulation at the time the His bundle is refractory and atrial tachycardia was excluded by the presence of intermittent V-A block at the beginning of the tachycardia (Figure 4). Paper speed 100 mm/s.

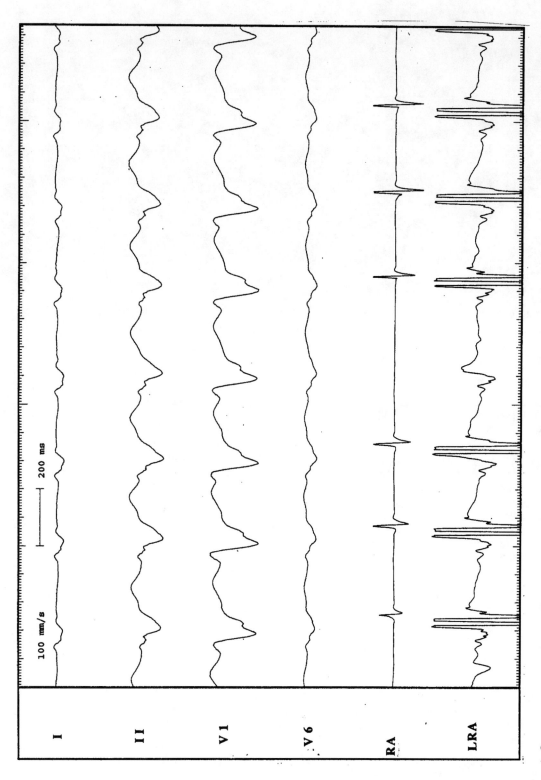

Figure 4. Same representation as Figure 3. Atrial tachycardia is excluded by the presence of intermittent V-A block at the beginning of the tachycardia. Paper speed 100 mm/s.

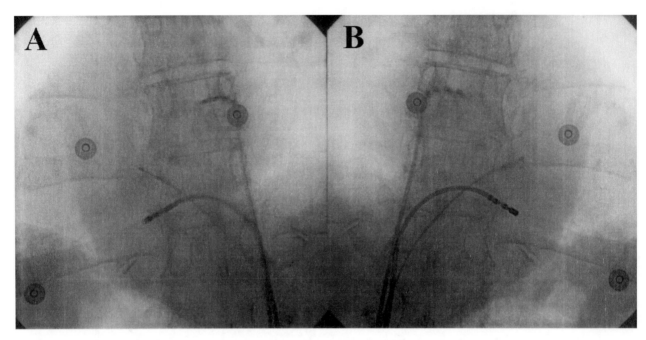

Figure 5. For catheter positioning in the presence of dextrocardia, single-plane fluoroscopy in the anteroposterior projection was used with simple left-right fluoroscopic image reversal. (**A**) Standard fluoroscopic image. (**B**) Left-right fluoroscopic image reversal. Control of the radiofrequency catheter position was made in the RAO 50° and in the LAO 30° positions. Identification of the optimal site for the slow pathway ablation was performed using anatomical and electrophysiological landmarks.

Suggested Reading

Kay GN, Epstein AE, Dailey SM, et al. Selective radiofrequency ablation of the slow pathway for the treatment of atrioventricular nodal reentrant tachycardia. Evidence for involvement of perinodal myocardium within the reentrant circuit. *Circulation* 1992;85:1675-1688.

Haïssaguerre M, Gaita F, Fischer B, et al. Elimination of atrioventricular nodal reentrant tachycardia using discrete slow potentials to guide application of radiofrequency energy. *Circulation* 1992;85:2162-2175.

Wu TJ, Chen SA, Chiang CE, et al. Radiofrequency catheter ablation of sustained intraatrial reentrant tachycardia in a patient with mirror-image dextrocardia. *J Cardiovasc Electrophysiol* 1994;5:790-794.

Hatala R, Weiss C, Koschyk DH, et al. Radiofrequency catheter ablation of left atrial tachycardia originating within the pulmonary vein in a patient with dextrocardia. *Pacing Clin Electrophysiol* 1996;19:999-1002.

Abe H, Araki M, Nagatomo T, et al. Radiofrequency catheter ablation of an accessory pathway in dextrocardia. *Pacing Clin Electrophysiol* 1997;20:2284-2285.

Levine JC, Walsh EP, Saul JP. Radiofrequency ablation of accessory pathways associated with congenital heart disease including heterotaxy syndrome. *Am J Cardiol* 1993;72:689-693.

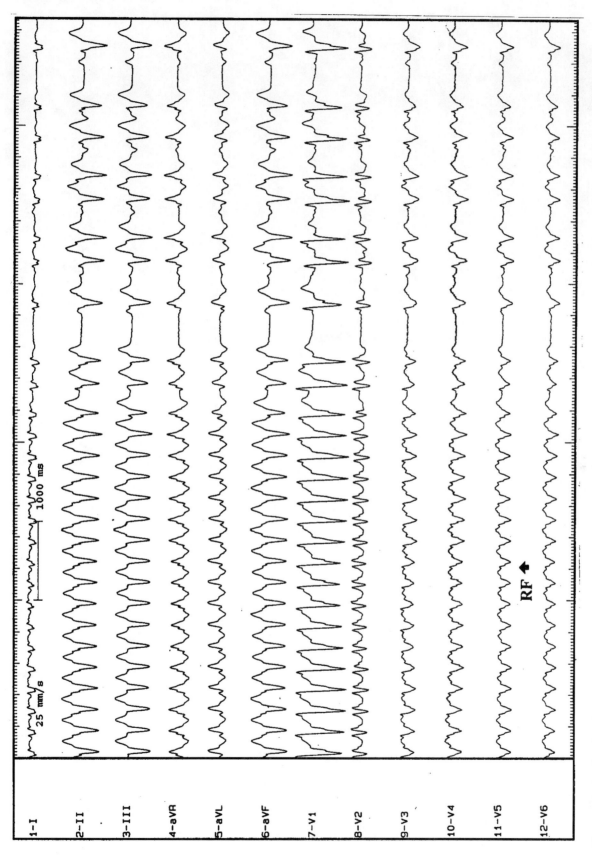

Figure 6. Twelve-lead ECG recorded during radiofrequency (RF) application at the successful site. Two seconds after RF application (arrow), the tachycardia is interrupted, and normal sinus rhythm is restored after several ectopic beats from the low right atrium and the atrioventricular junction. After this RF application, tachycardia was no more inducible even after isoproterenol, and only residual slow pathway conduction with one echo beat was observed. Paper speed 25 mm/s.

Chapter 33

Catheter Ablation of Typical and Atypical Atrioventricular Node Reentrant Tachycardia in the Same Patient

Medical History

A 39-year-old female with no structural heart disease had recurrent episodes of paroxysmal tachycardias for many years. Tachycardia has been resistant to several antiarrhythmics and restauration of sinus rhythm required intravenous administration of adenosine on several occasions. The 12-lead resting ECG was normal or sometimes showed an ectopic atrial rhythm with caudo-cranial atrial activation. Because of the occurrence of many tachycardia episodes during preg-

nancy, a decision was made to perform an EP study and a radiofrequency (RF) catheter ablation after delivery.

Comments

Both forms of atrioventricular node reentrant tachycardia (slow-fast and fast-slow AVNRT) may be present in the same patient but such a situation is rather unusual. No data exist to prove that the same reentrant circuits (but in the opposite direction) are

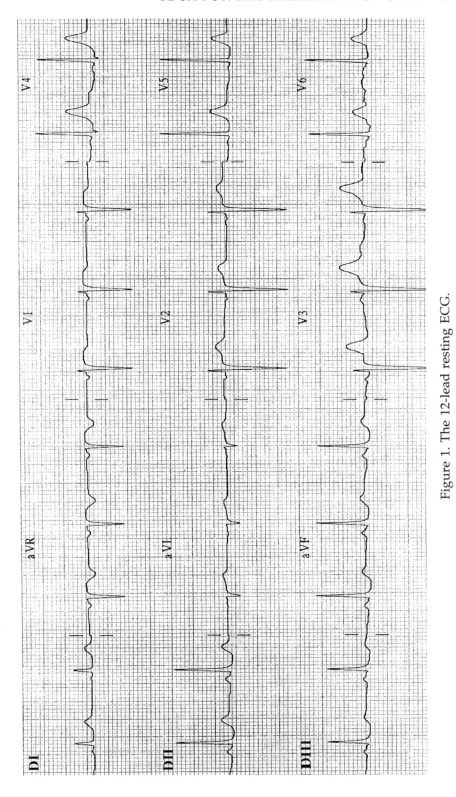

Figure 1. The 12-lead resting ECG.

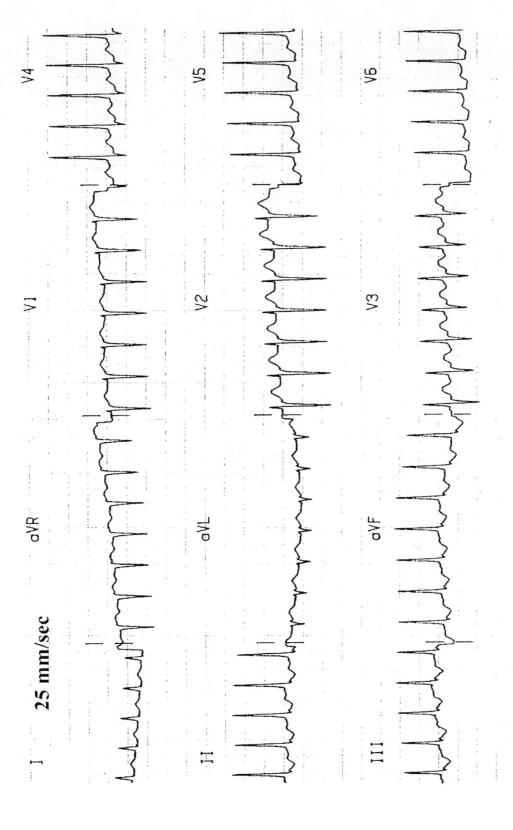

Figure 2. Twelve-lead ECG (25 mm/s) recorded during palpitations. The tracing shows a regular narrow QRS complexes tachycardia at a rate of 170 beats/min (cycle length 350 ms) with probable retrograde atrial activation occurring just after the QRS complex (R-P interval shorter than the P-R interval and a very short R-P interval): mechanism of the tachycardia may be either common atrioventricular node reentrant tachycardia (AVNRT) or atrioventricular reentrant tachycardia (AVRT) using a concealed bypass tract.

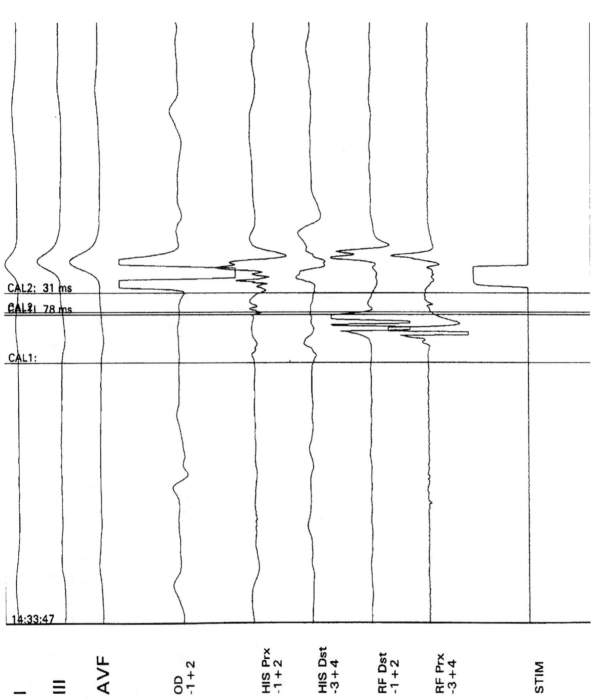

Figure 3. Intracardiac recordings (100 mm/s) at baseline. One catheter is positioned in the right atrium (OD) and one in the His bundle region (HIS Prx and Dst). The ablation catheter (RF Dst and Prx) is in the region of the coronary sinus os. A-H interval is 78 ms and H-V interval 31 ms.

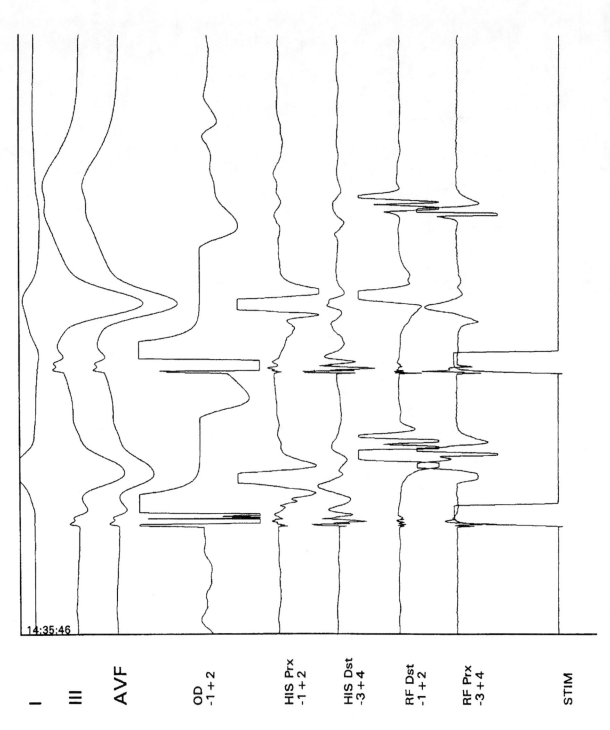

Figure 4. Intracardiac recordings (100 mm/s) showing decremental retrograde conduction during right ventricular programmed stimulation (differential diagnosis between retrograde conduction through the atrioventricular node compared to retrograde conduction over an accessory pathway).

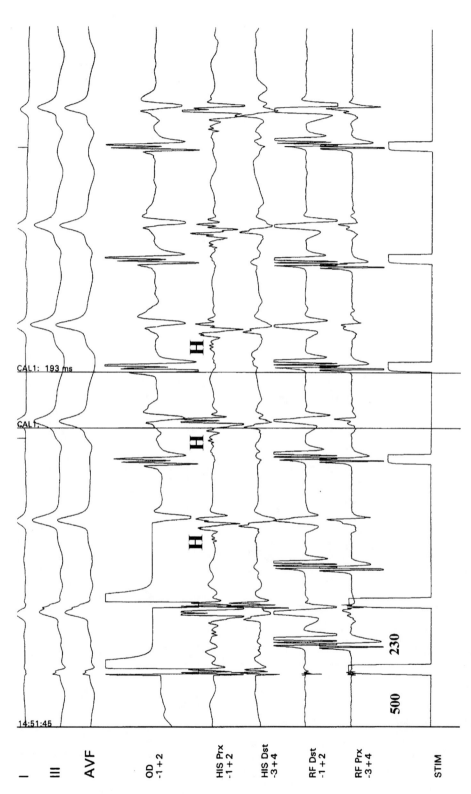

Figure 5. Intracardiac recordings (100 mm/s) showing induction of the tachycardia by atrial programmed stimulation (S1-S1 = 500 ms; S1-S2 = 230 ms). There was no jump anterogradely and during tachycardia there is anterograde conduction over the atrioventricular node (fast pathway) and retrograde conduction over a slow pathway. Note that the tachycardia is different from the clinical tachycardia shown in Figure 2. At this time the radiofrequency ablation catheter (RF Dst 1+2 and RF prx 3+4) was located in the coronary sinus.

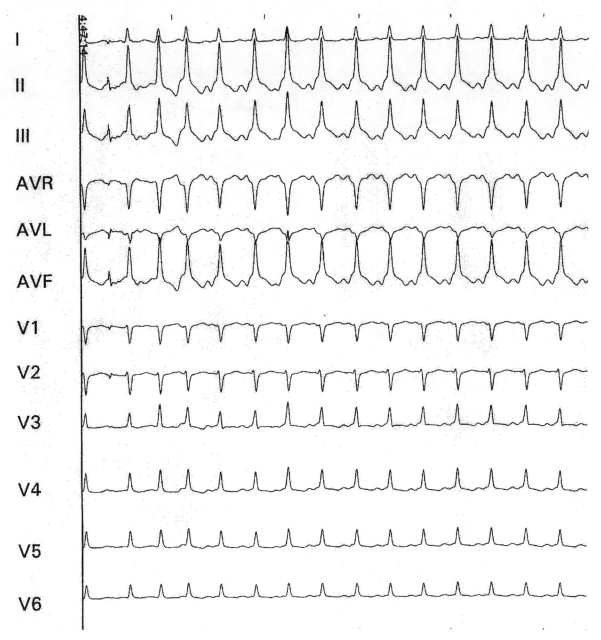

Figure 6. Twelve-lead ECG (25 mm/s) of the induced tachycardia. The R-P interval is long, longer than the P-R interval, and the P wave is negative in the inferior leads, suggesting an uncommon (or fast-slow) AVNRT, the presence of a concealed accessory pathway with decremental conduction properties (PJRT) or an atrial tachycardia.

used during theses two types of perinodal reentry. The initiation of the fast-slow type of AVNRT during atrial premature stimulation is usually not dependent on a critical A-H prolongation. Radiofrequency catheter ablation is the method of choice to abolish tachycardia recurrences. The location of the successful site for ablation of the slow pathway is often in the midseptal region, sometimes quite close to the compact AV node. During RF current application, junctional rhythm is frequently observed. During slow pathway ablation, complete AV block requiring pacemaker implantation may occur in 1% to 2% of cases. Transient AV block is sometimes observed, but the prognostic value of this type of findings is at present unclear.

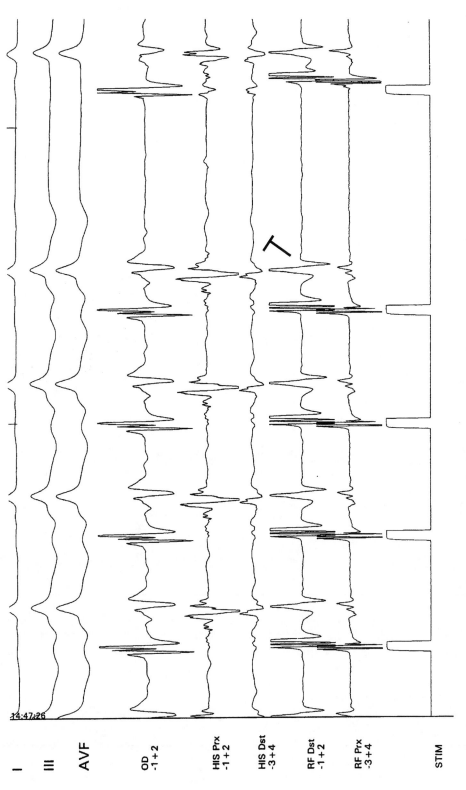

Figure 7. Intracardiac recordings (100 mm/s) showing the spontaneous termination of the tachycardia, which occurs on the retrograde slow pathway (arrow).

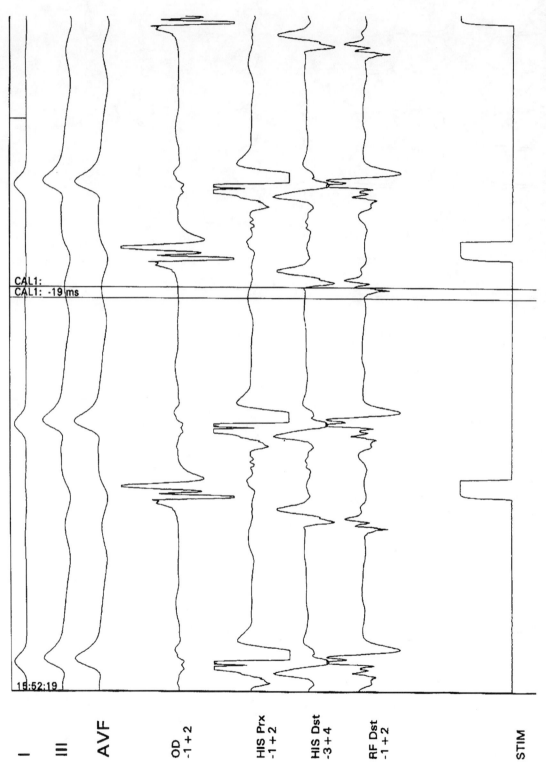

Figure 8. Intracardiac recordings (200 mm/s) during tachycardia. Mapping of the retrograde atrial activation shows a premature atrial potential occurring 19 ms before onset of the P wave on the surface ECG. This potential was recorded in the region of the coronary sinus os.

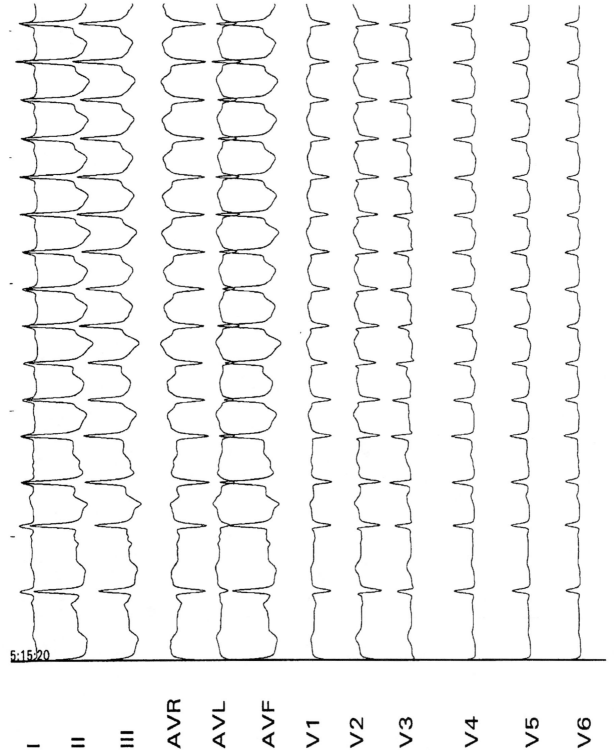

Figure 9. Twelve-lead ECG (25 mm/s) of the clinical tachycardia, induced by spontaneous atrial premature beats.

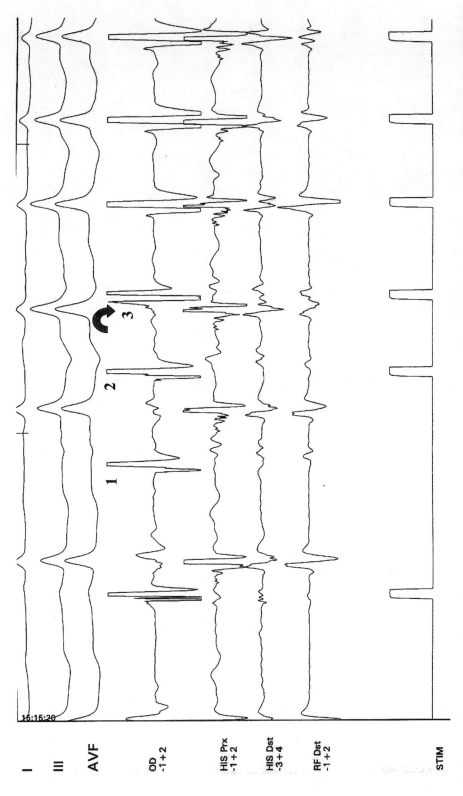

Figure 10. Intracardiac recordings (100 mm/s) of the initiation of the clinical tachycardia. The first premature atrial beat (1) is conducted over the fast pathway; the second premature atrial beat (2) is conducted over the fast pathway and induces an atrial echo beat; and the atrial echo (3) is conducted over a slow pathway with a jump in A-H interval and with initiation of a slow-fast atrioventricular node reentrant tachycardia.

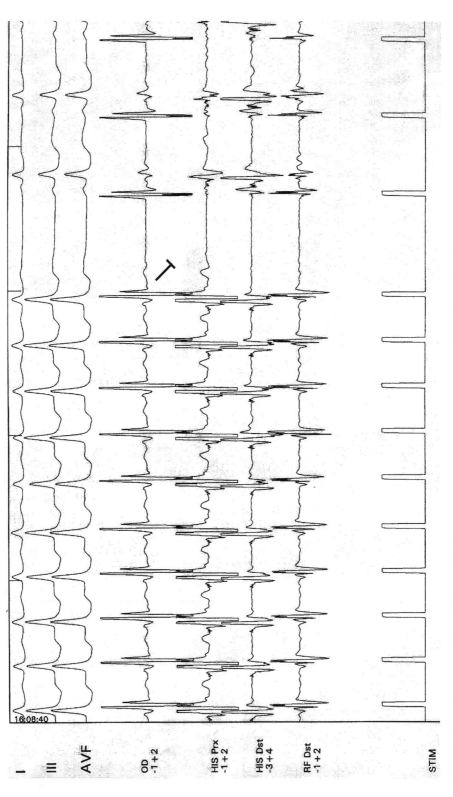

Figure 11. Intracardiac recordings (50 mm/s) during spontaneous termination of the clinical tachycardia. Termination occurs by anterograde block over the slow pathway.

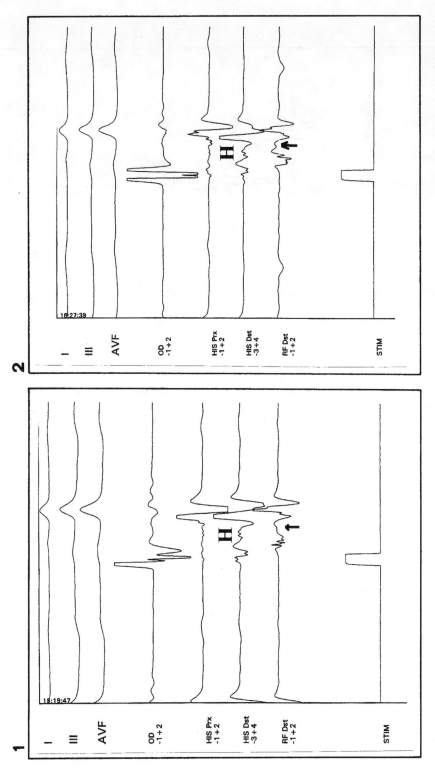

Figure 12. Intracardiac recording (100 mm/s) of the first two ablation sites (**1** and **2**), close to the coronary sinus os. A slow potential is clearly visible in RF Dst (arrow), but radiofrequency (RF) current application at those sites was not successful. The coronary sinus os was very close to the proximal His bundle region and no junctional rhythm was observed during RF current application at those sites.

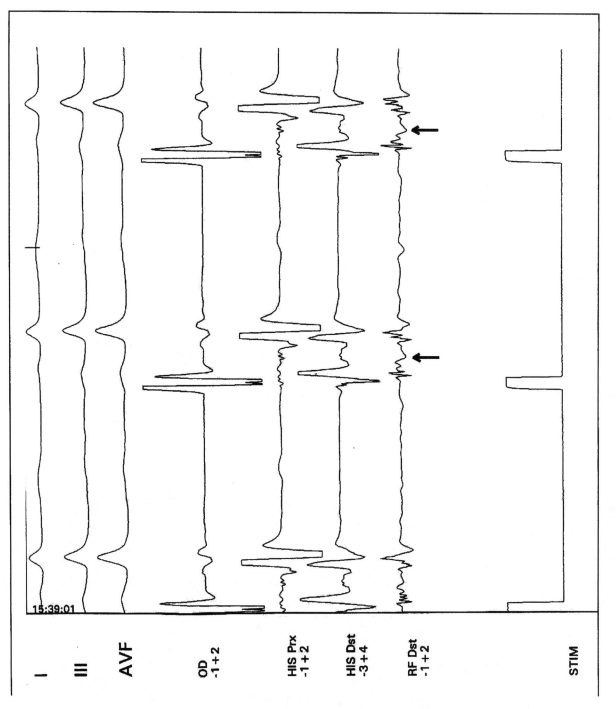

Figure 13. Intracardiac recording (100 mm/s) of the third ablation site, again in the close vicinity to the coronary sinus os. A slow potential is again clearly visible in RF Dst (arrow).

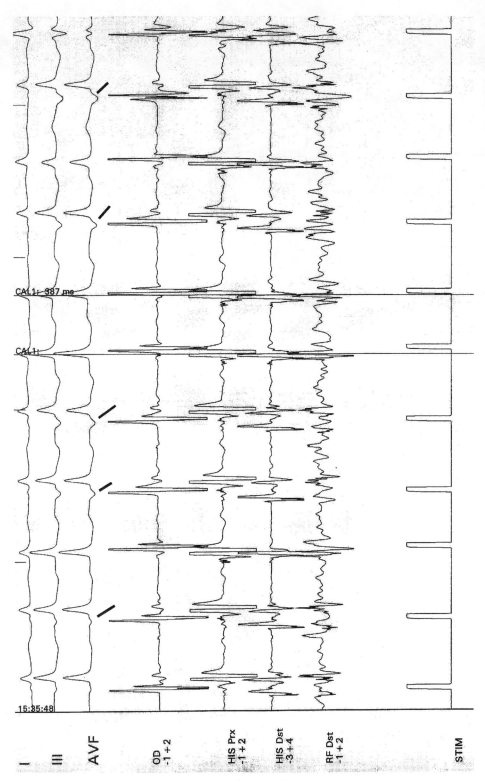

Figure 14. Intracardiac recordings (50 mm/s) during the third radiofrequency current application. No sustained junctional rhythm was observed, but isolated premature beats originating from the coronary sinus os region occurred (arrows). Radiofrequency current application was immediately interrupted.

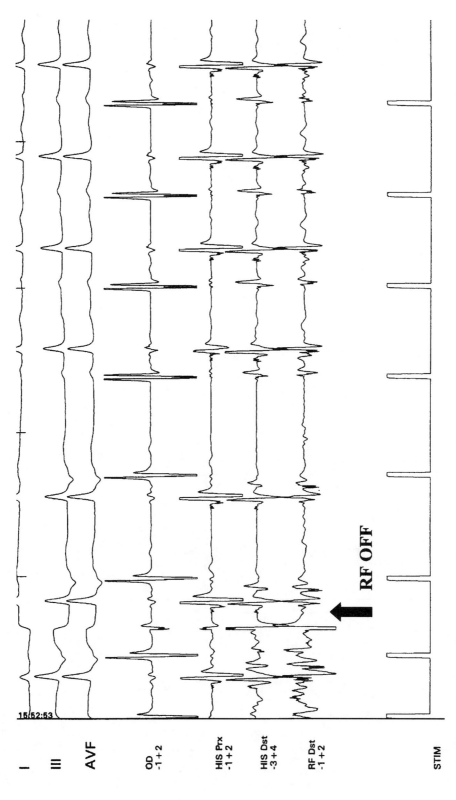

Figure 15. Intracardiac recordings (50 mm/s) just after interruption of the third radiofrequency current application (RF OFF). The first beat observed is a junctional beat conducted relatively slowly to the atrium (RA) suggesting fast pathway damage. After this junctional beat, sinus rhythm is restored, with a long P-R interval suggesting that the fast pathway has been ablated.

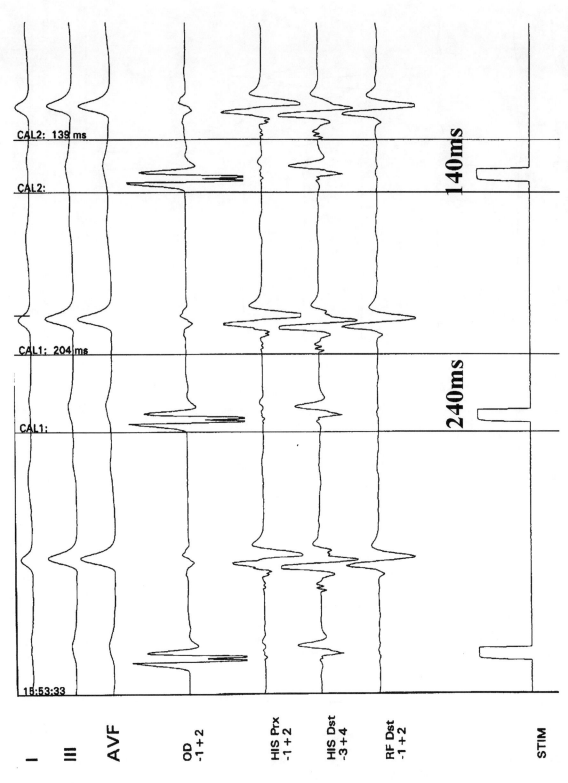

Figure 16. Intracardiac recording (100 mm/s) 30 seconds after the third radiofrequency current application showing partial recovery of anterograde conduction over the fast pathway (A-H interval decreasing abruptly from 240 ms to 140 ms). The slow-fast atrioventricular node reentrant tachycardia was then again easily inducible.

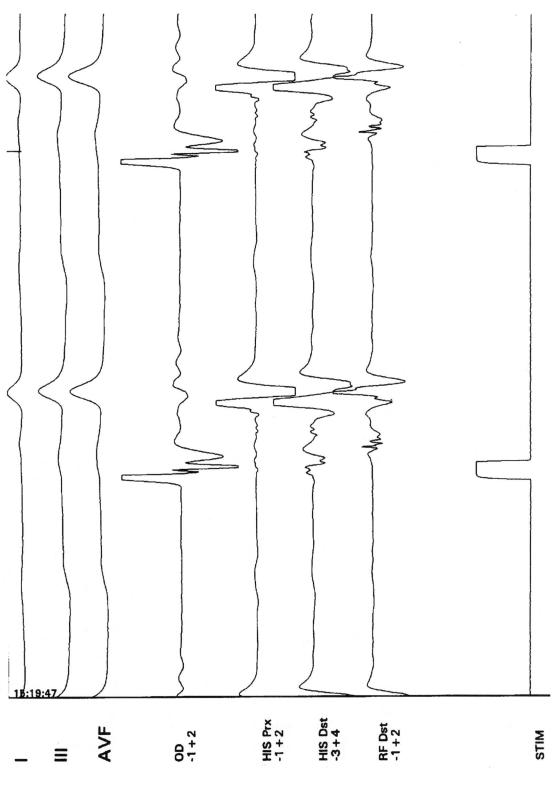

Figure 17. Intracardiac recording (100 mm/s) of the fourth ablation site, in the midseptal region. At this site, a slow but sustained junctional rhythm was observed during radiofrequency current application, and the slow pathway was successfully ablated. After this fourth application, no atrioventricular node tachycardia was inducible, even during isoproterenol infusion; no recurrence was observed during follow-up.

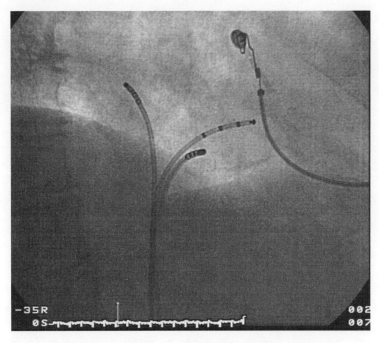

Figure 18. Chest X-ray showing catheter position.

Suggested Reading

Haïssaguerre M, Gaita F, Fischer B, et al. Elimination of atrioventricular nodal reentrant tachycardia using discrete slow potential to guide application of radiofrequency energy. *Circulation* 1992;85:2162-2175.

Jackmann WM, Beckman KJ, McClelland JH, et al. Treatment of supraventricular tachycardia due to atrioventricular reentry by radiofrequency catheter ablation of slow pathway conduction. *N Engl J Med* 1992;327:313-318.

Jaïs P, Haïssaguerre M, Gencel L, et al. Traitement par radiofréquence des tachycardies par réentrée intranodale: critères prédictifs de succès. *Arch Mal Coeur* 1995;88:1849-1854.

Poret P, Leclerc C, Gras D, et al. Junctional rhythm during slow pathway radiofrequency ablation with atrio nodal reentrant tachycardia: Beat to beat analysis and its prognostic value in relation to electrophysiologic and anatomic parameters. *J Cardiovasc Electrophysiol* 2000;11:405-412.

Chapter 34

Right Ventricular Outflow Tract Tachycardia

Medical History

A 71-year-old female patient was admitted for malaise and palpitations without loss of consciousness. She had been treated for hypertension for many years, but had no other medical problems. On admission, continuous electrocardiographic recording showed incessant runs of nonsustained ventricular tachycardia at a rate of 165 to 180 beats/min. The arrhythmia did not respond to lidocaine, and a treatment with amiodarone and β-blockers was started with partial success. However, one week later the ventricular arrhythmia recurred and the patient was transferred for an electrophysiologic evaluation. Coronary angiography was normal.

Comments

Repetitive monomorphic idiopathic ventricular tachycardia occurs typically in young patients with no structural heart disease. The main differential diagnosis is arrhythmogenic right ventricular dysplasia, and it is not always easy to exclude such a diagnosis. The arrhythmia is arising from the right ventricular outflow tract and is most commonly characterized by a left bundle branch block pattern with inferior axis. The arrhythmia is believed to be due to a cyclic AMP-mediated triggered activity related to catecholamine sensitivity. Clinically, the arrhythmia is nonsustained but frequently incessant, and depends on adrenergic situations (stress, after exercise). The trigger is probably a parasystolic focus incompletely protected from sinus rhythm and the repetitive response is maintained by triggered activity within the focus. The arrhythmia is considered as benign in patients with normal hearts. The arrhythmia is usually controlled by β-blockers or verapamil, but in drug-resistant cases radiofrequency catheter ablation is now the treatment of choice. The exact origin of the arrhythmia is based on the identifica-

From: RETAC: *Radiofrequency Catheter Ablation for the Treatment of Cardiac Arrhythmias: A Practical Atlas with Illustrative Cases.* © Futura Publishing Company, Inc. Armonk, NY, 2002.

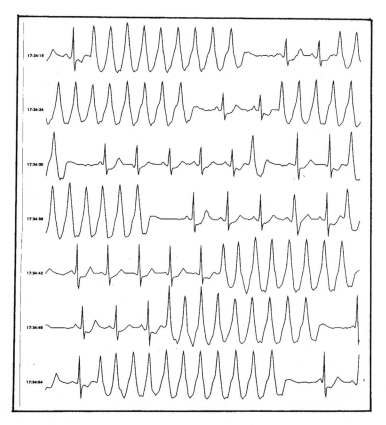

Figure 1. Continuous ECG recording on admission (25 mm/s) showing incessant runs of nonsustained ventricular tachycardia.

tion of the earliest site of ventricular activation, and on pace-mapping like in the present case.

Suggested Reading

Lerman BB, Stein KM, Markovitz SM, et al. Idiopathic right ventricular outflow tract tachycardia: A clinical approach. Review. *Pacing Clin Electrophysiol* 1996;19:2120-2137.

Morady F, Kadish AH, DiCarlo L, et al. Long-term results of catheter ablation of idiopathic right ventricular tachycardia. *Circulation* 1990;82:2093-2099.

Zimmermann M, Maisonblanche P, Cauchemez B, et al. Determinants of the spontaneous ectopic activity in repetitive monomorphic idiopathic ventricular tachycardia. *J Am Coll Cardiol* 1986;7:1219-1228.

Goy JJ, Tauxe F, Fromer M, et al. Ten-years follow-up of 20 patients with idiopathic ventricular tachycardia. *Pacing Clin Electrophysiol* 1990;13:1142-1147.

Gallavardin L. Extrasystolie ventriculaire à paroxysmes tachycardiques prolongés. *Arch Mal Coeur* 1922;15:928.

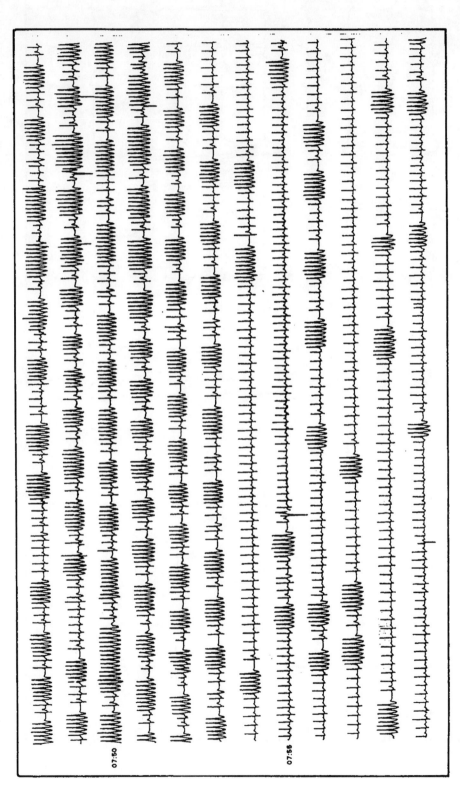

Figure 2. Fragment of the 24-hour Holter recording performed during treatment with amiodarone and β-blockers showing incessant short bursts of monomorphic ventricular tachycardia. Each line represents 1 minute of recording.

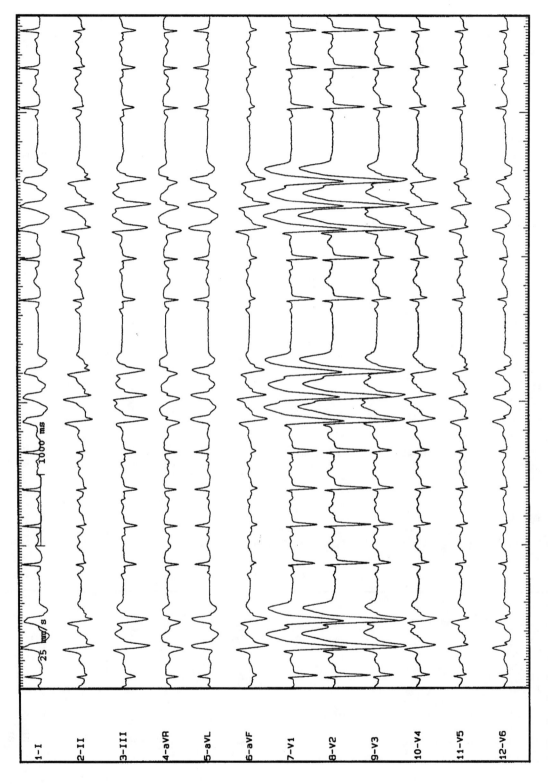

Figure 3. Twelve-lead resting ECG (25 mm/s) at the beginning of the electrophysiologic study showing normal sinus rhythm with incessant runs of nonsustained monomorphic ventricular tachycardia at a rate of 170 beats/min. The ventricular arrhythmia has a left bundle branch block morphology with transition in V_4 and a horizontal axis in the frontal plane.

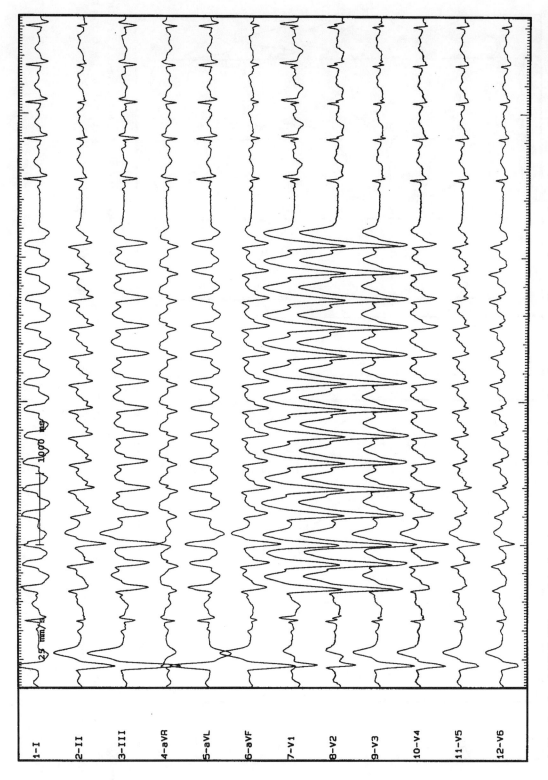

Figure 4. Twelve-lead ECG (25 mm/s) after isoproterenol infusion showing an increase in the number of ventricular tachycardia episodes, an increase in the length of the runs which remained nonsustained, and an increase in the tachycardia rate. The right bundle branch block observed during sinus rhythm is related to catheter manipulation during the procedure. Isolated ventricular premature beats with a different axis (left part of the figure) are present during sinus rhythm.

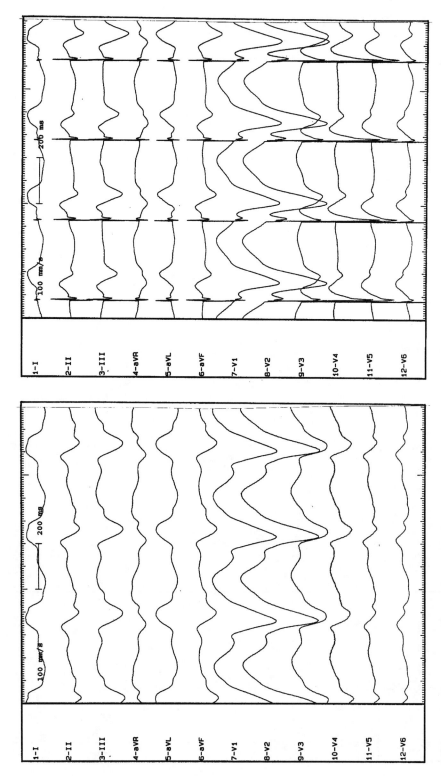

Figure 5. Twelve-lead ECG (100 mm/s) during pace mapping at the successful site of ablation (**right**) and during spontaneous ventricular tachycardia (**left**). An identical QRS morphology was observed in the anterolateral region of the right ventricular outflow tract, and eight radiofrequency current applications were necessary to completely abolish the ventricular arrhythmia.

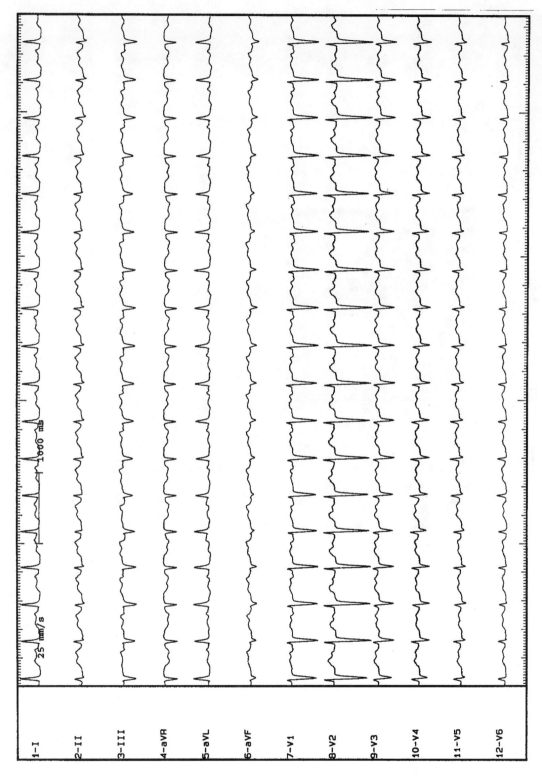

Figure 6. Twelve-lead ECG (25 mm/s) during isoproterenol infusion after the ablation procedure. The incessant ventricular arrhythmia has completely disappeared. During a follow-up of 2 years, no recurrence of ventricular tachycardia has been observed.

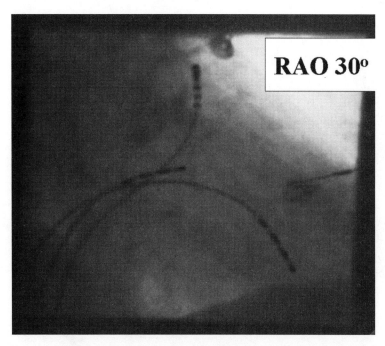

Figure 7. Chest X-ray showing catheter position.

Chapter 35

Idiopathic Left Ventricular Tachycardia:
Radiofrequency Catheter Ablation Guided by a Purkinje Potential

Medical History

This 37-year-old male patient without structural heart disease presented with 15-year history of three to five episodes per year of paroxysmal tachycardia. The longest episodes lasted more than 6 to 8 hours. For a couple of years, a treatment with sotalol could reduce the number of episodes significantly. In 1998, after having stopped the treatment with sotalol because of side effects, the episodes of tachycardia started to become more frequent again. In May 1998, a tachycardia with broad QRS complexes could be documented on a 12-lead ECG. It showed a cycle length of 300 ms and a right bundle branch block morphology with a left axis deviation typical of an idiopathic ven-

tricular tachycardia originating from the left ventricle and involving the left posterior fascicle.

After admission to the hospital, the tachycardia was terminated by an intravenous injection of verapamil. For a former episode of tachycardia several years ago, intravenous injection of ajmalin has also been shown to be effective. The tachycardia caused unpleasant palpitations, but was otherwise hemodynamically well tolerated by the patient.

Further examination showed no sign of structural heart disease and arrhythmogenic right ventricular dysplasia, dilated cardiomyopathy, and coronary artery disease were excluded.

Finally, on the basis of the medical history, the patient's age, and the patient's desire, an electrophysiologic study was proposed in order to perform radiofrequency catheter ablation of the clinical and well documented ventricular tachycardia.

Comments

There is a group of patients without structural heart disease who suffer from sustained ventricular tachycardia. The most common tachycardia in such patients originates from the right ventricular outflow tract, and shows a left bundle branch block morphology with an inferior axis. This type of tachycardia is often exercise-induced, or can be provoked by isoproterenol infusion during an electrophysiologic study. In these cases, arrhythmogenic right ventricular dysplasia must be excluded to confirm the diagnosis of an idiopathic ventricular tachycardia.

Left ventricular tachycardia without evidence of structural heart disease occurs mainly in young male individuals. The typical ECG aspect is a right bundle branch block morphology with left axis deviation. This type of tachycardia is also called "verapamil-sensitive VT," because verapamil has often a good success rate in treating this arrhythmia. The underlying mechanism of this type of tachycardia appears to be reentry involving the left posterior fascicle.

In the present case, the clinical tachycardia with right bundle branch block morphology and left axis deviation could be terminated several times by intravenous administration of verapamil.

Intracardiac mapping showed that the earliest ventricular activation during tachycardia was located in the left inferior midseptal region, close to the left posterior fascicle. At that site, a Purkinje potential was recorded on the mapping catheter positioned closed to the left posterior fascicle.

Radiofrequency catheter ablation at this site terminated the tachycardia and led to noninducibility.

After a follow-up of 7 months, the patient has had no recurrence of the tachycardia.

Suggested Reading

Nakagawa H, Beckman K, McClelland J, et al. Radiofrequency catheter ablation of idiopathic left ventricular tachycardia guided by a Purkinje potential. *Circulation* 1993;88:2607-2617.

Mont L, Seixas T, Brugada T, et al. The electrocardiographic, clinical and electrophysiological spectrum of idiopathic monomorphic ventricular tachycardia. *Am Heart J* 1992;124:746-753.

Okumura K, Matsuyama, Kmiyagi H, et al. Entrainment of idiopathic ventricular tachycardia of left ventricular origin with evidence for reentry with an area of slow conduction and effect of verapamil. *Am J Cardiol* 1988;62:727-732.

Ohe T, Simomura K, Aihara N, et al. Idiopathic sustained left ventricular tachycardia: Clinical and electrophysiologic characteristics. *Circulation* 1988;77:560-568.

Ohe T. Idiopathic verapamil sensitive sustained left ventricular tachycardia. *Clin Card* 1993;16:139-146.

Belhassen B, Rotmensch HH, Laniado S. Response of recurrent sustained ventricular tachycardia to verapamil. *Br Heart J* 1981;46:679-684.

Coggins DL, Lee RJ, Sweeney J, et al. Radiofrequency catheter ablation as a cure for idiopathic tachycardia of both left and right ventricular origin. *J Am Coll Cardiol* 1994,23:1333-1341.

Holt PM, Wainwright RJ, Curry PVL. Right ventricular outflow tract tachycardias in patients without apparent structural heart disease. *Int J Cardiol* 1986;10:99-106.

Gonzales RP, Scheinman MM, Lesh MD, et al. Clinical and electrophysiologic spectrum of fascicular tachycardias. *Am Heart J* 1994;128:147-155.

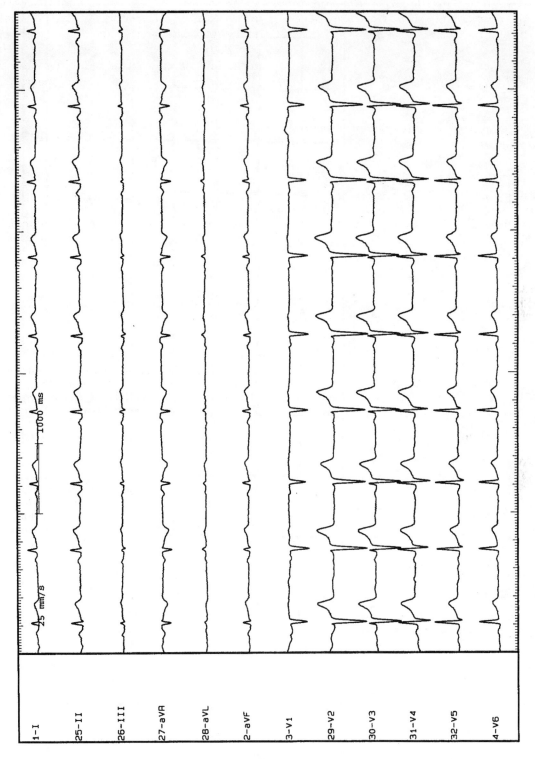

Figure 1. Normal resting 12-lead ECG at the beginning of the electrophysiologic study (paper speed 25 mm/s).

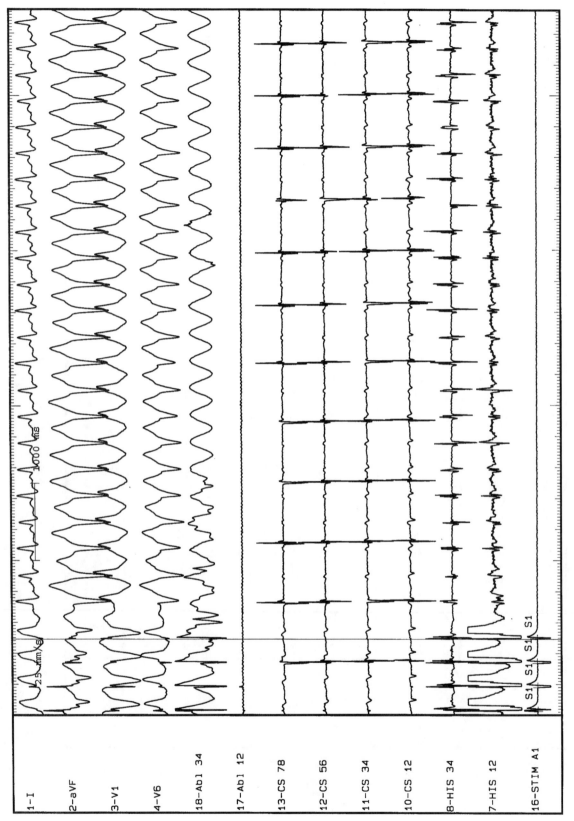

Figure 2. Induction of the clinical tachycardia by rapid ventricular pacing; the tachycardia has a right bundle branch block morphology with left axis deviation, a cycle length of 320 ms and 2:1 V-A conduction (paper speed 25 mm/s).

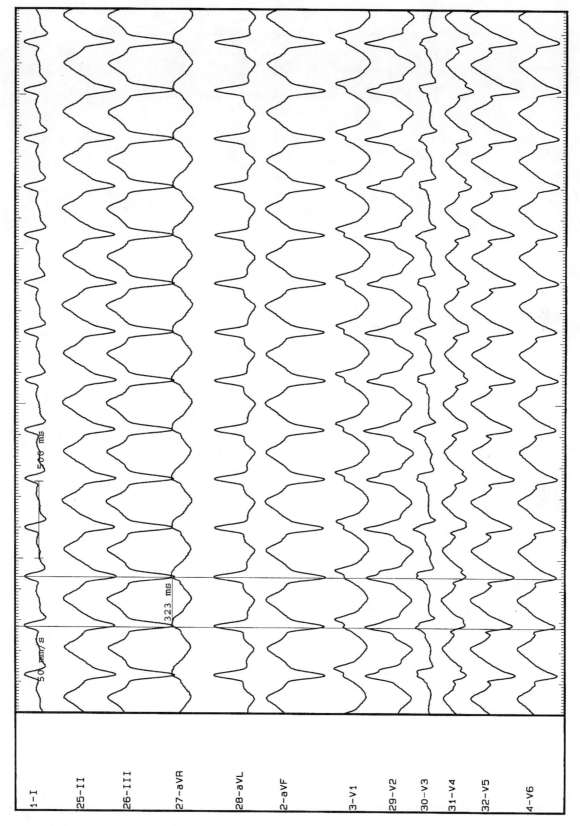

Figure 3. Twelve-lead ECG of the induced tachycardia (paper speed 50 mm/s). Cycle length is 323 ms.

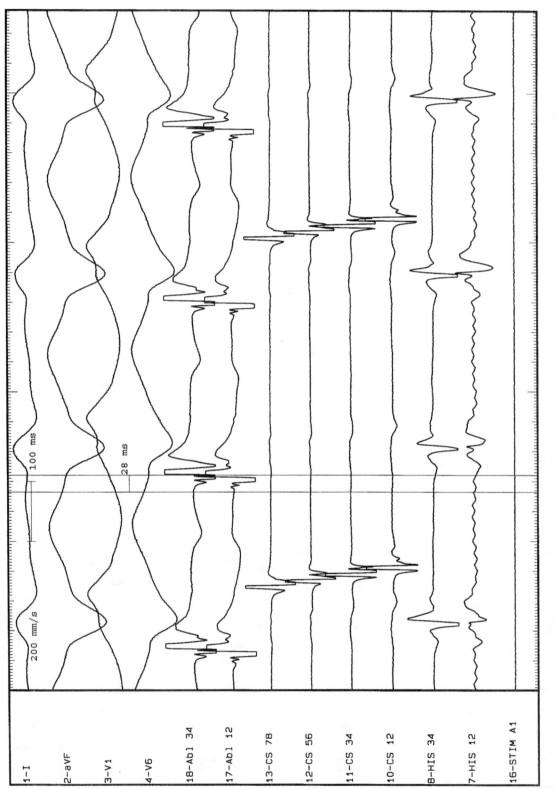

Figure 4. Intracardiac recordings during mapping. The mapping catheter (Abl 12 and Abl 34) is positioned in the left posterior region, and the earliest onset of intracardial ventricular potential (-28 ms) is recorded on the distal poles of the ablation catheter (Abl 12). On the figure are represented four surface ECG leads (I, aVF, V$_1$, V$_6$) and eight bipolar intracardiac recordings (Abl 12 and Abl 34 = distal and proximal poles of the ablation catheter; CS 12, CS 34, CS 56, CS 78 = coronary sinus catheter, from distal to proximal; HIS 12 and HIS 34 = distal and proximal His bundle recording). Paper speed 200 mm/s. The radiofrequency current application at this site was not successful on the tachycardia.

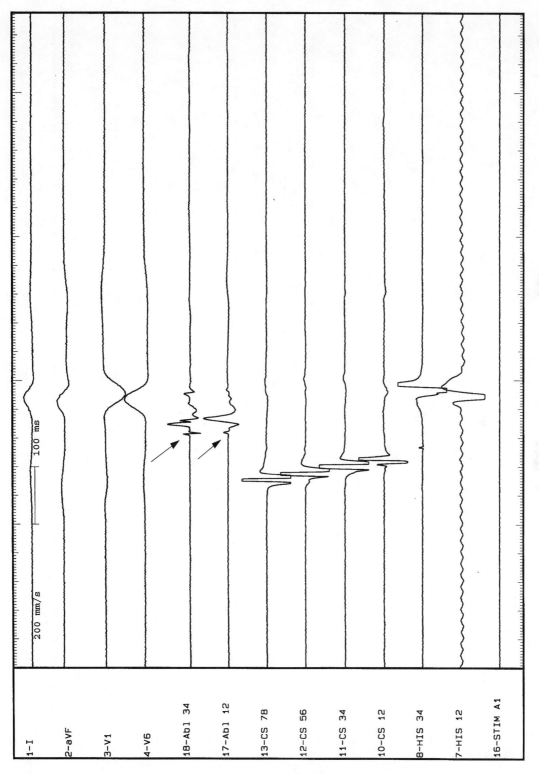

Figure 5. Intracardiac recordings during sinus rhythm. Purkinje potentials (arrows) originating from the left posterior fascicle are recorded during sinus rhythm while mapping the left inferior midseptal region (paper speed 200 mm/s). Same representation as Figure 4.

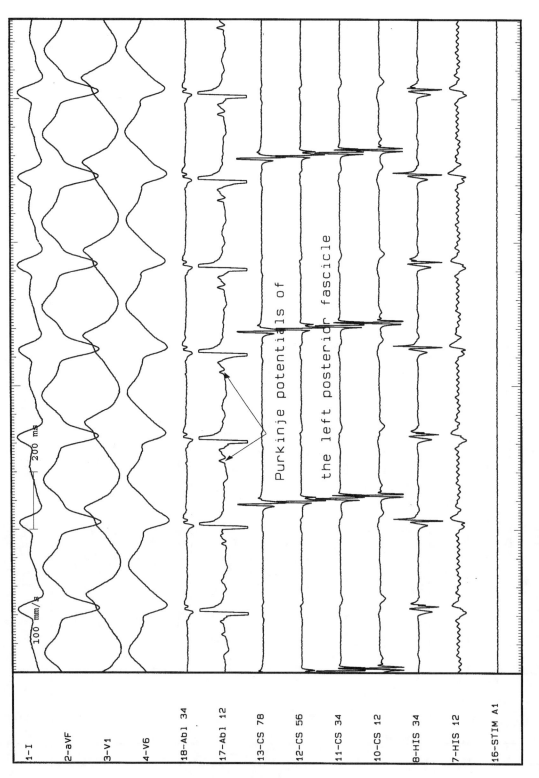

Figure 6. Intracardiac recording of the best map during tachycardia. The ablation catheter is located in the left inferior midseptal region, with Purkinje spike potentials clearly identified on Abl 34 and Abl 12 (paper speed 100 mm/s). Same representation as Figure 4.

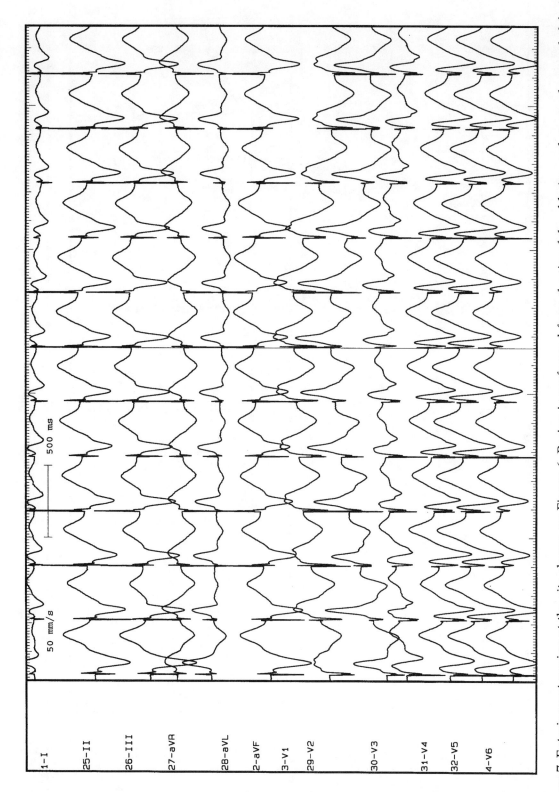

Figure 7. Entrainment-pacing at the site shown on Figure 6. Pacing is performed from the tip of the ablation catheter and concealed fusion is observed (paper speed 50 mm/s). Radiofrequency current application at this site terminated the tachycardia and resulted in noninducibility of the clinical tachycardia.

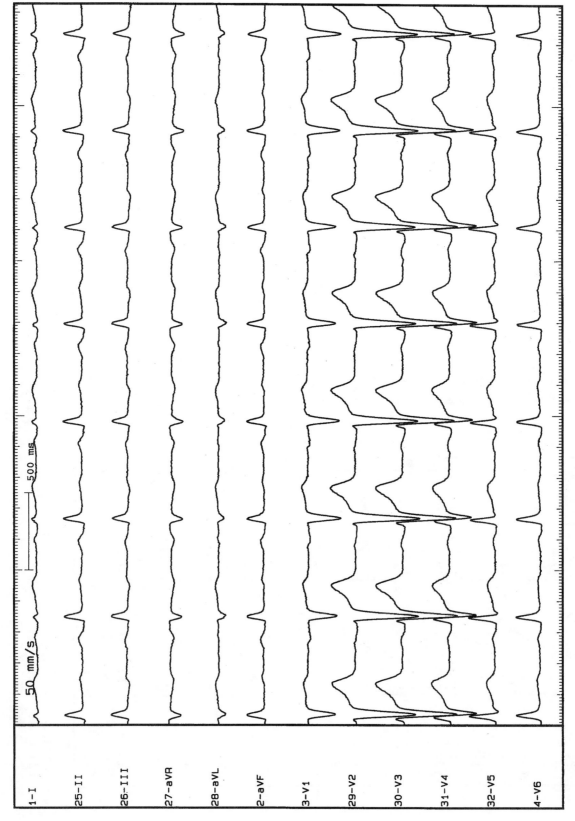

Figure 8. Twelve-lead ECG after successful ablation: note the shift of the axis in the frontal plane (paper speed 50 mm/s).

Chapter 36

Bundle Branch Reentrant Ventricular Tachycardia in a Patient With Steinert Disease

Medical History

A 28-year-old male patient with a history of palpitations for 3 years presented with a broad QRS complex tachycardia (cycle length 300 ms) with right bundle branch block morphology and left axis deviation. He was unresponsive to verapamil, adenosine, and amiodarone, and was referred to our institution 24 hours after the onset of the tachycardia. A diagnosis of ventricular tachycardia was made on the basis of an electrophysiologic study showing atrioventricular dissociation, and the tachycardia was easily terminated by programmed ventricular stimulation.

Comments

In the present case, echocardiography disclosed mitral valve prolapse with slight mitral insufficiency. Coronary angiography was normal and the diagnosis of myotonic muscular dystrophy was suspected on the basis of clinical examination and family history. The diagnosis of Steinert disease was finally confirmed by electromyography and genetic testing.

The patient's mother also suffered from myotonic muscular dystrophy and her resting 12-lead ECG showed sinus rhythm with slight prolongation of PR interval with left axis deviation. She also had presented

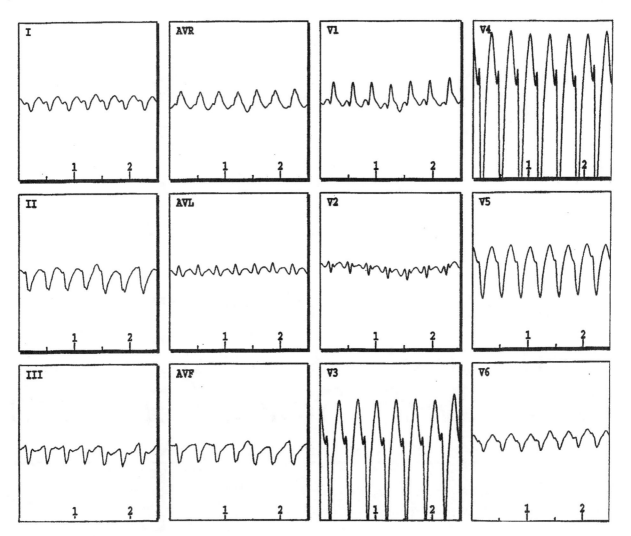

Figure 1. Twelve-lead ECG (25 mm/s) during palpitations, showing a broad complex tachycardia with right bundle branch block morphology and left axis deviation.

with a broad complex tachycardia with left bundle branch block morphology and left axis deviation. The suspected diagnosis was also bundle branch reentry, but the patient's mother refused an electrophysiologic evaluation.

Because of severe prolongation of H-V interval in association with major intraventricular conduction defects, a prophylactic permanent pacemaker was implanted.

Bundle branch reentry (BBR) is a rare arrhythmia (occurring in approximately 6% of patients with ventricular tachycardia) in which the His bundle, the right and left branches, and transseptal ventricular muscle conduction are the components of the reentrant circuit. The presence of a dilated cardiomyopathy together with slow conduction in the His-Purkinje system are common findings in patients who develop this form of ventricular tachycardia which frequently presents with syncope or sudden cardiac death. The mechanism of BBR should be included in the differential diagnosis of any sustained monomorphic ventricular tachycardia especially in the presence of a left bundle branch block morphology. The mechanism of BBR tachycardia is supported by one or more of the following previously published criteria:

1. Typical right or left bundle branch block morphology during tachycardia consistent with ventricular depolarization through the appropriate bundle branch.
2. During tachycardia, a His bundle potential preceeds each QRS complex which usually has a left bundle branch block pattern.

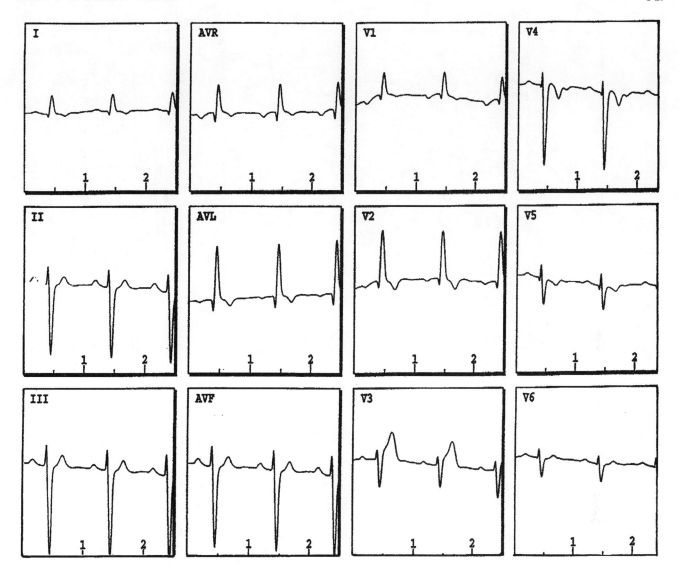

Figure 2. Twelve-lead surface ECG during sinus rhythm (25 mm/s) showing first-degree atrioventricular block, left axis deviation and intraventricular conduction defect mimicking right bundle branch block.

3. Spontaneous variations in V-V intervals are preceded by similar changes in H-H intervals.
4. Termination of the tachycardia occurs either spontaneously or by pacing-induced block in the His-Purkinje system.
5. BBR can no longer be induced after successful catheter ablation of the right bundle.

Catheter ablation is safe and effective to treat BBR, whereas pharmacologic options may expose patients with conduction defects and/or advanced structural heart disease to potentially serious side effects. The risk of excessive H-V prolongation after ablation of the right bundle may occasionally require implantation of a permanent pacemaker. In the presence of bundle branch reentry, the diagnosis of myotonic dystrophy should be excluded. In patients with myotonic dystrophy, an electrophysiologic evaluation (with programmed ventricular stimulation) should be proposed for symptomatic patients (dizzy spells or syncope) even if the presence of conduction defects may also explain the symptoms.

Suggested Reading

Caceres J, Jazayeri M, McKinnie, et al. Sustained bundle branch reentry as a mechanism of clinical tachycardia. *Circulation* 1989;79:256-270.

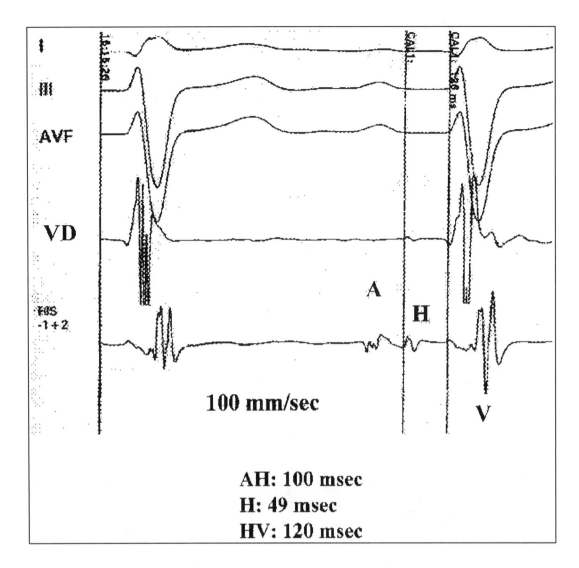

Figure 3. Intracardiac recordings at baseline. Paper speed 100 mm/s. Three surface ECG leads (I, III, aVF) are represented together with one bipolar recording from the right ventricular apex (VD) and one bipolar recording from the His bundle region (His –1+2). During sinus rhythm, A-H interval is 100 ms, and H-V interval is prolonged to 120 ms, with an H potential measuring 49 ms.

Blanck Z, Dhala A, Deshpande S, et al. Bundle branch reentrant ventricular tachycardia: Cumulative experience in 48 patients. *J Cardiovasc Electrophysiol* 1993;4:253-262.

Tchou O, Jazayeri M, Denker S, et al. Transcatheter electrical ablation of right bundle branch. A method of treating macroreentrant ventricular tachycardia attributed to bundle branch reentry. *Circulation* 1988;78:246-257.

Cohen TJ, Chien WW, Lurie KL, et al. Radiofrequency catheter ablation for treatment of bundle branch reentrant ventricular tachycardia: Results and long-term follow-up. *J Am Coll Cardiol* 1991;18:1767-1773.

Blank Z, Deshpande S, Jazayeri MR, et al. Catheter ablation of the left bundle branch for the treatment of sustained bundle branch reentrant ventricular tachycardia. *J Cardiovasc Electrophysiol* 1995;6:40-43.

Klein LS, Miles WM, Zipes DP. Ablation of idiopathic ventricular tachycardia and bundle branch reentry. In Zipes DP (ed): Catheter Ablation of Arrhythmias. Futura Publishing Co. Inc., Armonk, New-York, 1994.

Gallay P. Les Tachycardies ventriculaires par réentrée de branche à branche. *Arch Mal Coeur* 1992;85(IV):77-83.

Merino JL, Carmona JR, Fernandez-Lozano I, et al. Mechanisms of sustained ventricular tachycardia in myotonic dystrophy: Implications for catheter ablation. *Circulation* 1998;98:541-546.

Lagrange A, Lagrange P, Boveda S, et al. Tachycardie ventriculaire par réentrée de branche à branche. Cas familial avec maladie de Steinert. *Arch Mal Coeur* 2000;93:743-749.

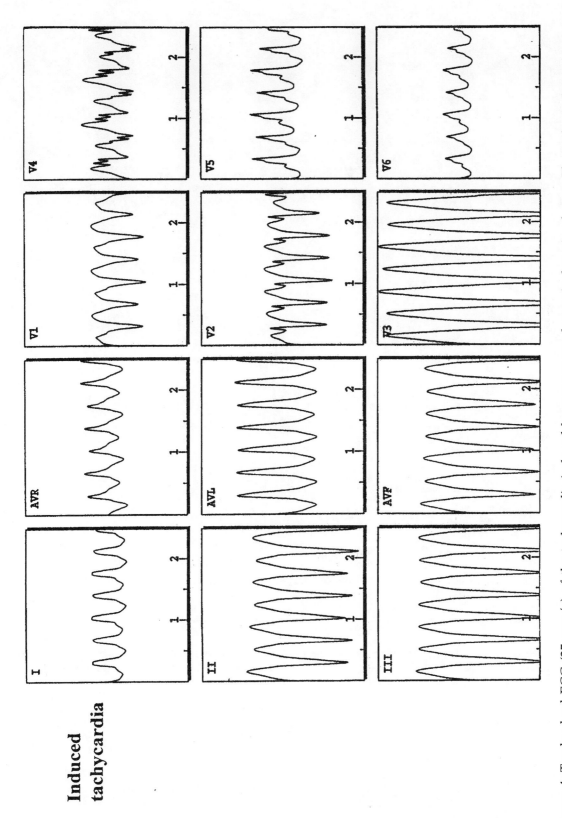

Figure 4. Twelve-lead ECG (25 mm/s) of the tachycardia induced by programmed ventricular stimulation. The tachycardia (cycle length 300 ms) has a left bundle branch block pattern with left axis deviation with a QRS complex which is positive in DI, V_5, and V_6.

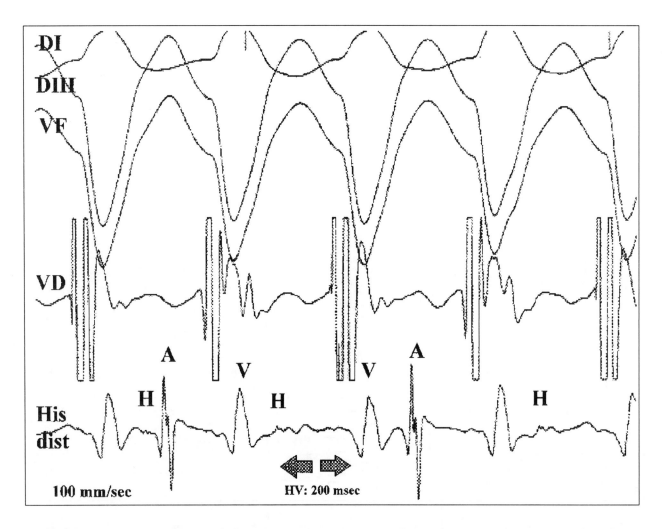

Figure 5. Intracardiac recordings (100 mm/s) during tachycardia. Same display as Figure 3. Each ventricular depolarization (V) is preceded by a His bundle deflection (H) with an H-V interval of 200 ms. Atrioventricular dissociation is present during the tachycardia.

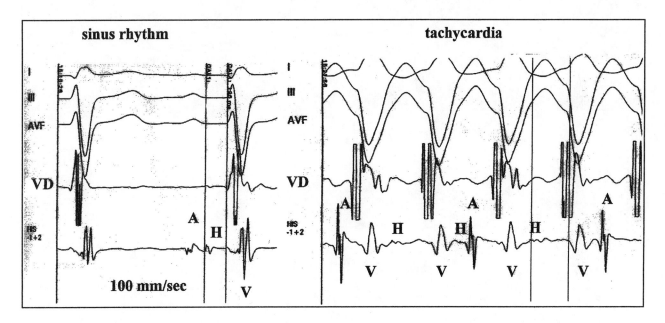

Figure 6. Intracardiac recordings (100 mm/s) during sinus rhythm and during tachycardia. Same display as Figures 3 and 5. H-V interval is longer during tachycardia (200 ms) than during sinus rhythm (120 ms).

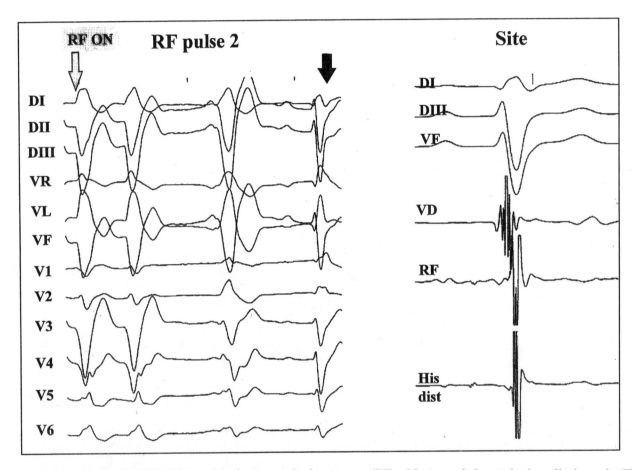

Figure 7. Twelve-lead ECG (50 mm/s) during radiofrequency (RF) ablation of the right bundle branch. The tachycardia was immediately interrupted (**left**) during the second RF current application (RF pulse 2) and sinus rhythm restored with right bundle branch block and left axis deviation. Intracardiac recording at the successful site (**right**) shows that the ablation catheter (RF) was located in the close vicinity of the His bundle. After ablation tachycardia was no longer inducible.

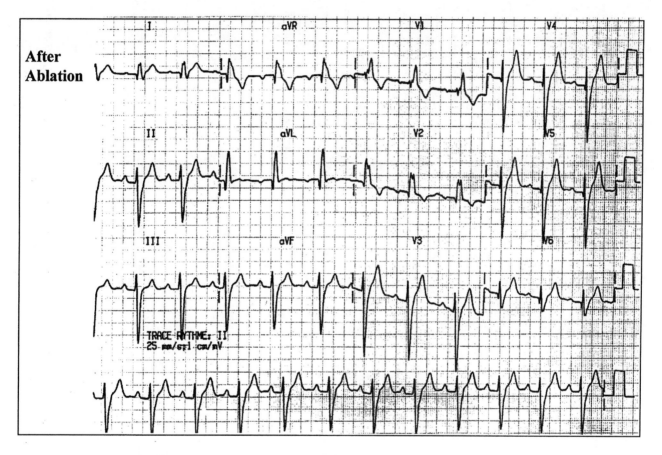

Figure 8. Twelve-lead ECG (25 mm/s) after radiofrequency ablation showing sinus rhythm with prolonged PR interval, right bundle branch block and left axis deviation.

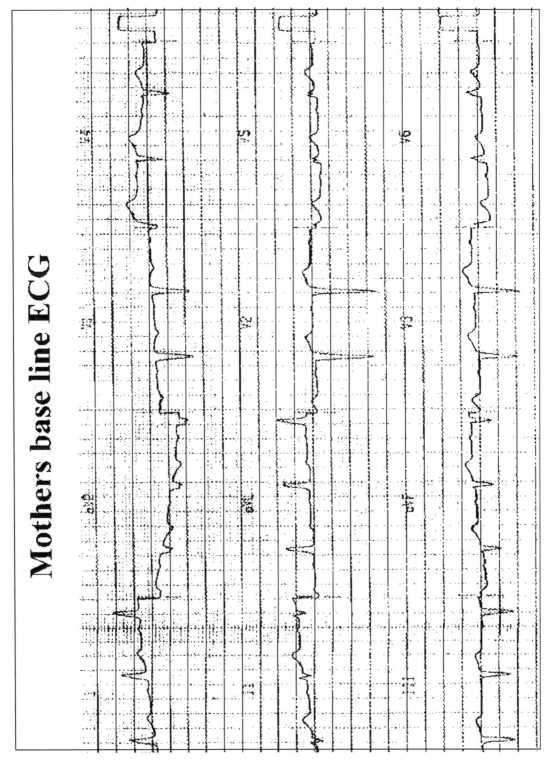

Figure 9. Results of a twelve-lead resting ECG (25 mm/s) performed on the patient's mother.

Mothers tachycardia

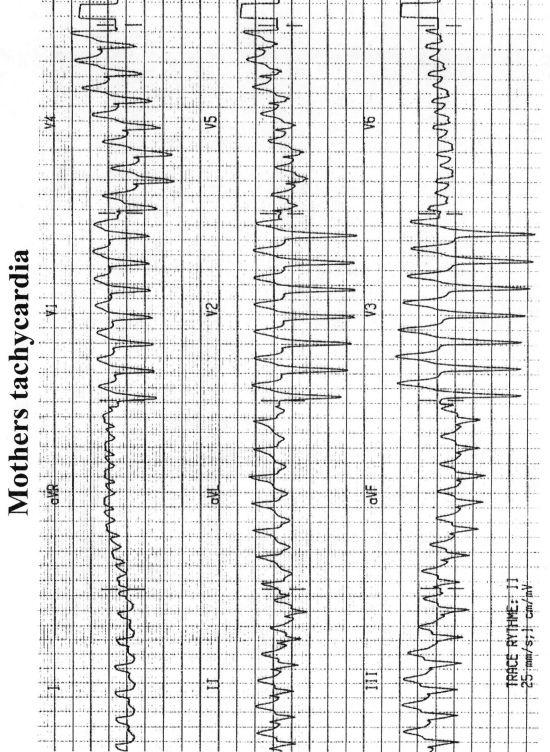

Figure 10. Twelve-lead ECG (25 mm/s) of the mother's tachycardia.

Chapter 37

Ventricular Tachycardia in Arrhythmogenic Right Ventricular Cardiomyopathy

Medical History

During vacation in Turkey, a 22-year-old male suffered from a first episode of rapid palpitations. The patient reported that the ECG in a local hospital revealed a wide QRS complex tachycardia with a rate of 240 beats/min. Because of being hemodynamically compromised (the patient almost fainted) external direct current (DC) shock was applied. The patient was discharged in sinus rhythm and was prescribed oral β-blocker therapy. After returning home again he was transferred for further investigation. No ECG of the event was available. Because of right precordial repolarization abnormalities during sinus rhythm and be-

cause of echocardiographically impaired right ventricular function with normal left ventricular function, an arrhythmogenic right ventricular cardiomyopathy (ARVC) was suspected and an electrophysiologic study was performed. During the electrophysiologic study, a sustained ventricular tachycardia with left bundle branch block morphology and a superior axis was induced at a rate of 180 beats/min. Ajmalin testing for Brugada syndrome was negative. After magnetic resonance imaging (MRI) confirmed the suspected diagnosis of ARVC, the patient was prescribed sotalol. The control study showed persisting inducibility of ventricular tachycardia with left bundle branch block (LBBB) morphology, but now with an inferior axis. Pharmacological treatment was changed to amiodarone. Ventricular tachycardia occurred despite this treatment and the patient underwent another electrophysiologic study with radiofrequency (RF) catheter ablation on the posterolateral ring of the tricuspid valve twice, at a site where the earliest activation was recorded. After ongoing episodes of ventricular tachycardia during follow-up the patient was scheduled to receive an implantable cardioverter defibrillator.

Comments

Symptomatic ventricular tachycardia with left bundle branch block morphology is commonly one of the first symptoms leading to the diagnosis of ARVC. Other symptoms consist of right (and later left) heart failure or sudden cardiac death. Repolarization abnormalities (mainly in right precordial leads as in the present case) reflect the electric disarray caused by fibrous or fibrofatty replacement of the right ventricular muscle proceeding from epi- to endocardial layers. Diagnosis of ARVC is made according to the criteria proposed by the Task Force of the World Health Organization and the International Society and Federation of Cardiology, which includes electrical and histomorphological features shown by ECG, signal-averaging, echocardiography, MRI, and endomyocardial biopsy as well as genetics and family history. Other etiologies for malignant ventricular arrhythmias, such as the Brugada syndrome, have to be excluded.

Antiarrhythmic therapy with sotalol or amiodarone with or without β-blockers and guided by electrophysiologic testing has been shown to be effective, although randomized placebo-controlled studies are lacking. Ablation therapy may be effective but can be dangerous because of the muscular thinning. Recurrences are quite often observed because of the progressive course of the disease. Implantable cardioverter-defibrillators are recommended in high risk subgroups. Family members should be evaluated on a regular basis.

Suggested Reading

Basso C, Thiene G, Corrado D, et al. Arrhythmogenic right ventricular cardiomyopathy. Dysplasia, dystrophy, or myocarditis? *Circulation* 1996;94:983-991.

Burke AP, Farb A, Tashko G, et al. Arrhythmogenic right ventricular cardiomyopathy and fatty replacement of the right ventricular myocardium: Are they different diseases? *Circulation* 1998;97:1571-1580.

Coonar AS, Protonotarius N, Tsatsopoulou A, et al. Gene for arrhythmogenic right ventricular cardiomyopathy with diffuse nonepidermolytic palmoplantar keratoderma and woolly hair (Naxos disease) maps to 17q21. *Circulation* 1998;97:2049-2058.

Ellison KE, Friedman PL, et al. Entrainment mapping and radiofrequency catheter ablation of ventricular tachycardia in right ventricular dysplasia. *J Am Coll Cardiol* 1998;32:724-728.

Fontaine G, Fontaliran F, et al. Arrhythmogenic right ventricular cardiomyopathies: Clinical forms and main differential diagnoses [editorial]. *Circulation* 1998;97:1532-1535.

Fontaliran F, Arkwright S, et al. Arrhythmogenic right ventricular dysplasia and cardiomyopathy. Clinical and anatomic-pathologic aspects, nosologic approach. *Arch Anat Cytol Pathol* 1998;46:171-177.

Harada T, Aonuma K, et al. Catheter ablation of ventricular tachycardia in patients with right ventricular dysplasia: Identification of target sites by entrainment mapping techniques. *Pacing Clin Electrophysiol* 1998;21:2547-2550.

Link MS, Wang PJ, Haugh CJ, et al. Arrhythmogenic right ventricular dysplasia: Clinical results with implantable cardioverter defibrillators. *J Interv Card Electrophysiol* 1997;1:41-48.

Pennell D, Casolo G. Right ventricular arrhythmia: Emergence of magnetic resonance imaging as an investigative tool [editorial]. *Eur Heart J* 1997;18:1843-1845.

Scheinman MM. Is the Brugada syndrome a distinct clinical entity? *J Cardiovasc Electrophysiol* 1997;80:332-336.

Valente M, Calabrese F, Angelini A, et al. In vivo evidence of apoptosis in arrhythmogenic right ventricular cardiomyopathy. *Am J Pathol* 1998;152:479-484.

Richardson P, McKenna WJ, Bristow M, et al. Report of the 1995 World Health Organization / International Society and Federation of Cardiology Task Force on the definition and classification of cardiomyopathies. *Circulation* 1996;93:841-842.

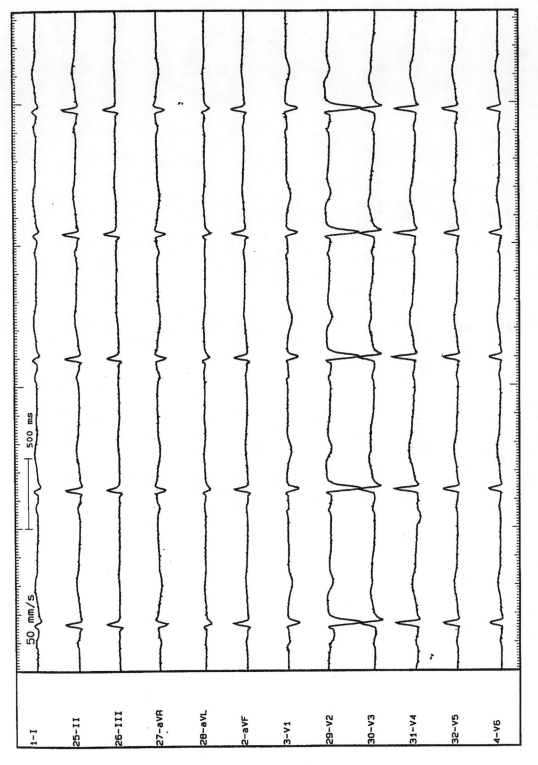

Figure 1. Twelve-lead resting ECG (50 mm/s) during sinus rhythm showing right precordial repolarization abnormalities.

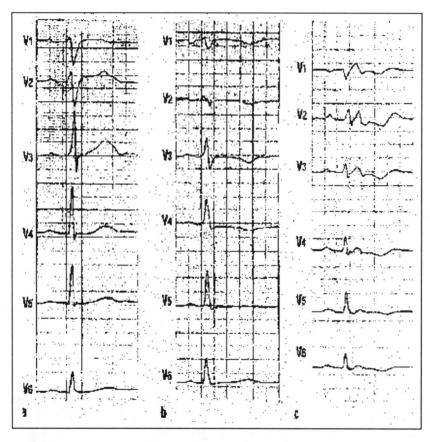

Figure 2. Another possible repolarization abnormalities in different patients with arrhythmogenic right ventricular cardiomyopathy.

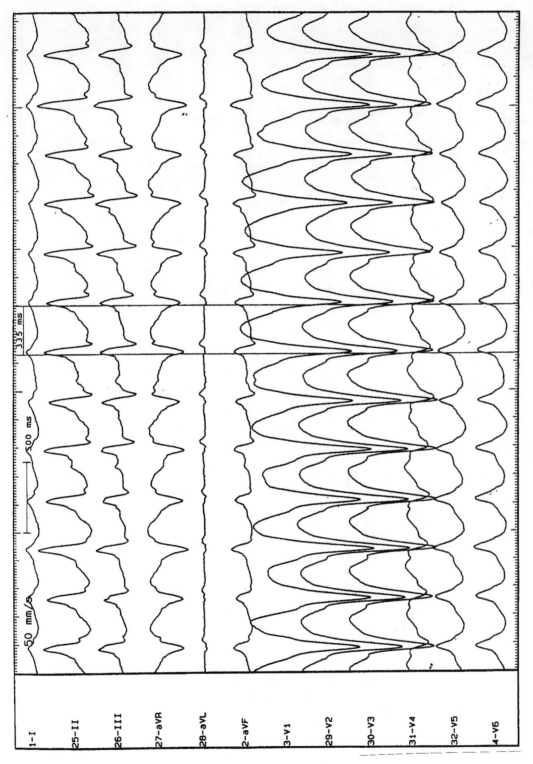

Figure 3. Twelve-lead ECG (50 mm/s) showing the electrocardiographic aspect of the ventricular tachycardia (cycle length 335 ms) with left bundle branch block morphology and superior axis induced during the first electrophysiologic study.

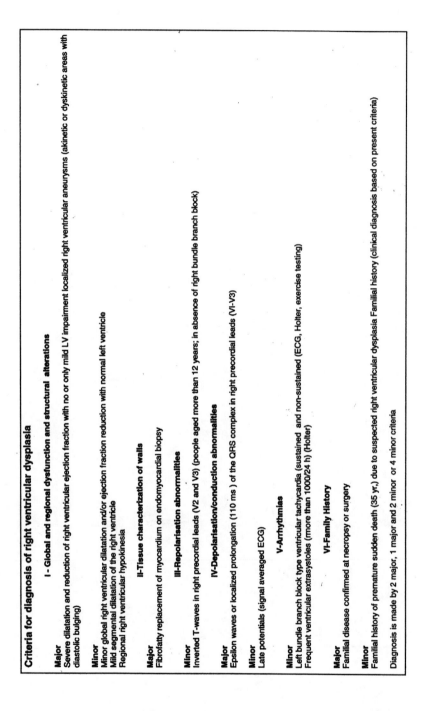

Figure 4. World Health Organization / International Society and Federation of Cardiology Task Force definition/classification of arrhythmogenic right ventricular cardiomyopathy.

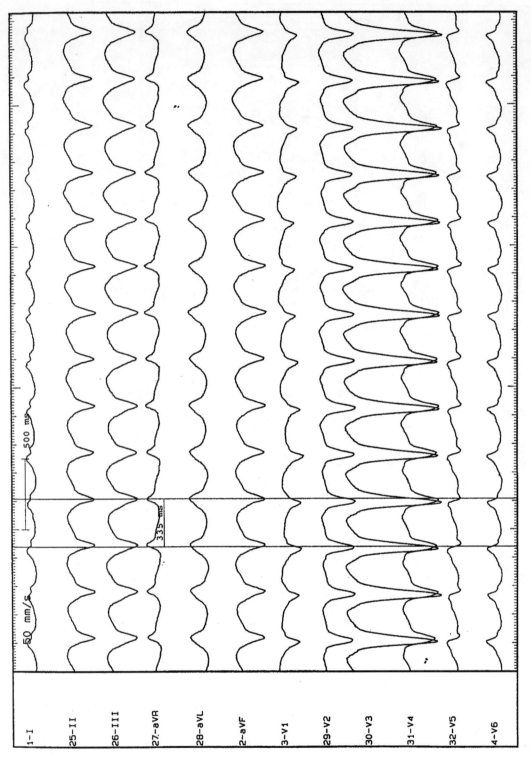

Figure 5. Twelve-lead ECG (50 mm/s) showing the electrocardiographic aspect of ventricular tachycardia (cycle length 335 ms) with left bundle branch block and superior axis recorded during the second electrophysiologic study.

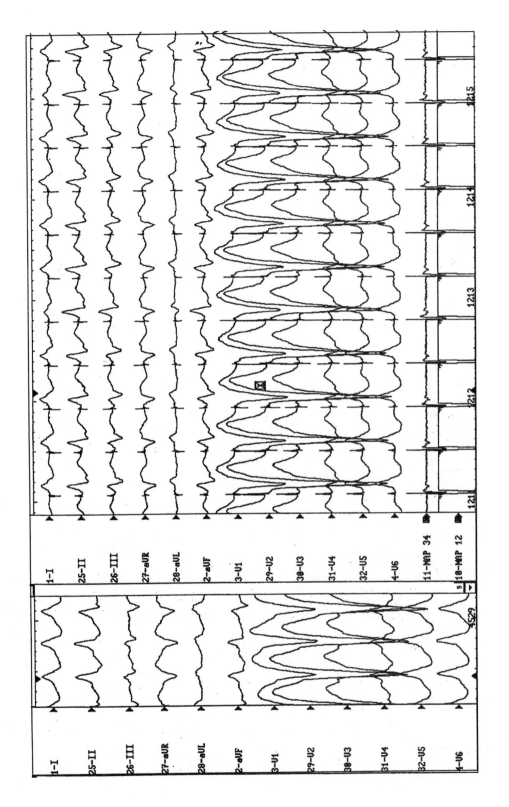

Figure 6. Twelve-lead ECG (50 mm/s) during pace-mapping. The ablation catheter is positioned at the posterolateral tricupid annulus. The morphology of the QRS complex during pace-mapping at this site (**right**) is identical to the morphology of the QRS complex observed during ventricular tachycardia (**left**).

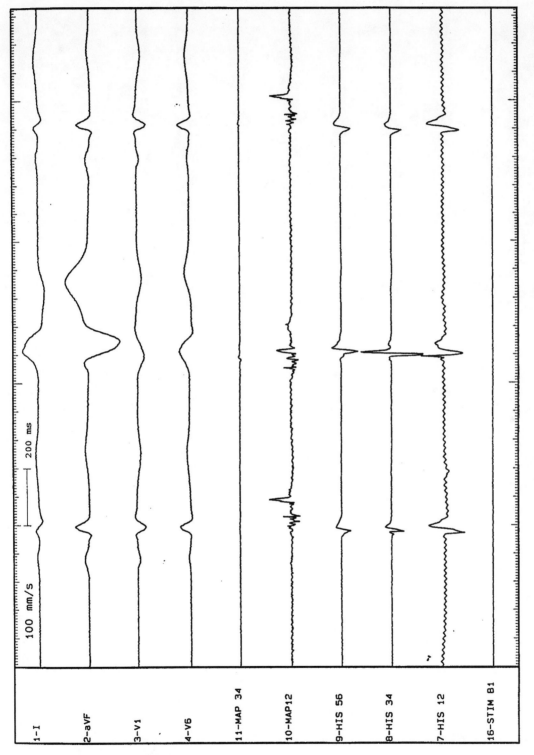

Figure 7. Intracardiac recordings (paper speed 100 mm/s) during sinus rhythm at the site of ablation. The local ventricular electrogram at this site shows late and fractionated ventricular potentials.

Chapter 38

Postinfarction Permanent Ventricular Tachycardia

Medical History

A 49-year-old diabetic patient, treated with insulin for 2 years, presented with an acute inferior myocardial infarction in 1992. Coronary angiography revealed 90% stenosis of the right coronary artery and successful percutaneous transluminal coronary angioplasty was performed a few days after infarction. Over the next 5 years the clinical course was uneventful, but in October 1997 an exercise stress test with Thallium 201 imaging showed signs of ischemia in the anteroseptal region. Coronary angiography was performed and severe stenosis were observed both on the right coronary artery and on the left anterior descending artery. Coronary artery bypass grafting was performed in December 1997, without complication. Eight months after surgery the patient complained of fatigue, shortness of breath, and palpitations. No chest pain was reported and the patient never experienced malaise or syncope. The patient was admitted at another institution.

At physical examination there was a rapid but regular pulse rate (125 beats/min), a normal blood pressure (110/80 mm Hg), and obvious signs of left heart failure including pulmonary rales and a third heart sound. On admission, potassium level was 5.0 mmol/L, blood sugar 18.7 mmol/L, and renal function tests were within normal limits. The 12-lead resting electrocardiogram showed a regular wide QRS complexes tachycardia at a rate of 128 beats/min. A chest X-ray showed the presence of cardiomegaly with radiologic evidence of left heart failure. Echocardiography revealed left ventricular dilatation, inferior and anterior hypokinesia, a left ventricular ejection fraction of 50%, and a slight mitral regurgitation.

Lidocaine, mexiletine, procainamide had no effect on the tachycardia, and high-dose amiodarone was instituted with progressive slowing of the tachycardia

From: RETAC: *Radiofrequency Catheter Ablation for the Treatment of Cardiac Arrhythmias: A Practical Atlas with Illustrative Cases.* © Futura Publishing Company, Inc. Armonk, NY, 2002.

367

rate from 128 to 100 beats/min. The patient was then discharged with amiodarone 200 mg/day, with a permanent tachycardia.

Three months later, because of symptoms worsening, the patient was referred to our institution for evaluation and treatment. The permanent tachycardia (100 beats/min) was still present, congestive heart failure was obvious (NYHA class IV), and left ventricular ejection fraction was 25%.

A radiofrequency catheter ablation of the ventricular tachycardia circuit was proposed.

Comments

Radiofrequency catheter ablation of ischemic ventricular tachycardia is a difficult task because the reentry circuit is frequently large and difficult to ablate with current technologies. The size of radiofrequency ablation lesions is relatively small, and in many instances most ablation lesions are not deep enough in the left ventricle to produce permanent modification of the reentrant circuit. Several techniques have been used to define the optimal site for ablation:

1. Pacemapping: a morphology of the QRS complex during ventricular pacing which is identical to the morphology of the spontaneous ventricular tachycardia suggests an optimal site for ablation but does not appear to be a sufficient criterion.
2. Identification of middiastolic potentials: these abnormal presystolic components are believed to represent slow conduction within the reentrant circuit and represent a good marker for successful ablation like in the present case.
3. Entrainment methods: these sophisticated pacing techniques are useful to determine if the

site is in the reentry circuit and if the ablation catheter is located in the proximal or in the distal isthmus. However, entrainment methods can be applied only if the ventricular tachycardia is slow and stable enough to allow pacing and analysis during tachycardia.

Even if radiofrequency catheter ablation of postinfarction ventricular tachycardia is usually long and difficult, such a therapy should be proposed to patients with drug resistant stable monomorphic ventricular tachycardia, to patients with incessant (or permanent) ventricular tachycardia, or to patients with ventricular tachycardia at a rate too slow to allow successful management by an internal cardioverter defibrillator.

Suggested Reading

Downar E, Harris L, Mickleborough LL, et al. Endocardial mapping of ventricular tachycardia in the intact human ventricle: Evidence of reentrant mechanisms. *J Am Coll Cardiol* 1988;11:783-791.

Frank R, Tonet JL, Kounde S, et al. Localization of the area of slow conduction during ventricular tachycardia. In Brugada P, Wellens HJJ (eds): Cardiac Arrhythmias: Where to Go From Here. Armonk, NY, Futura Publishing Co. Inc., 1987, pp 191-208.

Stevenson WG, Sager PT, Friedman PL. Entrainment techniques for mapping atrial and ventricular tachycardias. *J Electrophysiol Cardiovasc* 1995;6:201-216.

Wilber DJ, Kopp DE, Glascock D, et al. Catheter ablation of the mitral isthmus for ventricular tachycardia associated with inferior infarction. *Circulation* 1995;92:3481-3489.

Stevenson WG, Friedman PL, Sager PT, et al. Exploring postinfarction reentrant ventricular tachycardia with entrainment mapping. *J Am Coll Cardiol* 1997;29:1180-1189.

Borggrefe M, Chen X, Hindricks G, et al. Catheter ablation of ventricular tachycardia in patients with coronary heart disease. In Zipes DP, Jalife J (eds) Cardiac Electrophysiology: From Cell to Bedside, 2nd edition. WB Saunders Co, Philadelphia, 1995 : pp 1502-1517.

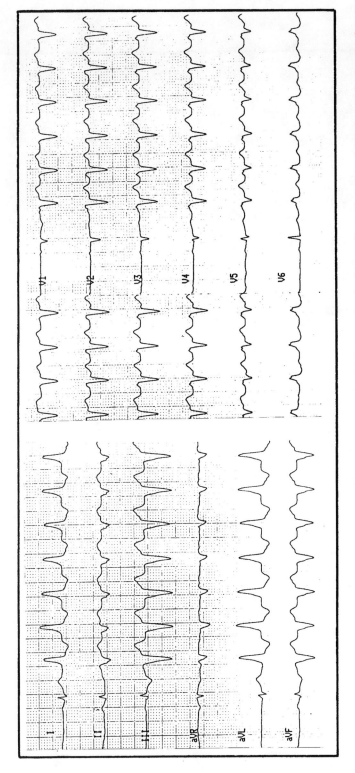

Figure 1. Twelve-lead resting ECG during sinus rhythm showing a wide QRS complex tachycardia, at a rate of 128 beats/min. Tachycardia is not permanent but shows spontaneous termination, return to sinus rhythm, and immediate reinitiation of the tachycardia. The tachycardia has a left bundle branch block morphology, QRS width is 140 ms, r-S interval is 120 ms in lead V$_5$, there is left axis deviation and 1:1 retrograde conduction. Paper speed 25 mm/s.

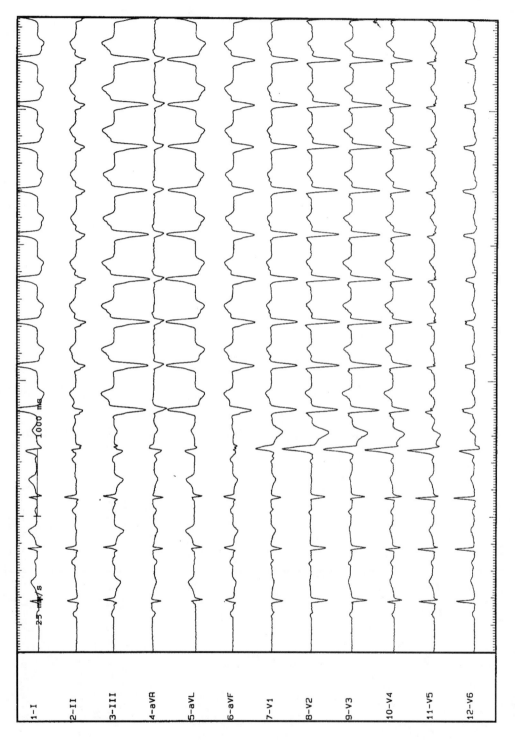

Figure 2. Twelve-lead resting ECG showing spontaneous initiation of the wide QRS complexes tachycardia. Rate is 100 beats/min because of amiodarone treatment. Paper speed 25 mm/s.

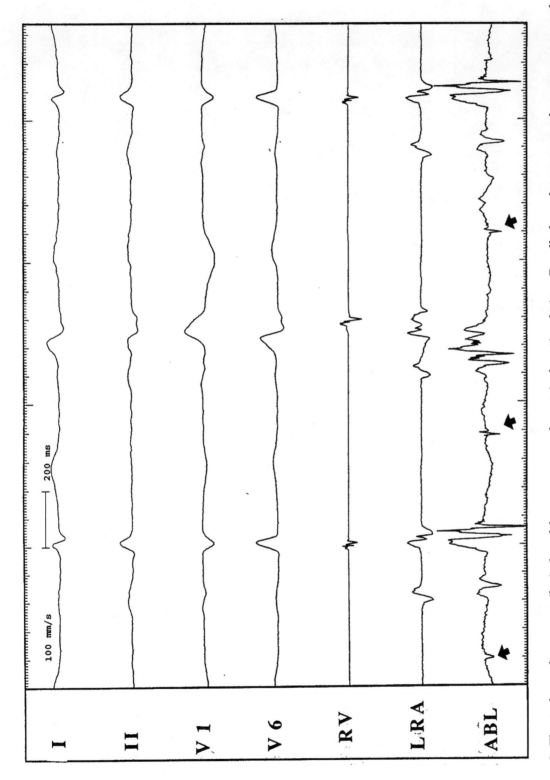

Figure 3. The tachycardia was easily induced by programmed ventricular stimulation. Bundle branch reentry and an accessory pathway were excluded. The ECG pattern of the tachycardia (left bundle branch block morphology, superior axis and increasing R-wave progression in precordial leads) suggested a left posteroseptal origin. The figure shows intracardiac recordings during tachycardia: represented are four surface ECG leads (DI, DII, V_1, V_6), one bipolar intracardiac electrogram from the right ventricular apex (RV), one bipolar intracardiac electrogram from the low right atrium (LRA), and one bipolar intracardiac electrogram from the left posteroseptal region (ABL). In that region, a middiastolic potential is clearly identified (arrows) preceding onset of QRS by 370 ms. Paper speed 100 mm/s.

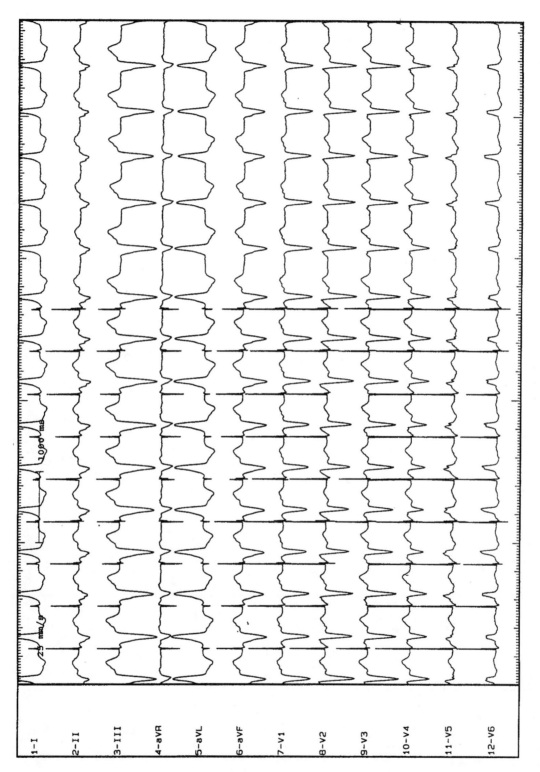

Figure 4. Twelve-lead electrocardiogram during pace-mapping. At the site middiastolic potentials were recorded, concealed entrainment was demonstrated with a short S1-QRS interval, and pace-mapping showed identical QRS morphology in 12/12 leads. Paper speed 25 mm/s.

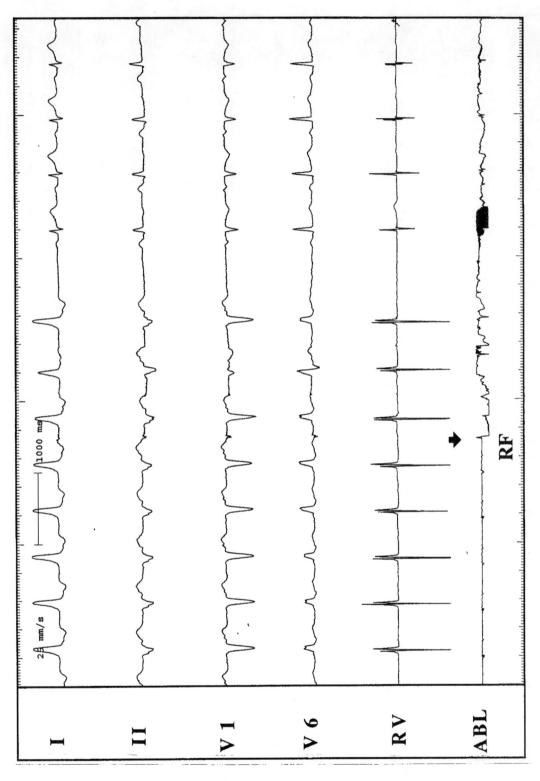

Figure 5. Recording during the first radiofrequency (RF) current application. Here are represented four surface ECG leads (DI, DII, V₁, V₆), one bipolar intracardiac electrogram from the right ventricular apex (RV) and one bipolar intracardiac electrogram from the tip of the ablation catheter (ABL). One second after RF application (RF, arrow), the ventricular tachycardia is interrupted, and normal sinus rhythm is restored. After this single RF application, tachycardia was no longer inducible even after isoproterenol infusion. Paper speed 25 mm/s.

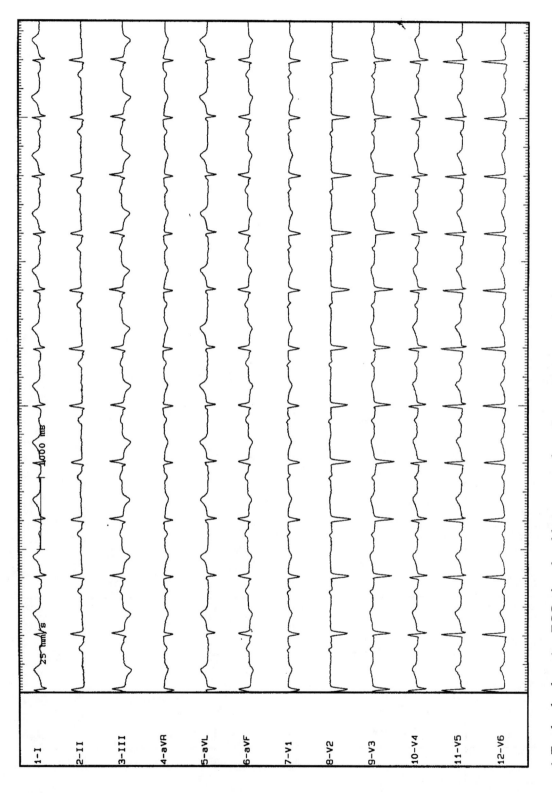

Figure 6. Twelve-lead resting ECG after the ablation procedure. Permanent sinus rhythm is present. Paper speed 25 mm/s. After a follow-up of 15 months, no recurrence of ventricular tachycardia has been observed, and signs of heart failure have disappeared (left ventricular ejection fraction 50%).

Index